D0154600

Orthopedic Taping, Wrapping, Bracing & Padding

Orthopedic Taping, Wrapping, Bracing & Padding

Joel W. Beam, EdD, ATC, LAT

Assistant Professor
Athletic Training Education Program
Brooks College of Health
University of North Florida
Jacksonville, Florida

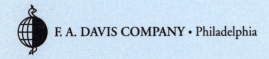

F. A. DAVIS COMPANY • Philadelphia

F. A. Davis Company
1915 Arch Street
Philadelphia, PA 19103
www.fadavis.com

Copyright © 2006 by F. A. Davis Company

All rights reserved. This product is protected by copyright. No part of it may be reproduced, stored in a retrieval system, or transmitted in any form or by any means, electronic, mechanical, photocopying, recording, or otherwise, without written permission from the publisher.

Printed in the United States of America

Last digit indicates print number: 10 9 8 7 6 5 4 3 2 1

Acquisitions Editor:	Christa A. Fratantoro
Developmental Editors:	Caryn Abramowitz, Jennifer A. Pine
Manager of Content Development:	Deborah Thorp
Photographers:	Linden Kinder Cannon IV, Joella Davis
Design and Illustration Manager:	Carolyn O'Brien
Illustration Coordinator:	Mike Carcel

As new scientific information becomes available through basic and clinical research, recommended treatments and drug therapies undergo changes. The author(s) and publisher have done everything possible to make this book accurate, up to date, and in accord with accepted standards at the time of publication. The author(s), editors, and publisher are not responsible for errors or omissions or for consequences from application of the book, and make no warranty, expressed or implied, in regard to the contents of the book. Any practice described in this book should be applied by the reader in accordance with professional standards of care used in regard to the unique circumstances that may apply in each situation. The reader is advised always to check product information (package inserts) for changes and new information regarding dose and contraindications before administering any drug. Caution is especially urged when using new or infrequently ordered drugs.

Library of Congress Cataloging-in-Publication Data

Beam, Joel W., 1963
    Orthopedic taping, wrapping, bracing & padding / Joel W. Beam.
        p. ; cm.
    Includes bibliographical references.
    ISBN-13: 978-0-8036-1212-9
    ISBN-10: 0-8036-1212-5
    1. Sports injuries—Treatment. 2. Bandages and bandaging.
  I. Title. II. Title: Orthopedic taping, wrapping, bracing and padding
techniques.
    [DNLM: 1. Athletic Injuries—therapy. 2. Athletic Injuries—
prevention & control. 3. Bandages. 4. Braces.   QT 261 B366o 2006]
RD97.B332 2006
617.1'027—dc22

                                    2006006776

Authorization to photocopy items for internal or personal use, or the internal or personal use of specific clients, is granted by F. A. Davis Company for users registered with the Copyright Clearance Center (CCC) Transactional Reporting Service, provided that the fee of $.10 per copy is paid directly to CCC, 222 Rosewood Drive, Danvers, MA 01923. For those organizations that have been granted a photocopy license by CCC, a separate system of payment has been arranged. The fee code for users of the Transactional Reporting Service is: 8036/1212/06 0 + $.10.

Dedication

This book is dedicated to several groups of people. To my family, without whose love and support I would not have been able to achieve my goals. To the many athletic trainers—several who have been true pioneers in our field—who took the time to share their knowledge and experience with me over the years. To the athletes I have been privileged to work with during the years. Finally, to the students who have inspired and allowed me to share my knowledge and experience with them, thank you.

"That's the thing. Sometimes when you sacrifice something precious, you're not really losing it. You're just passing it on to someone else."
The captain explaining the Second Lesson to Eddie in Mitch Albom's
The Five People You Meet in Heaven (Hyperion Books, New York, NY. 2003).

Acknowledgments

There are many people that I wish to thank for their time and willingness to assist in this project. At F.A. Davis, Christa Fratantoro, Acquisitions Editor, began by listening to the idea. She has been available to lend guidance and support throughout the entire process. Jennifer Pine provided the direction to bring the ideas from my head, to the inside of a front and back cover. Caryn Abramowitz gave me the necessary tools, wisdom, and confidence to complete each chapter successfully.

There are others I would also like to thank. Joella Davis and Kinder Cannon worked tirelessly to produce the photographs. The student models, John Kiddy, Maegan Mathisen, Julie Tribett, Chris Aubrey, Todd Guggisberg, Stephen Melnyk, Aimee Ragasa, Shane Miller, and David Libert performed like veterans during the photo shoot.

Lynne-Marie Young, MEd, ATC, and Bernadette Buckley, PhD, ATC, provided their expertise in the creation of the anatomy illustrations and instructor ancillaries. Melissa Anderson, ATC, provided another set of eyes in the early writing of each chapter. Heather Priest Gilchrist, ATC, and Rachel Daubenmire, ATC, conducted several literature reviews for the research briefs.

During the writing of this book, many allied health-care professionals served as chapter reviewers. I would like to thank each of them for their time and expertise. Their suggestions helped to strengthen the book.

A project such as this is not possible without the assistance of numerous manufacturers and others associated with taping, wrapping, bracing, and padding products. I want to thank the following people.

Johnson & Johnson
Ken Young Inc
Jack Weakley

3M
Dave Egemo

BSN-Jobst
Barbara Himmelein, Ernie Hahn,
Russ Kibler, Cindy Massey

Active Ankle
Scott Morton

Swede-O
Tom Traver

Silipos
Andrei Lombardi

Sports Health
John Miller, Tom Rokovitz, Amy Bauer

Breg
Jeff Regan, Jay Bassett

Dj Ortho
Brian Moore, Bob Rojahn

Med Spec
Scott Gaylord

Ultra Ankle
Rick Peters

Aircast
Dennis Mattessich, Bill Bartlett

Kinetic Innovations
Les Lundberg

Douglas Protective Equipment
Doug Douglass

Williams Sports Group
Fred Williams

Riddell
Kay Johnson

Sports Authority
Dan Davis

Medco
Don Laux

Hartmann Conco
Ernest Nelson

Sammons Preston Rolyan

Andover Coated Products
Julie Gatto, Ron O'Neil,
Christina Costanza

Impact Innovative Products
John Matechen

University of North Florida
Jim Scholler
Mark Power
Mike Munch
Bob Shepard
Mike Weglicki
Deborah Miller
David Wilson

Jacksonville University
Doug Frye
Tom Leonard

Florida Atlantic University
Mike Short

First Coast Orthotics and Prosthetics
Travis Richards
Carol Richards

Bailey Manufacturing Company
Brian Kolenich

Jacksonville Orthopaedic Institute
Matt Paulus

Episcopal High School
Mark Waybright
John Silkey

Dick's Sporting Goods
Ed Kish

Dr. Richard Salko
Terri Russ
Melissa Acevedo

Western Michigan University
Michael G. Miller

Stone Ridge School of the Sacred Heart
Jill Marks

Reviewers

David Berry, PhD, ATC
Assistant Professor of Athletic Training
Department of Health Promotion and Human
  Performance
Weber State University
Ogden, Utah

W. David Carr, PhD, ATC/L
Clinical Assistant Professor of Athletic Training
College of Business Administration
The University of Tulsa
Tulsa, Oklahoma

Tina Davlin, PhD, ATC
Assistant Professor and Director, Athletic Training
  Education Program
College of Social Sciences
Xavier University
Cincinnati, Ohio

Jean Fruh, MS, (ABD) ATC
Former Assistant Professor and Director of Athletic
  Training
Department of Exercise Science
West Virginia Wesleyan College
Buckhannon, West Virginia

Pete Koehneke, MS, ATC
Professor and Director, Athletic Training Education
  Program
Chair, Department of Sports Medicine, Health, and
  Human Performance
Canisius College
Buffalo, New York

Cynthia McKnight, PhD, ATC
Associate Professor of Physical Education
Chair, Department of Undergraduate Physical
  Education & Athletic Training
Azusa Pacific University
Azusa, California

Matthew Rothbard, MS, ATC
Clinical Assistant Professor of Athletic Training
Department of Kinesiology
Towson University
Towson, Maryland

Shannon Singletary, PT, ATC, CSCS
Supervisor of Sports Medicine
Department of Orthopedics/Sports Medicine
University of Mississippi Medical Center
Jackson, Mississippi

Chad Starkey, PhD, ATC
Visiting Professor, Athletic Training Program
School of Recreation and Sport Sciences
Ohio University
Athens, Ohio

Stacy Walker, PhD, ATC, LAT
Assistant Professor of Physical Education
School of Physical Education, Sport, & Exercise
  Science
Ball State University
Muncie, Indiana

Katie Walsh, EdD, ATC
Associate Professor and Director, Athletic Training
  Program
The Department of Health Education and Promotion
East Carolina University
Greenville, North Carolina

Preface

In the *Complete Book of Athletic Taping Techniques* (Parker Publishing Company, West Nyack, NY, 1972), J.V. Cerney describes taping as "the art and science of utilizing adhesive tape as a productive and functional tool." Today, this art and science also encompasses wrapping, bracing, and padding. The ability to apply the technique with proper tension and body contouring and placement, while avoiding gaps, wrinkles, and inconsistent layering and pressure is the *art*. Determining the needs of the healthy individual, the technique to use with a specific injury or condition, the effectiveness of the technique, and the knowledge of the allied health-care professional is the *science*. Taping, wrapping, bracing, and padding techniques can serve as *productive and functional tools* when properly applied within a comprehensive therapeutic exercise program. These techniques are designed to compliment range of motion, flexibility, muscular strength and endurance, neuromuscular, cardiorespiratory, and therapeutic modality goals in the prevention, treatment, and rehabilitation of injuries and conditions.

Taping, wrapping, bracing, and padding techniques are available in a variety of designs and are applied using many different methods. It is common for allied health-care professionals to have "their own way" with regards to technique use, construction, or application. These methods are often based on past experiences and anecdotal evidence. In addition, application of the same technique, on two different individuals with similar injuries, often results in different outcomes. The "one-size-fits-all" technique does not currently exist. Therefore, the use of taping, wrapping, bracing, and padding techniques should be based on the intended purpose of the technique, the individual, the injury, the activity, and the available evidence-based data. I wrote this text to provide allied health-care professionals multiple taping, wrapping, bracing, and padding techniques and alternatives. Differences among healthy individuals and their injuries and conditions, the skill and experience levels of allied health-care professionals, material availability, and facility budgets and sizes require a diverse set of strategies in the prevention, treatment, and rehabilitation of healthy individuals.

The overall goal of *Orthopedic Taping, Wrapping, Bracing, and Padding* is to facilitate learning of the cognitive, psychomotor, and affective skills required to effectively tape, wrap, brace, and pad healthy individuals. The book is intended for entry-level undergraduate and graduate athletic training students, practicing athletic trainers, and other allied health-care professionals responsible for technique application. Among students, the text is

designed to first be used in the didactic setting, then taken to the clinical setting for practice and skill development. The material in the text covers the National Athletic Trainers' Association (NATA) Role Delineation Study and the NATA Education Council Educational Competencies and Proficiencies related to taping, wrapping, bracing, and padding. Among practicing athletic trainers and other allied health-care professionals, the text can serve as a practical resource guide.

The text is designed for use in a semester-length course or course component normally taught early in an athletic training education program curriculum. The all-inclusive, step-by-step technique focus of the text requires that students possess a general knowledge of anatomy, biomechanics, injury evaluation, treatment, and rehabilitation. This general knowledge can be obtained through either prerequisite or concurrent courses in an education program. Several techniques can be performed during the first day of instruction, while others require advanced knowledge and skill levels obtained through years of clinical experience.

Chapter 1 introduces tapes, wraps, braces, and pads and includes types, objectives, and recommendations for application. Chapter 2 provides information on current and long-range needs and structural considerations of the application area. Chapter 3 includes the foot and toes, Chapter 4, the ankle; Chapter 5, the lower leg; Chapter 6, the knee; Chapter 7, the thigh, hip, and pelvis; Chapter 8, the shoulder and upper arm; Chapter 9, the elbow and forearm; Chapter 10, the wrist; Chapter 11, the hand, fingers, and thumb; and Chapter 12, the thorax, abdomen, and spine. These chapters begin with a general review of injuries and conditions that are common to the body region(s). Next, the chapters present step-by-step taping, wrapping, bracing, and padding techniques used in the prevention, treatment, and rehabilitation of these injuries and conditions. Chapter 13 discusses liability issues, standards and testing, and construction and application of NCAA and NFHS mandatory and standard equipment and padding.

Several pedagogical features are used throughout the text to enhance the material, to assist the reader in developing critical thinking skills, and to further explain the use and application of the techniques.

Injuries and Conditions

Chapters 3 through 12 contain a brief discussion of common injuries and conditions for the particular body region. This feature allows readers to further develop an understanding of the purpose of the technique for each injury and condition.

Photographs and Line Drawings

The photography in each chapter plays an integral role in the presentation and learning of the techniques. The photographs are arranged to provide the reader with visual representation of the specific instructions for each technique step. The line drawings illustrate the basic anatomy of each body region to assist the reader in developing an understanding of the purpose and effect of each technique on bone and soft tissue.

Key Words

Anatomical structures and positions, injuries and conditions, and important terms are boldfaced to assist readers in recognizing key words.

Helpful Hints

Helpful hints, identified by the icon ʄ, provide quick tips and other "tricks of the trade" to assist in technique application.

Research Brief Boxes

Research brief boxes offer evidence-based information on the techniques.

IF/THEN Boxes

IF/THEN boxes guide the student in choosing the most appropriate technique in a given situation.

Details Boxes

Details boxes offer additional information on technique origin, construction, and application.

Critical Thinking Boxes

Critical thinking boxes are located throughout each chapter to allow the reader the opportunity to critically synthesize technique use and application. Answers to the questions are provided in the Appendix Solutions section.

Case Study

Case studies promote critical thinking and allow the reader the opportunity to select appropriate techniques within an actual injury prevention, treatment, and rehabilitation protocol. Answers to the questions are provided in the Appendix Solutions section.

Wrap-Up

The wrap-up summarizes the most important content of each chapter.

Web References

Web references provide resources for supplemental information on the prevention, treatment, and rehabilitation of injuries and conditions, on-line journals, surgical procedures, photographs, and other educational materials.

References

Each chapter contains a list of cited references to give both the reader and instructor the opportunity to locate additional information.

Glossary

Key words from each chapter are located at the end of the book.

Index

The index allows for cross-referencing to locate specific techniques and information within the chapters.

Instructor's CD-ROM

The CD-ROM provides multiple choice questions, clinical activities, and real-world situations for each chapter. The questions and activities encompass the NATA Role Delineation Study and NATA Education Council Educational Competencies and Proficiencies associated with taping, wrapping, bracing, and padding techniques.

This text does not intend to include every taping, wrapping, bracing, and padding technique that allied health-care professionals currently utilize. I wrote the text to provide athletic training students a comprehensive look into and practicing allied health-care professionals a resource of "the art and science" of taping, wrapping, bracing, and padding. I hope that after each has had the opportunity to read the text, both groups will develop the necessary skills to effectively use the techniques in the prevention, treatment, and rehabilitation of injuries and conditions among healthy individuals. I would appreciate any ideas or suggestions for the improvement of this text in future editions. Please feel free to contact me with your suggestions through F.A. Davis Company, my Publisher, or directly.

Joel W. Beam, EdD, ATC, LAT

Brief Contents

Contents

Tapes, Wraps, Braces, and Pads

1. Discuss and explain the types, objectives, and application recommendations for taping, wrapping, bracing, and padding techniques used when preventing, treating, and rehabilitating injuries.
2. Discuss and demonstrate the ability to select the appropriate types of tapes, wraps, braces, and pads used when preventing, treating, and rehabilitating various injuries.

Taping, wrapping, bracing, and padding techniques have been used for many years by health-care professionals in the prevention, treatment, and rehabilitation of injuries. Athletic trainers, the allied health-care professionals who typically apply the techniques, are skilled in technique application as a result of instruction and practice. For example, in a day, a typical athletic trainer may tape 20 ankles, wrap two adductor strains, apply three knee braces, and construct two protective pads. With appropriate didactic instruction in anatomy, biomechanics, injury evaluation, treatment, and rehabilitation, students can become proficient in the application of these techniques. In fact, practice may be the only hurdle to becoming proficient.

Current research investigating the effectiveness of taping, wrapping, bracing, and padding techniques has demonstrated conflicting results among various populations. Many researchers have examined the influence of taping and bracing techniques on the reduction of injuries, functional performance, proprioception, balance, and joint position sense. Although these studies have provided useful empirical data, much remains unknown. Summaries of relevant studies will be presented in "Research Brief" boxes and accompany specific taping, wrapping, bracing, and padding techniques in later chapters.

TAPES

The use of tape in preventing, treating, and rehabilitating injuries and conditions has been and continues to be popular with health-care professionals. Many intercollegiate and professional sport medical staffs allot large proportions of their budgets to tape and associated supplies necessary for application. There are many different types of tape, and decisions regarding which type to purchase and use should be based on the desired objective of the technique.

Types

Tapes fall into three main categories: non-elastic, elastic, and cast (Fig. 1–1). Non-elastic and elastic tapes have an adhesive backing that can adhere directly to the skin and other materials.

Non-Elastic

As the name implies, non-elastic tape does not possess elastic properties, so conformability to body contours can be difficult. Non-elastic tape is manufactured in a variety of sizes and colors. The most commonly used is white, which is available in $\frac{1}{2}$, 1, $1\frac{1}{2}$, 2, and 3 inch widths by 10 to 15 yard lengths (see Fig. 1–1A).

Non-elastic tape is made of cotton and/or polyester with a zinc oxide adhesive mass backing. Some types possess a high adhesive backing designed for application directly to the skin. The number of longitudinal and vertical fibers per inch in the backing determines the quality of the tape.[5] High quality tapes have 85 or more longitudinal fibers and 65 vertical fibers per square inch. Lesser quality tapes have 65 or fewer longitudinal fibers and 45 vertical fibers. The quality of the tape will determine the amount and durability of the adhesive backing and the roll tension. The adhesive mass should be of a quality to withstand moisture, perspiration, and body and joint movements of the individual, and allow for easy removal. High quality tapes typically possess the greatest amount of adhesive backing. Roll tension refers to how the tape comes off the roll. The tension ideally should be even and fluid when removing the tape from the roll.

Elastic

Elastic tape, commonly referred to as stretch tape, is manufactured in heavyweight and lightweight designs. The tape is available in 1, 2, 3, and 4 inch widths by 5 yard length in two commonly used colors, white and tan (see Fig. 1–1B).

Elastic tape is made of twisted cotton with an adhesive backing. The quality of elastic tapes is determined in a similar fashion as non-elastic tapes. The heavyweight tape is thicker than the lightweight design and provides more tensile strength and support when applied to the body. Several of the heavyweight designs require taping scissors to cut the tape from the roll during technique application. Elastic tapes have the ability to conform to the contour of the body while providing support.

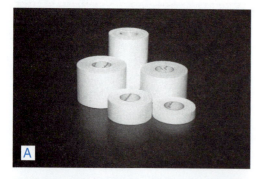

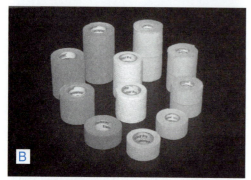

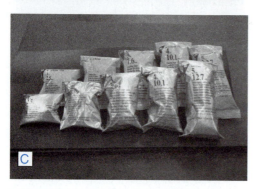

Figure 1-1 **A** Variety of non-elastic tape.
B Variety of heavyweight and lightweight elastic
tape. **C** Variety of semirigid and rigid cast tape.

Cast

Unlike non-elastic and elastic tapes, cast tape is a fiberglass
fabric containing a polyurethane resin that reacts to water
and air, causing a chemical reaction. This reaction makes
the fiberglass set, or become hard. The tape is manufactured
on a roll in semirigid and rigid types, and is available in 1,

2, 3, 4, and 5 inch widths by 4 yard length (see Fig. 1–1C).
Semirigid tape provides support while allowing range of
motion of the body parts; rigid tape provides complete
immobilization. Both types conform to the contour of the
body. Taping scissors are needed to cut cast tape.

Objectives of Taping

Use taping techniques to:

• Provide support and reduce range of motion in prevent-
ing injuries
• Provide support and reduce range of motion in treating
and rehabilitating existing injuries
• Secure elastic wraps when preventing, treating, and
rehabilitating injuries
• Secure pads in preventing and treating injuries
• Secure dressings in treating wounds

Recommendations for Tape Application

Applying tape is more than simply "placing the sticky
side down." The following recommendations will assist in
effectively applying taping techniques.

Preparation of Individual

Clean and dry the skin of the individual. Body oils from
perspiration, lotions, and dirt/grass will lessen the adhesive properties of the tape. In some cases, shave the body
hair over the area for effective application and removal of
the tape. The position of the individual during application
is important. As a general rule, when applying non-elastic
and cast tapes, position the joint in the range of motion in
which the joint will be stabilized. The position of the
joint when applying elastic tape will vary because of the
stretch qualities of the tape. There are exceptions to these
rules, which will be illustrated in subsequent chapters.

Tearing Tape

Learning how to tear non-elastic and elastic tapes is the
first step in becoming proficient in technique application.
There are many methods to tear tape, but all have two
commonalities: becoming comfortable with a method and
practicing it to become efficient. Below is a description of
one successful method. It can be altered to accommodate
individual preference (Fig. 1–2).

STEP 1: Hold the roll of non-elastic tape in one
hand. Place the third finger of the hand through the
roll to provide stabilization (see Fig. 1–2A). The roll
should rest on the **proximal** phalanx of the finger
and slightly on the palm.

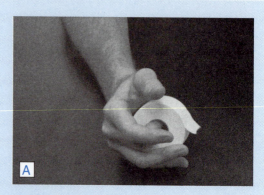

Figure 1-2

STEP 2: Place the tape extending from the roll between the tips of the thumb and second finger (see Fig. 1–2B).

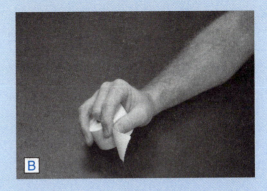

STEP 3: With the thumb and second finger of the other hand, hold the extended tape between the fingertips in close proximity to the fingers of the first hand (see Fig. 1–2C).

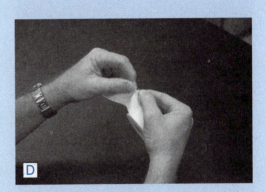

STEP 4: Following this placement, pull both hands in straight, opposing directions with a slight downward motion (see Fig. 1–2D). Pressure on the fingertips with this movement will begin to tear the horizontal fibers of the tape.

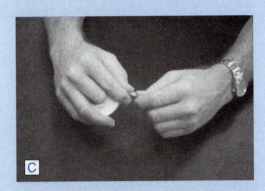

STEP 5: As the tape begins to tear, quickly **supinate** the hand holding the roll and **pronate** the other hand in a tearing motion (see Fig. 1–2E). The hands will rotate in opposite directions. Avoid twisting or crimping the tape. With practice, these two movements become synchronized into one movement.

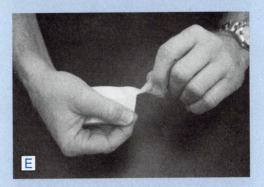

Figure 1-2 *continued*

Practice this method to become proficient at tearing all sizes of non-elastic tape. Without this skill, smooth and efficient application of non-elastic tape will not be possible. The roll of tape should remain in one hand during application, in order to avoid the time it would take to set the tape down and pick it up again repeatedly. Note, however, that the ability to tear most sizes of lightweight elastic tape should come with skill in tearing non-elastic tape. The ability to tear heavyweight elastic tape requires experience and variation of hand and finger positions on the roll (Fig. 1–3). Do not become overly concerned if tearing heavyweight elastic tape is difficult; most health-care professionals use taping scissors to cut heavyweight elastic tape during application. If the position of the individual allows, have him or her cut the tape with scissors during technique application. This procedure will lessen the application time and involve the individual in the technique.

> **Helpful Hint:** Hold the roll of elastic tape in one hand without placing a finger through the roll (see Fig. 1–3A). Instead of placing the extended tape between the fingertips of the thumbs and second fingers, grasp the tape between the distal thumbs and second, third, fourth, and fifth fingers of each hand (see Fig. 1–3B). The fingers will push the tape into the palms of the hands. Pull the tape tight to remove the elastic properties and rotate the hands in opposite directions (see Fig. 1–3C). As the hands rotate, use the forearms and upper arms to assist with the rotating movement.

Application of Tape

These general recommendations will guide the application of non-elastic and elastic taping techniques (Fig. 1–4). The recommendations for cast tape are discussed at the end of this section. Individual variations of the techniques are presented in each chapter.

Non-Elastic and Elastic

Once the individual is positioned on the taping table or bench with the skin clean and dry, begin the taping technique. Decide whether non-elastic or elastic tape will be applied directly to the skin or over pre-tape material. Applying tape directly to the skin will provide the greatest support, but may cause skin irritation with daily use.

- Regardless of which method is used, applying adherent tape spray prior to taping should lessen migration of the tape (see Fig. 1–4A).
- Pre-tape material, referred to as underwrap or prewrap, is a thin, porous foam material wrapped on 3 inch rolls (see Fig. 1–4B). Apply one layer of the material in an overlapping fashion, covering the body area.

Tape techniques applied over bony prominences and high friction areas should receive extra attention. Use thin foam pads on the heel and lace areas with ankle and foot techniques. For individuals who require daily taping, provide additional protection by using skin lubricants and foam pads.

- Use thin foam pads over bony prominences and high friction areas to reduce irritation, which can lead to cuts or blisters of the skin (see Fig. 1–4C).

The objective of the technique and the size of the individual will dictate the type of the tape to use. As previously mentioned, non-elastic tape does not have elastic properties and will adhere to the body at the specific angle in which the tape is applied. Non-elastic tape also provides more stability than elastic tape. Applying non-elastic tape over body contours can be difficult, however, especially

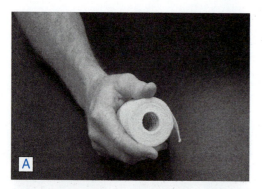

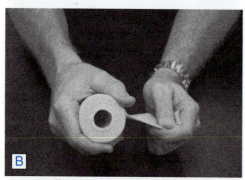

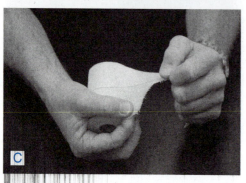

Figure 1-3

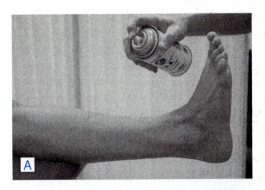

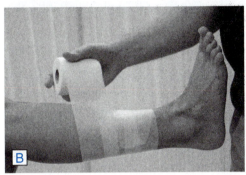

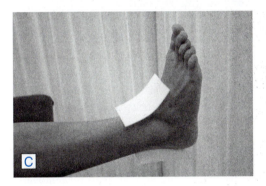

Figure 1-4

with small joints. With practice and experience, the correct angles of application will be obtained. Do not force non-elastic tape to fit body contours. Place non-elastic tape over the belly of a muscle carefully to avoid causing constriction. Focus attention on restricting range of motion affecting normal body movements such as gait. In these cases, use elastic tape to provide support while allowing normal body movement.

Allergic reactions and trauma to the skin can occur when tape is applied. A reaction to taping materials, such as adherents or zinc oxide, can appear immediately or days following contact. Redness, swelling, and itching may indicate an allergic reaction. Protect the area from further injury and treat accordingly. If taping materials

are shown to be the cause, discontinue their use. Replace the closed basketweave technique (see Fig. 4–1), for example, with a lace-up ankle brace (see Fig. 4–14) to limit inversion, eversion, plantar flexion, and dorsiflexion until the skin is asymptomatic. Refer the individual to a physician if symptoms persist.

Blisters and lacerations are often the result of gaps, wrinkles, or inconsistent roll tension during application. Proper management of the wound includes cleansing, debridement, and dressing. If the wound is open, maintain a sterile wound environment. Use foam, felt, lubricants, or hydrogel wound dressings to protect a blister or laceration during tape application. Cut a felt or foam donut pad (see Fig. 3–27) to lessen the amount of stress and impact over the wound. Applying skin lubricants either under or over a donut pad to further reduce friction is possible. Hydrogel wound dressings not only provide a moist wound environment but also reduce friction. Use adhesive gauze material (see Fig. 3–13) to attach the dressing to the skin.

Follow these recommendations when applying non-elastic and elastic tapes:

- Gather the equipment and supplies needed (which may include adherent tape spray, pre-tape material, taping scissors, and various tapes, wraps, and pads) prior to beginning technique application.
- As a general rule, each technique begins and ends with anchor strips.
- To avoid gaps, overlap each strip of tape by at least ½ of its width.
- To avoid wrinkles, smooth each strip of tape with the fingers or hands as it is applied.
- Avoid gaps, wrinkles, or inconsistent roll tension, which may lead to skin irritations such as cuts and blisters.
- Follow the sequence of strips in each technique, avoiding multiple wraps or turns around a muscle or joint.
- Exercise caution when applying tape on individuals with broken skin, rashes on the skin, or known allergies to taping materials.

DETAILS

Use non-elastic and elastic tapes of ½ and 1 inch widths by 5 and 15 yard lengths on the foot, toes, hand, and fingers; 1½, 2, and 3 inch widths by 5 and 15 yard lengths on the ankle, lower leg, knee, thigh, hip/pelvis, upper arm, elbow, forearm, wrist, hand, and fingers; and 3, 4, and 6 inch widths by 5 and 15 yard lengths on the knee, thigh, hip/pelvis, shoulder, upper arm, elbow, chest/abdomen, and spine.

Helpful Hint: If ½ inch or 1 inch non-elastic or elastic tapes are not available, create a roll from 1½ inch or 2 inch non-elastic or 2 inch elastic tape. Begin a longitudinal tear down the extended end of the tape at the desired width. Continue to tear this strip around the roll one time, leaving the other strip anchored on the roll. Strips in the same (¾ inch or 1 inch) or different (½ inch and 1 inch) widths on the same roll of non-elastic and elastic tapes may be made.

Cast

Applying cast tape requires several pieces of equipment: gloves, taping scissors, water, self-adherent wrap, stockinet, or padding material. Position the individual on the taping table or bench. The objective of the technique and size of the individual will determine the type and width of tape to use.

Rigid tape is normally applied by an orthopedic technician or physician following acute fractures. Application guidelines for rigid casting are beyond the scope of this text and can be found elsewhere. Semirigid tape, on the other hand, is used by many health-care professionals when total immobilization is not required. In the athletic setting, this tape is often used to provide support and protection when treating various injuries.

Generally, cast tape is applied over stockinet and soft cast padding, Gore-Tex padding, or self-adherent wrap. Apply the cast tape over one layer of stockinet placed directly on the skin and covered with two to three layers of soft cast padding material. This technique is commonly used with rigid tape techniques that require extended periods of wear. Protect the padding material under the cast tape from excessive moisture to prevent skin **maceration** and itching. An alternative to use with rigid tape is a Gore-Tex cast padding, which repels water, allowing any type of water activity, including bathing. Moisture underneath the cast tape evaporates, and the skin dries completely. In the athletic setting, apply three to four layers of self-adherent wrap underneath semirigid cast tape to allow reuse of the cast upon removal.

Applying semirigid cast tape requires experience and skill (see Fig. 11–12). The following recommendations apply to cast tape techniques:

- Wear examination or surgical gloves coated with petroleum jelly or silicone to protect the hands from tape resin and prevent the tape from adhering to the gloves during application.
- Open the sealed foil pouch and remove the roll of tape. Most rigid and semirigid tapes require immersion in water of 70° to 75°F to begin the chemical reaction. Approximately three to five minutes is allowed to apply, mold, and shape the tape before setting occurs.
- Apply the tape in a spiral or circular pattern with slight roll tension.
- Overlap each layer by $\frac{1}{3}$ to $\frac{1}{2}$ of the width of the tape. The number of layers applied will determine the amount of support.
- Avoid gaps, wrinkles, inconsistent roll tension, or direct contact of the tape with the skin to lessen irritation.
- Use taping scissors to make partial cuts in the material to fit the contours of the body. Pad bony prominences to lessen the occurrence of irritation.
- Place the last 8–10 inches of tape on the body without roll tension. Smooth and mold the tape to the body part with the hands to achieve adhesion of the layers.
- Approximately 10–15 minutes after removal of the tape from its pouch, curing is complete.

DETAILS

Use cast tape of 1 inch width by 4 yard length on the toes and fingers; 2 inch width by 4 yard length on the foot, ankle, forearm, wrist, and hand; 3 inch width by 4 yard length on the ankle, lower leg, upper arm, elbow, and forearm; 4 inch width by 4 yard length on the ankle, lower leg, knee, thigh, hip/pelvis, shoulder, upper arm, elbow, chest/abdomen, and spine; and 5 inch width by 4 yard length on the ankle, knee, thigh, hip/pelvis, shoulder, chest/abdomen, and spine.

Removing Tape

Removing tape can cause injury to the individual and should be performed in a controlled manner.

Non-Elastic and Elastic

There are several ways to remove non-elastic and elastic tapes (Fig. 1–5). Manually, remove the skin from the tape in a direct line with the body.[5]

- One hand grasps the tape and pulls it across the skin while the other hand pulls the skin in the opposite direction (see Fig. 1–5A). Do not rip the tape from the skin.
- Tape removal solvents in spray or liquid forms work as well. Apply the solvent between the skin and tape to dissolve the adhesive (see Fig. 1–5B).

If using tape removal solvents, thoroughly wash the area and monitor for possible skin reactions to the chemicals. Taping scissors and cutting tools used for removal allow individuals to perform the task themselves.

- Taping scissors are designed with a blunt end to reach under the tape and reduce the chance of damage to the skin (see Fig. 1–5C).[5]
- Tape cutters are molded plastic tools with a single-edged metal blade located at the end (see Fig. 1–5D). These tools fit into the hand and also have a blunt end. Purchase replacement blades for tape cutters as needed.
- To remove tape, slip the blunt end of the scissors or cutter under the tape and cut in a **proximal-to-distal** direction away from the body. Keep the scissors or cutter parallel to the skin, following the contour of the body and avoiding bony prominences (see Fig. 1–5E).

Cast

Remove semirigid cast tape with taping scissors or a cast saw and spreaders, or by unwrapping. Rigid tape requires the use of a cast saw, cast spreaders, and scissors (see Fig. 1–5F). Guidelines for cast saw use can be found elsewhere. Exercise care when operating a cast saw.

Chapter 1: Tapes, Wraps, Braces, and Pads   7

Tapes, Wraps, Braces, and Pads

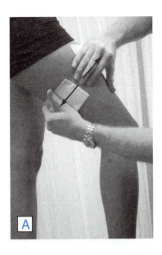
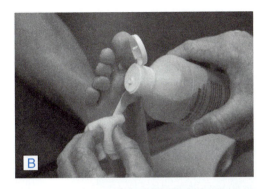
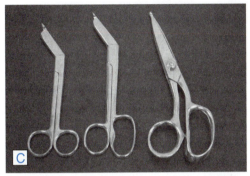
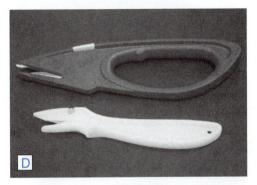
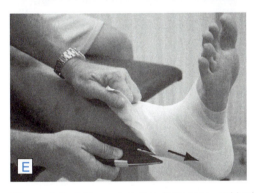
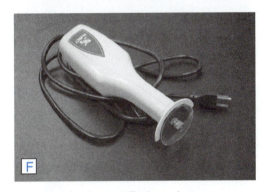

Figure 1-5 **A** Removing skin from tape. **B** Liquid tape-removal solvent. **C** Taping scissors. (Left) Single ring. (Middle) Double ring. (Right) Heavy duty. **D** Tape cutters. **E** Removing tape with cutters. **F** Cast saw.

Critical Thinking Question 1

During football practice, several players begin to complain of a burning sensation over the **posterior** heel area. Prior to practice, you applied a preventive taping technique to their ankles. You remove the tape and discover irritation of the skin over the posterior heel of each player.

▶ **Question: How can you treat and prevent skin irritation?**

...IF/THEN...

IF the scissors or cutter cannot be easily placed between the tape and skin, **THEN** apply a skin lubricant to the blunt end of the scissors to assist in cutting the tape in tight areas.

WRAPS

Wraps are used for a variety of purposes and can be reused for multiple applications. Similar to tapes, many different types of wraps are available; their use should be based on the objective of the technique.

Types

Wraps, similar to tape, can be divided into three basic types: elastic, self-adherent, and cloth (Fig. 1–6).

Elastic

Elastic wraps allow for adjustments of compression during application. These wraps also conform well to body

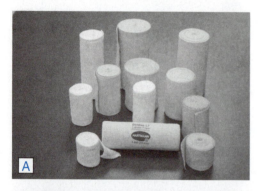

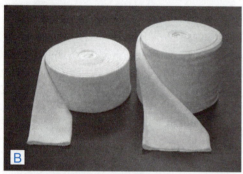

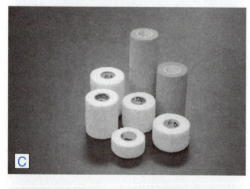

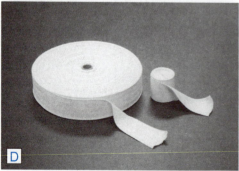

Figure 1-6 A Variety of elastic wraps. **B** Variety of elastic sleeves. **C** Variety of self-adherent wrap. **D** Cloth wrap. (Left) Roll. (Right) Individual wrap.

contours, providing multidirectional compression. Use Velcro fasteners, metal clips, or tape to anchor the wraps. Wash and dry elastic wraps after each use and reuse them. Similar to elastic wraps, elastic sleeves provide compression to the extremities. No additional anchor is required. Elastic wraps are made of cotton, rubber latex, or nylon in white and tan in 2, 3, 4, and 6 inch widths by 5 yard length and 4 and 6 inch widths by 10 yard length (see Fig. 1–6A). The sleeves are made of cotton and rubber latex in 3 and 5 inch widths by 11 yard length (see Fig. 1–6B).

Self-Adherent

Self-adherent wraps have elastic properties and the ability to adhere to themselves without irritation to hair or skin. These wraps come in a variety of colors, and tear manually. Self-adherent wraps conform to body contours easily and provide adjustable compression. The wraps are intended for single use. Made of elastic yarn, they are available in 1, 1½, 2, 2¾, 3, 4, and 6 inch widths by 6 yard length (see Fig. 1–6C).

Cloth

Cloth wraps, referred to as ankle wraps, are made of strong cotton weaves in a 2 inch width by 36 or 72 yard length roll. Cut individual wraps in 72–96 inch lengths from the roll (see Fig. 1–6D). Use cloth wraps in a **prophylactic** manner to prevent medial and lateral ankle sprains. The wraps provide mild support. Wash and dry cloth wraps after each use and reuse.

Objectives of Wrapping

Use wrapping techniques to:

- Provide compression to reduce effusion and swelling when treating and rehabilitating injuries
- Provide support and reduce range of motion when preventing, treating, and rehabilitating injuries
- Secure pads when preventing and treating injuries
- Secure dressings when treating wounds

Recommendations for Wrap Application

The following recommendations apply generally to all wrapping techniques.

Preparation of Individual

The objective of the wrapping technique will determine the position of the individual. For example, when applying a wrap over a muscular area, sustain muscular contraction during the technique to lessen the chance of constriction. To provide support and reduction in range of motion, position the joint in the range of motion in which the joint will be stabilized. Because wraps do not possess adhesive properties, wraps may be applied directly to the skin or, for cloth wraps, over socks.

Application of Wraps

After determining the technique objective and positioning the individual, choose the appropriate type of wrap.

Tapes, Wraps, Braces, and Pads

Elastic

Elastic wraps have the potential to cause injury and should be used with care. Improper application can cause impairment in circulation, abnormal accumulation of swelling or effusion, or irritation of the skin. Use these recommendations for assistance when applying elastic wraps.

- Apply elastic wraps with firm, constant tension.
- Overlap each successive turn of the wrap by ½ of its width, while being careful to eliminate gaps, wrinkles, or inconsistent roll tension, which may cause skin irritation.
- Apply the compression wrap technique in a **distal-to-proximal** sequence to assist in venous return (see Fig. 3–15). Never cover the **distal** aspects of the extremities with the wrap. Keep the tips of the fingers and toes visible and monitor for impairment of circulation.
- Anchor elastic wraps with Velcro fasteners, metal clips, or non-elastic or elastic tapes.
- Place the end of the wrap and anchor on the dorsal or **anterior** aspect of the body part for comfort and easy removal.

Detailed elastic wrap application techniques are presented in individual chapters.

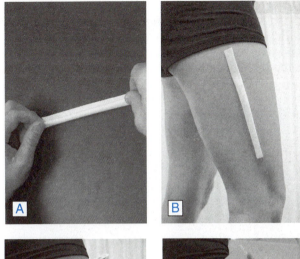
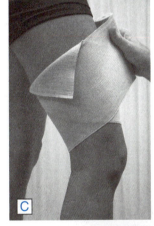
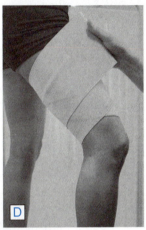
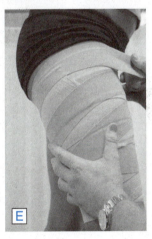

Figure 1-7

DETAILS

Use elastic wraps of 2 inch width by 5 yard length on the foot, toes, wrist, hand, and fingers; 3 inch width by 5 yard length on the foot, ankle, wrist, and hand; 4 inch width by 5 yard length on the foot, ankle, lower leg, upper arm, elbow, forearm, and wrist; 6 inch width by 5 yard length on the lower leg, knee, thigh, shoulder, upper arm, elbow, and chest/abdomen; 4 inch width by 10 yard length on the knee, thigh, hip/pelvis, shoulder, chest/abdomen, and spine; and 6 inch width by 10 yard length on the knee, hip/pelvis, shoulder, chest/abdomen, and spine.

Migration, slippage, or bunching of the elastic wrap may lessen the effectiveness of the technique (Fig. 1–7). To prevent this from happening, use one of several methods. Apply adherent tape spray to the area prior to applying the wrap. Placing non-elastic or elastic tape strip(s) directly on the skin under the wrap is also possible.

- Tear a 6–8 inch piece of tape and double the strip onto itself, leaving the adhesive mass exposed on both sides (see Fig. 1–7A).
- Place the strip(s) in a **longitudinal** position directly on the skin and then apply the wrap (see Fig. 1–7B).

Adjusting anchors may also lessen migration, slippage, and bunching. Begin the wrapping technique by placing the loose end of the wrap on the skin.

- When applying the first wrap or turn around the body part, fold the loose end over by ⅓–½ of the wrap's width (see Fig. 1–7C).
- When applying the next wrap or turn, cover the folded end and continue with the technique (see Fig. 1–7D).

Another method involves placing an elastic tape anchor directly on the skin.

- When the wrapping technique is completed, apply the anchor partially on the wrap and partially on the skin in an overlapping manner (see Fig. 1–7E).

To fit different areas of the body, cut different lengths of elastic sleeves from a roll. Apply the elastic sleeve directly to the skin by simply pulling the sleeve onto the extremity (see Fig. 4–11). Use the sleeves during athletic, work, and casual activities.

...IF/THEN...

IF an elastic wrap loses its stretch characteristics and fails to conform to body contours, which is common with repeated use and cleaning, **THEN** use the elastic wrap only during treatments to anchor an ice bag to a body part.

Self-Adherent

Self-adherent wrap is manufactured on a roll and is applied with the same technique as elastic tape. The wrap has similar uses as elastic tape and wraps. In many taping techniques, the wrap may be used in place of pre-tape material to provide protection from irritation and additional support to a joint.

- Apply the wrap with firm and consistent tension, following body contours.
- Anchoring does not require fasteners, clips, or additional tape, an advantage of the wrap.
- Avoid gaps, wrinkles, or inconsistent roll tension.

The use of self-adherent wrap is discussed further in individual chapters.

DETAILS

Use self-adherent wrap in 1 inch width by 6 yard length on the toes and fingers; 1½ inch width by 6 yard length on the foot, ankle, wrist, and hand; 2 inch width by 6 yard length on the foot, ankle, wrist, and hand; 2¾ and 3 inch widths by 6 yard length on the foot, ankle, lower leg, upper arm, elbow, forearm, and wrist; 4 inch width by 6 yard length on the lower leg, knee, thigh, upper arm, elbow, and forearm; and 6 inch width by 6 yard length on the knee, thigh, hip/pelvis, shoulder, chest/abdomen, and spine.

Cloth

Use cloth wraps to provide support to the ankle. Apply a cloth wrap over a sock (see Fig. 4–13). Place thin foam pads over high friction areas under the wrap to reduce irritation. Apply these wraps with firm, constant tension.

During technique application, roll an elastic or cloth wrap onto the body part. (Fig. 1–8).

STEP 1: Holding the wrap in one hand, remove a portion with the other hand and place on the body part (see Fig. 1–8A).

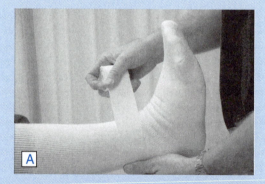

STEP 2: Hold the extended end and encircle the body part with the wrap (see Fig. 1–8B).

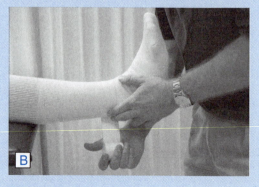

Figure 1-8

STEP 3: As the wrap encircles the body part, proceed over the extended end to anchor the wrap (see Fig. 1–8C).

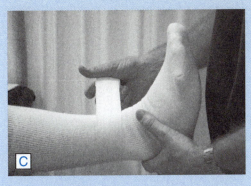

Figure 1-8 *continued*

Continue the specific steps of the application technique. During application, keep constant pressure on the wrap as it is passed between the hands.

Removal of Wraps

Remove elastic and cloth wraps by unwrapping the material after use. Use taping scissors to cut tape anchors.

Remove an elastic sleeve by pulling it off the extremity in a distal direction. Use taping scissors or tape cutters to remove self-adherent wraps. Wash and dry elastic and cloth wraps after each use and reuse.

Critical Thinking Question 2

A professor at the local university participating in an intramural basketball league on campus sustains a first degree **inversion sprain** of the left ankle. He is taken to the Athletic Training Room for treatment. After applying an ice bag, you decide to use a wrap to provide compression to reduce effusion and swelling.

▶ **Question: What type of wrap can you use?**

...IF/THEN...

IF small amounts of non-elastic and/or elastic tape, pre-tape material, and/or self-adherent wrap are left on rolls, **THEN** collect the unused rolls in a box; soccer athletes use the tape to anchor shin guards, others use the pre-tape material and wrap to tie their hair up, and some use tape and wrap cores to construct heel lifts (see Fig. 6–2) and teardrop thumb spica supports (see Fig. 11–9).

BRACES

Advances in the research and development of bracing techniques provide an opportunity to select among a variety of types. Braces are designed to be used for specific injuries and conditions, and are available for the majority of body areas and joints.

Types

Braces will be classified according to their fit, purpose, and body area design (Fig. 1–9).

Fit

The fit of a brace refers to the sizing and manufacturing, either off-the-shelf or custom-made. Off-the-shelf braces come in predetermined sizes, such as small, medium, large, and extra large (see Fig. 1–9A). Off-the-shelf braces are ready to use upon purchase and are generally less expensive than custom-made designs. Although braces are manufactured in predetermined sizes, many companies provide circumference measurements of body areas on the package to assist in proper fitting. Most off-the-shelf braces allow for small size adjustments during wear.

Custom-made braces are fitted and manufactured for specific individuals. Manufacturer representatives or orthopedic technicians typically perform the fitting procedures prior to construction of the braces (see Fig. 1–9B). The type of injury, surgical procedure, and rehabilitation, as well as the limb girth, height, weight, and sport/occupation of the individual often determine which model of brace to purchase. Because of the custom fitting, increases in muscular girth from the development of strength or length of bones from growth periods may need to be considered.

Purpose

Braces are used for dynamic purposes and can be grouped as prophylactic, functional, and rehabilitative.[1] A prophylactic brace is designed to protect an uninjured joint and the surrounding soft tissue structures. Use ankle braces as alternatives to ankle taping to protect against abnormal ranges of motion (see Fig. 1–9C).[6]

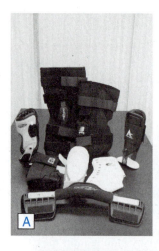
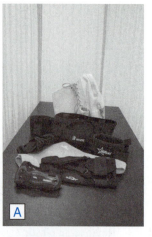
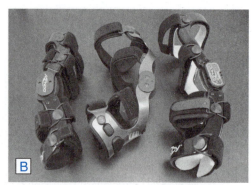
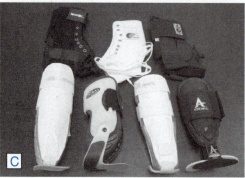
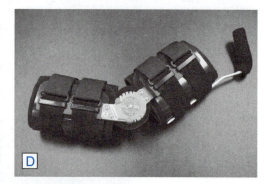
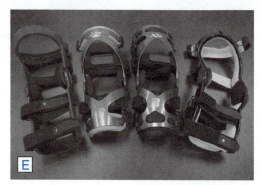

Figure 1-9 **A** (Left) Variety of off-the-shelf lower extremity braces. (Right) Variety of off-the-shelf upper extremity braces. **B** Custom-made braces. (Left) Elbow. (Middle and Right) Knee. **C** Variety of prophylactic ankle braces. **D** Rehabilitative elbow brace. **E** Variety of functional ACL knee braces.

A rehabilitative brace is used following a surgical procedure to provide immobilization. Many designs allow for control of range of motion for the individual through the use of adjustable hinges. Use hinged elbow braces for the progression of passive and active **flexion** and **extension** during rehabilitation following **ulnar collateral ligament** reconstruction (see Fig. 1–9D).

Functional braces are used to provide support and protection for existing injuries or postsurgical repairs or reconstructions.[1] Use off-the-shelf and custom-made brace designs, for example, to reduce anterior translation of the tibia on the femur to protect an injured **anterior cruciate ligament (ACL)** or ACL graft following reconstruction (see Fig. 1–9E).[2]

Body Area

Braces are designed to provide compression, protection, support, and limitations in range of motion for many areas of the body. For example:

- Orthotics are used for many foot injuries and conditions.
- Braces commonly referred to as walking boots provide immobilization and control of range of motion for foot and ankle fractures and sprains.
- Night splints are used as nocturnal braces to assist in the treatment of plantar fasciitis by keeping the foot in dorsiflexion.
- Prophylactic, functional, and rehabilitative braces for the ankle in lace-up, semirigid, air/gel bladder, and

wrap designs provide support and limit range of motion.

- Neoprene sleeves, rubber material commonly coated with elastic nylon, provide compression and support of muscular strains for the lower leg.
- Braces for the knee are available in prophylactic, functional, and rehabilitative designs.
- Neoprene sleeves and shorts support muscular strains of the thigh and hip/pelvis.
- Functional braces worn on the body or attached to football shoulder pads can reduce range of motion with glenohumeral instabilities and rotator cuff pathologies.
- Functional braces are used to lessen medial and lateral stresses and range of motion with ligamentous injuries in the elbow. Rehabilitative elbow braces are used for postsurgical conditions.
- Wrist braces made of neoprene or semirigid plastic are available in prophylactic, functional, and rehabilitative designs.
- Braces for the hand and fingers can provide immobilization, support, and compression.
- Functional and rehabilitative braces for the chest/abdomen and spine can provide support and immobilization for a variety of injuries and conditions.

Illustrations and further discussions of these and other braces are found in subsequent chapters.

Braces are constructed from a variety of materials. The materials used vary as much as the types of braces. Many braces are constructed from tempered and aircraft aluminums and carbon composites. Other braces use semirigid plastic, layered nylon, polyester Lycra, and air and gel bladders. Neoprene, porous nylon, and polyester materials are also used in many brace designs.

Objectives of Bracing

Use bracing techniques to:

- Provide support and protection when preventing injuries
- Provide support and protection when treating and rehabilitating existing injuries
- Provide compression to reduce effusion and swelling when treating and rehabilitating injuries
- Provide control of range of motion when treating and rehabilitating injuries

Recommendations for Brace Application

Braces are designed to provide compression, support, and protection for the individual during sport, work, and casual activities. The following recommendations will assist in achieving these objectives. Keep in mind that braces are similar to footwear in that a few days of wear are required for a break-in period.

Preparation of Individual

Clean and dry the skin of the individual for brace application. The position of the individual is determined by the type of brace worn. For example, place the individual in a seated position to apply an ankle brace and in a standing position to apply a shoulder brace.

Application of Braces

When purchased, each brace will have specific instructions for application. For proper application and fit, follow the step-by-step procedure carefully. Deviation from the steps may cause injury to the individual. One advantage of bracing techniques is that it is possible to teach the individual the application procedure, which will lessen the time required for health-care professionals to assist. Several brace designs allow for adjustments in the outer shell or frame, straps, inner pads, and hinges to achieve proper fit. Follow manufacturer guidelines when performing any adjustments to the brace.

Brace migration is a common problem that may occur even with proper fit. The easiest method to correct migration is to stop the activity and reapply the brace in the step-by-step procedure. Using a neoprene sleeve under the brace can also help lessen migration. However, the additional girth of the sleeve may affect the original fitting measurements of the brace. Applying adherent tape spray over the body area that makes contact with the brace can also lessen migration. If adherent tape spray is used, monitor brace straps for damage from the adherent and chemical components in the spray. This disadvantage of bracing (migration) is also one of its advantages; bracing allows for adjustability and reuse.

Intercollegiate and high school athletic associations provide rules governing the use of braces in practices and competitions. The National Collegiate Athletic Association (NCAA)[3] and the National Federation of State High School Associations (NFHS)[4] allow braces to be worn if no metal or **nonpliable** substance is exposed. If a metal or nonpliable substance is exposed, high-density, closed-cell foam or similar material of at least $\frac{1}{2}$ inch thickness must cover the areas. Padded covers for many braces may be purchased through the manufacturer. For a more comprehensive discussion of NCAA and NFHS rules, see Chapter 13.

Removal of Braces

The majority of braces can be removed by the individual after use. Release the straps and lift the brace from the body part. Several braces, such as shoulder instability designs and designs attached directly to the skin with tape, do require assistance.

Care of Braces

Clean braces and allow them to dry in a well-ventilated area between uses. Clean and inspect braces regularly. Rinse the frames and hinges of rigid braces with clean, fresh water, then drain and air-dry them. Hinge lubrication is typically not required; instead, use a dry lubricant such as Teflon spray. Hand wash straps and frame liners in cold water with mild detergent, then rinse and air-dry.

Wash neoprene and other soft brace materials in cold water with mild detergent, rinse and air-dry. Do not heat straps, liners, or neoprene materials in a dryer. Monitor hinge screws and movable parts for loosening and excessive wear. Replacement straps and frame liners are available for many brace designs.

Critical Thinking Question 3

A metal fabricator returns to work following surgery and rehabilitation of the right knee. The surgeon has placed her in a custom-made functional knee brace for all work activities. During the past week in the afternoons, the brace gradually migrates distally.

▶ **Question: What can you do to prevent the migration?**

...IF/THEN...

IF a brace is no longer needed by an individual to provide protection, support, and/or immobilization, **THEN** wash and retain the brace for use in the future or use for spare parts as recommended by the manufacturer.

PADS

Pads are used to provide protection from injury or further injury for the individual. Many sports require padding during play. Padding techniques range from a simple piece of felt or foam to advanced protective gear such as a football helmet.

Types

Pads are categorized into two basic types: soft, low-density materials and hard, high-density materials (Fig. 1–10).[1] Soft, low-density materials are light and comfortable on the body because of the presence of air in the material. These materials only protect the individual from impact forces at low intensity levels. By contrast, hard, high-density materials are less comfortable on the body but protect the individual from forces at high impact levels. These materials have the ability to absorb energy through deformation, resulting in less force at the area of impact.

Soft, Low-Density

Soft, low-density materials used by health-care professionals include cotton, gauze, moleskin, felt, foam, and viscoelastic polymers. These materials come in a variety of lengths, widths, and thicknesses (see Fig. 1–10A). Cotton is found in most facilities and is used to provide a mild padding effect.[5] Apply gauze in various thicknesses to lessen friction or impact forces. Use adhesive gauze material in 2, 4, and 6 inch widths and 2 and 10 yard lengths to lessen friction, cover wound dressings, and attach pads to the body. Moleskin is available in heavyweight and lightweight elastic and non-elastic designs in 1½, 2, 3, 7, 9, and 12 inch widths by 1, 4, 5, and 25 yard lengths. Use the material on high friction areas to lessen the chance of skin irritations. Moleskin

may also be used with many taping techniques to provide additional support. Made from matted wool and rayon fibers, felt comes in thicknesses of ⅛, ¼, ½, and 1 inch sheets and 36–108 inch rolls. Many types are

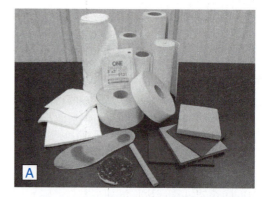

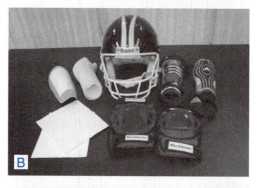

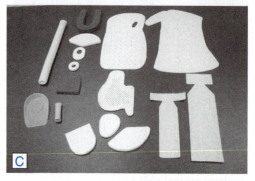

Figure 1-10 A Variety of soft, low-density pads. **B** Variety of hard, high-density pads. **C** Variety of pre-cut and pre-formed pads.

available, with and without an adhesive backing, to provide support, protection, and compression. Felt has absorbent properties that allow the material to remain in place during activity.

Foam is available in thicknesses of ⅛, ¼, ⅜, ½, ⅝, ¾, and 1 inch sheets and 36–108 inch rolls, with and without an adhesive backing. Foam is perhaps the most widely used material for padding. Foam material that allows air to transfer from cell to cell is referred to as **open-cell foam.** These foams deform quickly as stress is applied, providing minimal shock-absorbing qualities.[1] Open-cell foam is commonly used as a liner in the construction of custom-made pads. **Closed-cell foam** does not allow transfer of air from cell to cell. These foams are not as comfortable on the body, but the material regains its original shape quickly following impact. Closed-cell foams provide less cushioning at low levels of impact.[1] Manufacturers combine both open- and closed-cell foams in the construction of various pads. These padding techniques will be discussed in Chapter 13.

Thermomoldable foams are materials that allow custom-fitting to the individual for protection. The material is available in sheets of 3/16, ¼, ⅜, ½, and ⅝ inch thicknesses. Heat the material first in a conventional oven and then fit to a body part. After cooling, the material retains its shape and can be reheated and remolded if necessary. These foams can be used anywhere on the body, especially as outer padding of rigid casts.

Viscoelastic polymers, used in the design of inner soles, strips, squares, patches, and discs, protect against shear, pressure, and friction forces. Many of these materials have an adhesive backing or are incorporated into elastic sleeves or tubing to reduce migration during activity. Use viscoelastic polymers anywhere on the body, such as the foot, hand, and fingers.

Hard, High-Density

Hard, high-density pads are constructed from polycarbonate, plastic, thermoplastic, and casting materials. Polycarbonate materials are used in many helmet designs for construction of the outer shell. Off-the-shelf padding designs, such as shoulder pads, use high-density plastics for the outer shell. These materials are available in off-the-shelf designs or can be used for custom-made padding techniques (see Fig. 1–10B).

For custom-made pads, purchase thermoplastic materials made from plastic or rubber with varying amounts of conformability and resistance in thicknesses of 1/16, 1/32, 3/32, ⅛, and 3/16 inch sheets. Heat these materials at temperatures ranging from 150° to 170°F for 35 seconds to 1 minute for the materials to become pliable for molding to the body part. Use heating sources such as water, a conventional or microwave oven, or a heat gun. The most commonly used source of heat is a hydrocollator. Professionals have between one and six minutes to mold and shape the material before the thermoplastic cools and becomes rigid. The materials used

in the manufacturing process and the material's thickness will affect heating and molding times. Use thermoplastics to protect, support, and splint multiple areas of the body.

Casting materials made from fiberglass or plaster can also be used to protect, support, and splint various areas of the body. Fiberglass material is preferred over plaster by most health-care professionals because of the ease of use and less clean-up time required.

Many soft, low-density and hard, high-density pads come in off-the-shelf designs. Moleskin, felt, foam, viscoelastic polymers, and thermoplastic materials are available in pre-cut and pre-formed designs (see Fig. 1–10C). For example, moleskin plantar fascia and turf toe straps, felt heel lifts and arch pads, foam blister and corn pads, viscoelastic polymer digit covers and orthotics, and thermoplastic thumb spica and wrist cock-up splints are available from manufacturers in a variety of sizes and thicknesses. These pre-cut and pre-formed materials can lessen application and fabrication time and perhaps eliminate wasted materials.

Resilience

The resilience of soft and hard materials will determine their ability to withstand impact forces.[1] Following impact, highly resilient materials regain their shape. Use these materials over body areas that receive frequent impact. Slow-recovery resilient materials provide optimal protection and are useable over body areas that receive sporadic impact.

Objectives of Padding

Use padding techniques to:

- Provide support and protection when preventing injuries
- Provide support and protection when treating and rehabilitating existing injuries
- Provide compression to reduce effusion and swelling when treating and rehabilitating injuries

Recommendations for Pad Application

The following recommendations will assist in applying padding techniques.

Preparation of Individual

Because most padding techniques require tapes and/or wraps to secure pads to the body, preparation of the individual should follow the guidelines for taping and wrapping applications.

Application of Pads

Off-the-shelf and custom-made pads may be attached to the body with a variety of methods (Fig. 1–11). The three techniques discussed briefly here are covered in more detail in later chapters.

Tapes, Wraps, Braces, and Pads

STEP 1: When using tape, apply one layer of pre-tape material or self-adherent wrap directly to the skin over the area in an overlapping manner (see Fig. 1–11A). Apply adherent tape spray if necessary.

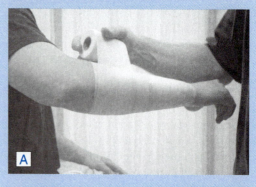

STEP 2: Place the pad on the body part over the material or wrap (see Fig. 1–11B).

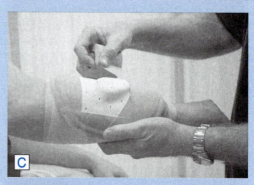

STEP 3: Anchor 2 inch or 3 inch elastic tape directly on the pad and proceed around the body part in a circular or spiral pattern, overlapping the tape by ½ of its width with each pass (see Fig. 1–11C). Avoid gaps, wrinkles, or inconsistent roll tension.

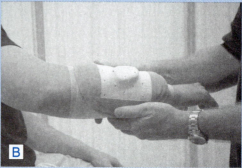

STEP 4: Cover the entire pad and anchor the tape on the top of the pad to prevent irritation during activity (see Fig. 1–11D).

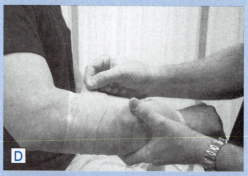

STEP 5: A final anchor of 1 inch or 1½ inch non-elastic tape may be applied loosely around the pad, but this is not necessary (see Fig. 1–11E).

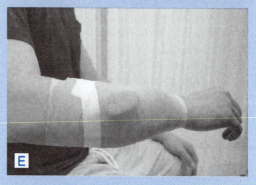

Figure 1-11

Elastic wraps are also used to apply pads (Fig. 1–12). The size of the pad and body part involved will determine the width and length of the wrap. Use adherent tape spray if necessary.

STEP 1: Place the pad directly on the skin over the body part (see Fig. 1–12A).

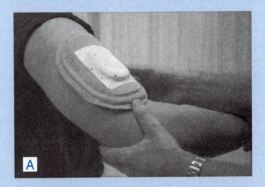

A

STEP 2: Anchor the wrap below the distal pad and proceed in a circular or spiral pattern, overlapping the wrap by ½–¾ of its width with each pass (see Fig. 1–12B).

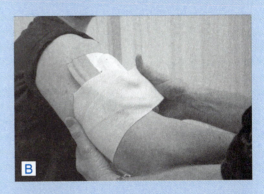

B

STEP 3: Continue with the entire length of the wrap (see Fig. 1–12C). Avoid gaps, wrinkles, or inconsistent roll tension.

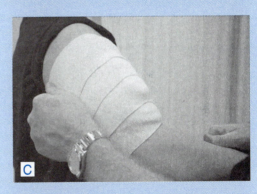

C

STEP 4: To anchor the wrap, apply one circular or spiral pattern of 2 inch or 3 inch elastic tape over the wrap (see Fig. 1–12D).

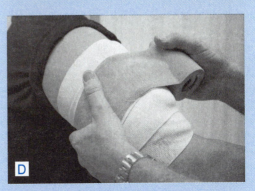

D

Figure 1-12

Tapes, Wraps, Braces, and Pads

STEP 5: Start and finish the tape on the top of the pad, overlapping the tape ends by 3–4 inches to ensure adhesion (see Fig. 1–12E). The pad may be loosely anchored with non-elastic tape, but this is not required.

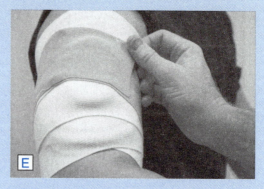

Figure 1-12 *continued*

With some techniques, apply pads directly to the skin (Fig. 1–13).

STEP 1: Apply adherent tape spray over the pad area and 4–6 inches beyond (see Fig. 1–13A). Allow the spray to dry ⚡.

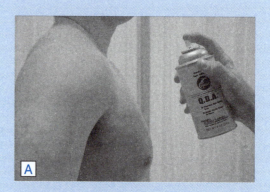

STEP 2: Place the pad directly on the skin over the body part (see Fig. 1–13B).

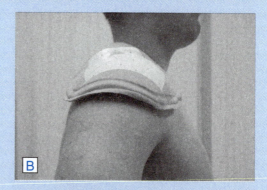

STEP 3: Cut several strips of 2 inch or 3 inch heavyweight elastic tape in lengths that will cover the pad and extend 4–6 inches beyond the pad on two sides. Anchor a tape strip to the skin 4–6 inches from the edge of the pad and pat down (see Fig. 1–13C). Do not stretch the tape as the anchor is applied.

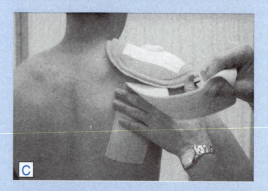

Figure 1-13

STEP 4: Continue to apply the anchor to the edge of the pad. At the edge, hold the anchor on the skin with one hand and pull the strip over the pad with tension on the tape (see Fig. 1–13D).

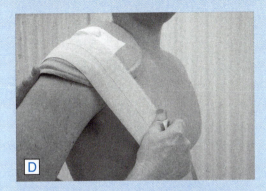

STEP 5: When the strip completely covers the pad, release the tension in the tape and anchor the tape to the skin as before (see Fig. 1–13E). Not allowing stretch in the anchor portions of the strip placed directly on the skin improves adherence of the tape. Applying tension and stretch to the portion of the strip placed over the pad secures the pad to the body. This technique can be thought of as a release-stretch-release sequence.

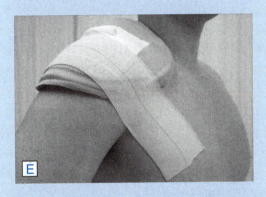

STEP 6: Continue with additional strips in the same manner, overlapping each by ½ the width of the tape (see Fig. 1–13F).

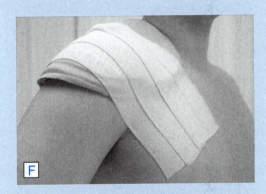

STEP 7: Apply enough strips to cover the majority of the pad (see Fig. 1–13G).

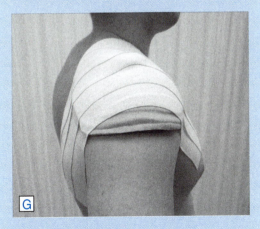

Figure 1-13 *continued*

Helpful Hint: You can quickly dry adherent tape spray by patting the area with a full roll of pre-tape material. When the roll begins to adhere to the skin during patting, the area is ready for application of tape.

Custom-Made Pads

Custom-made pad designs may be constructed for a variety of body areas. Begin the designs with a paper pattern to avoid wasting materials (Fig. 1–14).

STEP 1: Cover the area to be padded with paper (see Fig. 1–14A).

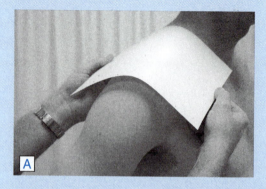

STEP 2: Draw, cut, and shape the pattern based on the objectives of the technique (see Fig. 1–14B).

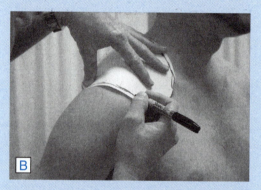

STEP 3: Lay the paper on the padding material and outline the pattern with a felt tip pen (see Fig. 1–14C).

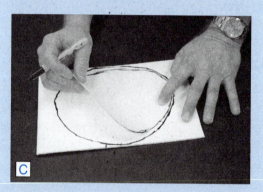

Figure 1-14

Some manufacturers include paper patterns with the materials to assist with construction. Pads may also be designed by outlining the body part directly on the material, then cutting the material with taping scissors. For example, position an individual on a piece of felt or foam and outline the foot.

Construction of a custom-made thermoplastic pad requires several types of materials and equipment (Fig. 1–15). Select the appropriate thermoplastic material based on conformability, resistance, and thickness. Use soft, low-density foam to line the inside of the pad. Additional equipment includes taping scissors, a heating source, 1 inch or 1½ inch non-elastic tape, 2 inch or 3 inch elastic tape, an elastic wrap, ¼ inch or ½ inch felt, and rubber cement.

STEP 1: Cut a piece of ¼ inch or ½ inch felt slightly larger than the injured area (see Fig. 1–15A).

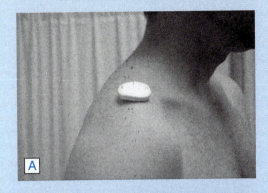

A

STEP 2: Attach the felt directly to the skin over the injured area with a strip of non-elastic tape (see Fig. 1–15B).

If no paper pattern is available, construct the design of the pad. Using the paper pattern, cut a piece of thermoplastic material. With partial heating of the material, cutting is made easier. Heat the material following the manufacturer's instructions. If using water as the heating source, remove the material when heated and place it on a towel to remove excess water.

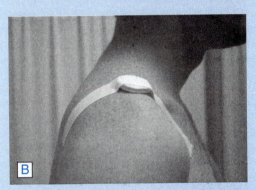

B

STEP 3: Apply the pliable thermoplastic material to the body part over the felt pad and lightly mold the material around the contours and felt pad with the hands (see Fig. 1–15C).

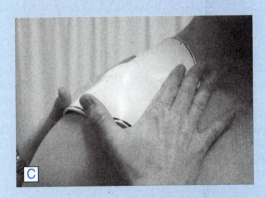

C

STEP 4: Apply an elastic wrap in a circular or spiral pattern over the body part and thermoplastic material to assist with molding (see Fig. 1–15D).

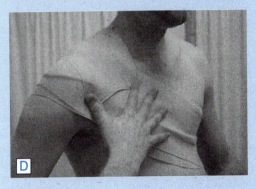

D

Figure 1-15

STEP 5: Continue to mold the material to the body with the hands (see Fig. 1–15E). Pay attention to the recommended amount of time before the material cools. Apply an ice bag or pack over the material to decrease the cooling time.

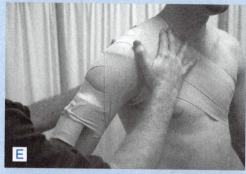

STEP 6: After the material cools, carefully remove the elastic wrap. Inspect the thermoplastic material to ensure proper shape and contour before removing. Use a felt tip pen to mark on the material any areas that require trimming (see Fig. 1–15F).

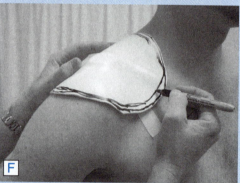

STEP 7: Remove the thermoplastic material and felt from the body part. Trim the material with taping scissors to remove sharp edges (see Fig. 1–15G). Place the material once again on the body part to make certain of the fit. Additional trimming may be necessary.

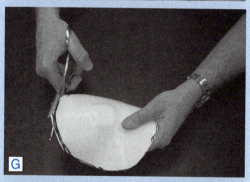

STEP 8: Completely dry the inside surface of the thermoplastic material. Place the thermoplastic material on soft, low-density foam and outline an area ½ inch larger than the material (see Fig. 1–15H). Cut the piece of foam.

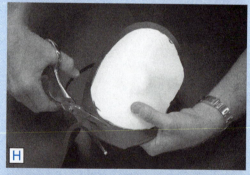

STEP 9: If using adhesive foam, remove the backing and attach the foam to the inside surface of the thermoplastic material. Otherwise, apply rubber cement or another non-toxic cement on the inside surface of the thermoplastic material and on the foam side that will be in contact with the material. When the cement is ready, attach the foam to the inside surface of the material (see Fig. 1–15I). The foam should extend ½ inch from each side of the thermoplastic material. This extra padding prevents irritation and possible injury from the semirigid thermoplastic material.

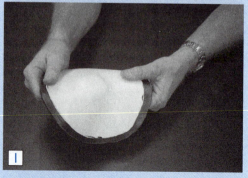

Figure 1–15 *continued*

STEP 10: Use taping scissors to cut the foam away from the raised area shaped by the felt pad (see Fig. 1–15J). This raised area will disperse the impact force away from the injured area to the outer edges of the pad, preventing further damage.

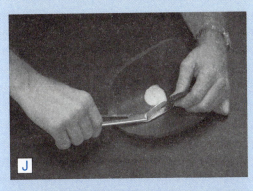

J

STEP 11: Cut strips of elastic tape to line the edges of the pad. Place strips on the top edges of the pad in a square pattern, then on the bottom edges (see Fig. 1–15K).

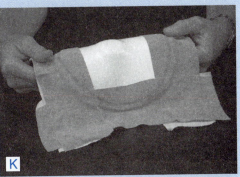

K

STEP 12: The tape strips should be applied on the thermoplastic material and extend beyond the foam by at least ¼ inch (see Fig. 1–15L). Use the fingers to adhere the top and bottom tape strips together.

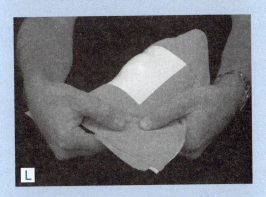

L

STEP 13: Trim the edges of the tape around the pad to provide a uniform edge, leaving enough of the tape to maintain adherence (see Fig. 1–15M). The elastic tape prevents separation of the foam from the thermoplastic material following repeated use.

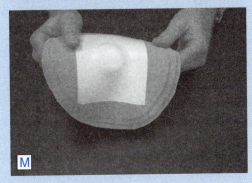

M

Figure 1-15 *continued*

...IF/THEN...

IF mistakes are made in the design and/or construction of custom-made, thermoplastic material pads, causing an irregular fit, **THEN** save the materials in order to use them again, potentially in the design of another pad.

Mandatory Padding

The NCAA[3] and NFHS[4] have rules that govern the use of mandatory injury prevention and injury protection padding for practices and competitions. Sports that require the use of mandatory protective equipment include baseball, fencing, field hockey, football, ice hockey, lacrosse, rifle, soccer, skiing, softball, water polo, and wrestling. Currently, basketball, gymnastics, swimming and diving, track and field, and volleyball do not have rules regarding mandatory protective equipment. Chapter 13 provides a more in-depth examination of protective equipment.

Rules[3,4] governing protective pads prohibit the use of fiberglass, plaster, metal, or other nonpliable materials unless they are covered by high-density, closed-cell foam or similar material of at least ½ inch thickness. Moreover, these hard, unyielding materials may only be used to protect an existing injury. Written verification from a physician may be required. Protective pads cannot create a hazard for the athlete or his/her opponent. The on-site referee or official has the authority to judge whether or not the protective pad is allowed for use in competition. Seek out the referee or official prior to the start of the competition to obtain approval of the pad. That way, if the pad is found unacceptable, there is time available to make the necessary changes before the competition.

Removal of Pads

The removal of mandatory protective equipment is typically done by the athlete following use, although custom-made pads secured to the body part with tape or an elastic wrap may require assistance for removal. Use taping scissors or tape cutters to cut pads secured with tape. Unwrap elastic wraps and reuse them. Remove pads applied directly to the skin with tape as described earlier. Moleskin adheres to the skin more tightly than other materials, especially when used on weight-bearing surfaces of the body. Use particular caution when removing moleskin from the plantar surfaces of the feet. Remove moleskin in the same manner as tape. Using a tape removal solvent may prove helpful.

Critical Thinking Question 4

The starting right offensive tackle on your football team has a second degree **ulnar collateral ligament** sprain of the left thumb. Your team physician will allow him to return to play if placed in a semirigid thumb spica cast.

▶ **Question: What should you do to meet NCAA and NFHS rules?**

STICKING POINTS

This information focuses on "what not to do" or "things to watch out for" when applying taping, wrapping, bracing, and padding techniques (Fig. 1–16). Use these pointers to avoid common mistakes.

Tapes

- Always overlap tape by ½ of the width to avoid gaps or inconsistent layering.
  - Gaps between strips of tape can pinch the underlying skin and result in a blister or abrasion (see Fig. 1–16A). These wounds are referred to as tape cuts.
  - Inconsistent layering can allow the underlying skin to bulge through the tape and cause a blister or abrasion (see Fig. 1–16B). Generally, the application of at least two layers of tape is sufficient.
- Avoid wrinkles in the layer of tape that is applied next to the skin.
  - Wrinkles in the tape can increase the amount of tension over a small area of the skin and result in a blister or abrasion (see Fig. 1–16C).
- When applying tape, focus attention on the correct angles of application.
  - Application angles must follow the contours of the body to prevent constriction of soft tissue or abnormal restriction of range of motion (see Fig. 1–16D).
- Continually monitor roll tension during application. Students often ask, "How tight does the tape need to be?" The finished technique should fit snugly to the body part and be comfortable to the individual given the objectives of the technique. For example, while the correct application of the elbow **hyperextension** taping technique will limit elbow extension, the elastic tape anchor placed around the proximal upper arm may cause mild constriction of the biceps.

Wraps

- Similar to tape, overlap wraps to avoid gaps and inconsistent layering.
  - Gaps or inconsistent layering can affect the mechanical pressure over the injured area (see Fig. 1–16E). As a result, swelling or effusion can accumulate in these areas, lessening the effectiveness of the technique.

Braces

- Closely follow the manufacturer's instructions when applying braces.
  - The omission or reversal of just one step in the application process may alter the intended purpose or fit of the brace. For example, improperly applying a functional knee brace may allow range of motion beyond the limits of the healing process, possibly predisposing the individual to further injury (see Fig. 1–16F).
- Use caution when making adjustments or alterations to braces.
  - Cutting or repositioning straps, applying tape anchors, or trimming the brace shell may affect the structural design of the brace (see Fig. 1–16G). Consult the brace manufacturer if questions arise.

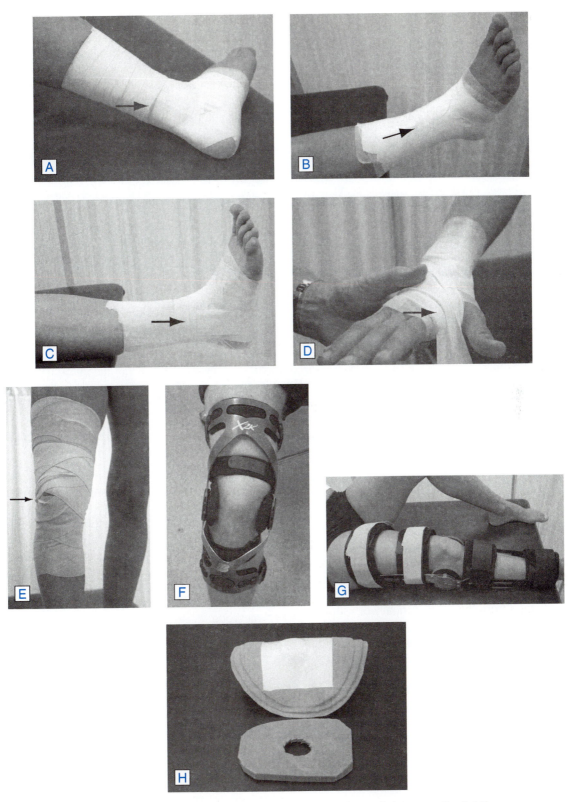

Figure 1–16 A Gap in the closed basketweave ankle taping technique over the Achilles tendon. **B** Inconsistent layering in the closed basketweave ankle taping technique over the anterior lower leg. **C** Wrinkle in the third horseshoe strip of the closed basketweave ankle taping technique. **D** Incorrect angle in the figure-of-eight wrist taping technique over the thenar web space. **E** Gap in the knee compression wrapping technique over the patella. **F** Low positioning of a custom-made functional ACL knee brace on the femoral condyles. **G** Tape anchors on the thigh straps of a rehabilitative knee brace. **H** AC joint pads. (Top) Custom-made, hard, high-density. (Bottom) Low-density foam.

Pads

• Use appropriate materials in the design and construction of protective pads. Select the materials based on the density, resiliency, and thickness.
• Padding of the **acromioclavicular joint (AC)** following a sprain or **contusion** requires several types of

materials. Construct the outer shell from hard, high-density thermoplastic material and line the inside of the pad with low-density foam (see Fig. 1–16H). Using only low-density foam will not provide effective protection from high impact forces.

CASE STUDY

Amanda Womack is a driver for Sanville Package Delivery Service. Two weeks ago, as Amanda was exiting her delivery van, she stepped into a large hole in a parking lot, inverting her right ankle. She immediately felt pain over the lateral aspect of the ankle and was unable to ambulate normally because of pain. Upon her return to the warehouse, her supervisors scheduled an appointment with a physician for an examination. Radiographs were negative; the physician diagnosed her with a first degree inversion ankle sprain. She has completed rehabilitation at Scholler Orthopedic Clinic and has been cleared to return to work. What types of tapes, wraps, braces, and pads could you apply to provide support and protection for Amanda's right ankle to prevent further injury?

Mark Cook is a senior running back at East Miflorclem High School participating in fall football practice. During a full-contact scrimmage, Mark caught a pass and was tackled by a defensive back. The helmet of the defensive back struck Mark in the left anterior thigh. The ATC at East Miflorclem High School, Jessica Rose, evaluated Mark on the field. Mark demonstrated full bilateral strength and range of motion and successfully completed all functional tests. Jessica determined that Mark had sustained a mild anterior left thigh contusion. Which types of tapes, wraps, braces, and pads could Jessica use to provide Mark protection from further injury upon his return to the scrimmage? Which types of tapes, wraps, braces, and pads can Jessica use following the scrimmage to provide compression and support to Mark's left thigh?

WRAP UP

- Apply non-elastic, elastic, and cast tapes to support and reduce range of motion, and secure wraps, pads, and dressings.
- Tapes are torn manually or cut with taping scissors.
- Tapes are commonly applied directly to the skin or over pre-tape material, self-adherent wrap, or cast padding.
- Remove tape from the body manually or with taping scissors or cutting tools.
- Use wraps to provide compression and support, reduce range of motion, and secure pads and dressings.
- Several methods may be used to prevent migration, slippage, or bunching of wraps.
- Wraps are rolled onto the body and removed by unwrapping or cutting.

- Off-the-shelf and custom-made braces provide support, protection, and compression, and control range of motion.
- Follow the manufacturer's step-by-step procedures when applying braces.
- Soft, low-density and hard, high-density padding materials provide support, protection, and compression.
- Pads may be applied to the body in a variety of methods.
- NCAA and NFHS rules mandate padding of all exposed nonpliable materials for practices and competitions.
- Before applying tapes, wraps, braces, and pads, clean and dry the skin of the individual, then position the body part according to the technique objective.
- Overlap tapes and wraps and avoid gaps, wrinkles, or inconsistent roll tension during application.

■ ## WEB REFERENCES

Active Ankle Systems
http://www.activeankle.com
· This Web site is an online catalog for the brace manufacturer and provides injury care, fitting, and ordering information.

Andover
http://www.andovercoated.com
· This site provides information about a variety of tapes and self-adherent wraps as well as resources for college professors and students.

Aircast
http://www.aircast.com
· This site is an online catalog for the brace manufacturer and provides sizing and ordering information and educational materials.

Breg
http://www.breg.com
· This Web site is an online catalog for the manufacturer and provides sizing information and research on prophylactic, rehabilitation, and functional braces.

BSN-Jobst
http://www.bsnmedical.com/BSNmedical/Corporate/home.htm
· This site allows you access to information on tapes, wraps, braces, pads, and wound care products.

dj Orthopedics
http://www.djortho.com
· This site is an online catalog for the manufacturer and provides research and development and fitting information about prophylactic, rehabilitation, and functional braces, and pads.

Hartmann-Conco
http://us.hartmann.info
· This Web site is an online catalog for the manufacturer and provides information about a variety of tapes, wraps, braces, pads, and wound care products.

Impact Innovative Products
http://www.zoombang.com
· This Web site allows access to information about viscoelastic polymer padding techniques used in athletic, work, and casual activities.

Johnson & Johnson
http://www.jnj.com/home.htm
· This site provides access to information on tapes, wraps, pads, and wound care products and educational resources for patients and students.

Kinetic Innovations
http://www.kineticinnovations.com
· This Web site is an online catalog for the brace manufacturer and provides sizing and ordering information.

Medco
http://www.medcosupply.com/
· This Web site is an online catalog for sports medicine products, including tapes, wraps, braces, and pads.

MedSpec
http://www.medspec.com
· This site is an online catalog for the brace manufacturer and provides fitting and ordering information.

Silipos
http://www.silipos.com
· This site is an online catalog for gel bracing and padding techniques and provides injury care, fitting, and ordering information.

Sports Health
http://www.esportshealth.com/shop/default.asp
· This Web site is an online catalog for sports medicine products and provides fitting and ordering information and educational materials and resources.

Swede-O
http://www.swedeo.com
· This site is an online catalog for the brace manufacturer and provides injury care, sizing, and ordering information.

3M
http://www.mmm.com
· This site provides access to information on tapes, wraps, pads, and wound care products and educational materials and resources.

Ultra Ankle
http://www.ultraankle.com
· This Web site is an online catalog for the brace manufacturer and provides fitting and ordering information.

■ REFERENCES

1. Anderson, MK, Hall, SJ, and Martin, M: Sports Injury Management, ed 2. Lippincott Williams & Wilkins, Philadelphia, 2000.
2. Fleming, BC, Renstrom, PA, Beynnon, BD, Engstrom, B, and Peura, G: The influence of functional knee bracing on the anterior cruciate ligament strain biomechanics in weightbearing and nonweightbearing knees. Am J Sports Med 28:815–824, 2000.
3. http://www.ncaa.org/library/sports_sciences/sports_med_handbook/2003-04/2003-04_sports_med_handbook.pdf, Sports medicine handbook, 2003–2004.
4. National Federation of State High School Associations. 2004 Football Rules Book. Indianapolis, IN: National Federation of State High School Associations, 2004.
5. Prentice, WE: Arnheim's Principles of Athletic Training, ed 11. McGraw-Hill, Boston, 2003.
6. Wilkerson, GB: Biomechanical and neuromuscular effects of ankle taping and bracing. J Athl Train 37:436–445, 2002.

Facility Design for Taping, Wrapping, Bracing, and Padding

LEARNING OBJECTIVES

1. Describe ergonomic principles of an application area for taping, wrapping, bracing, and padding.

2. Describe common program and structural considerations in the design of an application area for taping, wrapping, bracing, and padding.

3. Explain and demonstrate the ability to design an application area for taping, wrapping, bracing, and padding.

In a health-care facility, the space designated for taping, wrapping, bracing, and padding techniques should receive careful consideration. Whether the space is developed within new or existing structures, several design aspects need to be addressed. In scholastic, inter-collegiate, and professional sport facilities, this space is commonly referred to as the **taping area.** Other health-care facilities, such as clinics, typically do not have dedicated space for a taping area because of a lower patient demand for technique application. For our discussion, **application area** will refer to the facility space dedicated to taping, wrapping, bracing, and padding techniques.

The design of the application area should be based upon ergonomic principles. Ergonomics is defined by *Taber's* (p. 733)[4] as "the science concerned with fitting a job to a person's anatomical, physiological, and psychological characteristics in a way that enhances human efficiency and well-being." Health-care professionals who are responsible for applying taping, wrapping, bracing, and padding techniques come in many different sizes and shapes. Accordingly, spaces and tables should be designed to accommodate these differences. The goal of ergonomics is to provide an efficient, healthful, and safe working environment. This goal can be achieved with careful planning of new facility construction or existing facility renovations.

Planning for new construction or renovation of a facility's application area should direct thought to current and future program needs, as well as structural considerations. Program needs, such as the number of individuals requiring daily technique application, available time and staff, and long-range plans, will assist in deciding on furniture and space. Application areas in scholastic, intercollegiate, and professional sport facilities are typically the most congested spaces, especially during peak periods prior to practices and competitions. Application areas in these facilities should be located close to an entrance and exit for easy access. The time available to complete taping, wrapping, bracing, and padding techniques is often influenced by predetermined

practice, competition, and appointment schedules. Note that adequate staffing of health-care professionals who are proficient in applying the techniques is also an important consideration.

After determining current needs, attempt to make long-range projections based on the organization's strategic plan, such as future renovations to the facility or the addition of staff or sport teams. As interest in the health care of the active population continues to grow, the space required to apply taping, wrapping, bracing, and padding techniques will also increase.

After assessing program needs, consider structural needs in the application area. Structural factors include table design; storage areas; benches; seating; floor, wall, and ceiling coverings; and the design of electrical, plumbing, ventilation, and lighting systems.

TABLES/BENCHES

Tables and benches used in the application area can be purchased or constructed in a variety of sizes and shapes to accommodate individual differences and space restrictions (Fig. 2–1).

• Use multiple individual tables or benches in areas without space constraints (see Fig. 2–1A).

• Use custom-made tables or benches in areas with irregular or limited spaces to fit into corners between walls or as an island around a support beam in a multi-floor facility (see Fig. 2–1B).

When applying ergonomic principles, vary the height of the tables and benches between 30–40 inches to accommodate the different heights of health-care professionals and positions of individuals. Some taping, wrapping, bracing, and padding techniques require the individual to be placed in a seated position, while other techniques mandate a standing position on a table or bench. Vary the width of the tables and benches between 2–3 feet with individual and custom-made designs. The table and bench tops should be constructed of durable, easy-to-clean

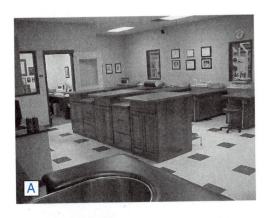

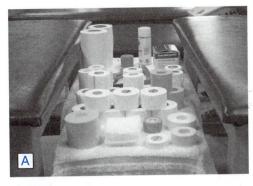

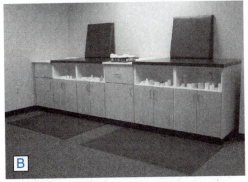

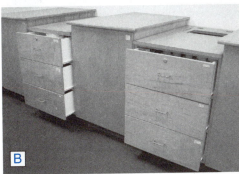

Figure 2-1 **A** Multiple taping tables in an athletic training room. (Courtesy of Bailey Manufacturing Company, Lodi, Ohio). **B** Custom-made taping bench positioned between two walls.

Figure 2-2 **A** Cart positioned between two individual taping tables. **B** Pull-out drawers in a taping bench.

material such as Formica. Many facilities use vinyl material with padding for added comfort.

An important feature to include with tables and benches is storage space for taping, wrapping, bracing, and padding supplies (Fig. 2–2).

- When using individual tables and benches, built-in storage underneath or carts placed between the tables provide easy access to materials (see Fig. 2–2A).
- Countertops with pull-out drawers positioned between individual tables and benches present another option (see Fig. 2–2B).

Adequate countertop space allows supplies to be arranged and readied prior to daily technique application. Custom-made tables and benches are commonly built with storage space. Design features that allow for storage of specific sizes or types of tapes, wraps, braces, and pads assist with timely, efficient technique application. Design all storage spaces in tables and benches with easy access in mind.

Clean and disinfect tables and benches immediately after completing taping, wrapping, bracing, and padding technique application. Use **disinfectant** agents to clean the tables, benches, and countertops. While most facilities do not use the application area to treat open wounds, exposure to **bloodborne pathogens** should be a consideration. The Occupational Safety and Health Administration (OSHA)[5] has developed standards for bloodborne pathogens, and facilities should develop and adhere to a plan of universal precautions to protect the health-care professional and individuals.

DETAILS

OSHA[5] Guidelines state, "Employers shall ensure that the worksite is maintained in a clean and sanitary condition. The employer shall determine and implement an appropriate written schedule for cleaning and method of decontamination based upon the location within the facility, type of surface to be cleaned, type of soil present, and tasks or procedures being performed in the area.... Contaminated work surfaces shall be decontaminated with an appropriate disinfectant after completion of procedures; immediately or as soon as feasible when surfaces are overtly contaminated or after any spill of blood or other potentially infectious materials; and at the end of the work shift if the surface may have become contaminated since the last cleaning."

STORAGE

The following recommendations should assist in the proper storage of tapes, wraps, braces, and pads.

Tape

Intercollegiate and professional sport teams may purchase 100–500 cases of tape per year, which requires a large

Critical Thinking Question 1

You are developing plans for the renovation of the application area in your facility. The available space allows you to consider using multiple individual taping tables.

▶ **Question: What ergonomic principles should you consider in the design of the tables?**

...IF/THEN...

IF individual table heights need to be adjusted to accommodate different heights of a staff, **THEN** consider placing wood blocks or boards underneath the legs or table, forming a stable base for the desired height.

amount of storage space. The type of storage space is key. The storage and handling of non-elastic and elastic tapes can determine their effectiveness when they are ready to be used (Fig. 2–3). Store tape in a cool, moisture-free environment. The room or area used for storage should also have an adequate ventilation system, as discussed later in this chapter. Tape is normally purchased by the box or case—depending on the type and size—and packaged 16 to 24 rolls per box or case. Store tape in its original box or case and stack the boxes or cases with the tops facing up and the bottoms facing down. Stacking boxes or cases on their sides or down side up may cause indentations in the rolls. These indentations can be thought of as "bruises" and may affect roll tension during application (see Fig. 2–3A). When removing tape from boxes or cases, handling prior to application can also cause damage. Squeezing or haphazard storage can cause excessive pressure on the side of the roll and produce indentations.

• Many manufacturers place tape dividers or roll holders in boxes or cases to protect individual rolls from damage during storage (see Fig. 2–3B).
• Stack tape stored in taping tables and benches individually or place onto custom-made wooden dowels (see Fig. 2–3C).

When traveling with tape, store it in its original box or case, or in an area protected from excessive pressure and heat. Many intercollegiate and professional teams use trunks that are designed to store tape in compartments. Protect tape carried in personal medical kits from direct sunlight. Heat and humidity will also damage the tape.

Limit the storage of non-elastic and elastic tapes to a one-year period. While tape does not have an expiration date, time can adversely affect the adhesive mass and roll tension, resulting in difficult application. Inventory regularly and rotate the tape stock when necessary.

Store rolls of cast tape in the original sealed pouch in a cool, dry area. Unlike non-elastic and elastic tapes, cast tape does have an expiration date. Using cast tape after the expiration date may result in shortened setting times,

incomplete curing, or premature hardening of the fiberglass material on the roll.

Wraps

Elastic and cloth wraps are typically stored in taping tables and benches in the application area. Drawers in the

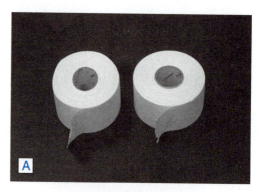

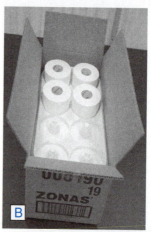

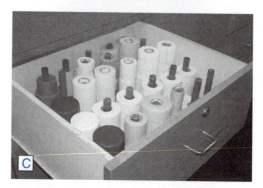

Figure 2-3 **A** (Left) Roll with indentation. (Right) Normal roll. **B** Case of non-elastic tape with dividers/holders. **C** Taping bench drawer with wooden dowels.

tables or benches may be divided to store wraps by different sizes or lengths, allowing for easy access. Store and handle self-adherent wrap in the same manner as non-elastic and elastic tapes.

Clean elastic and cloth wraps by following OSHA[5] standards for bloodborne pathogens. After proper washing and drying, roll the wraps for the next application (Fig. 2–4A). Hand-driven devices can be purchased to roll the wraps and are recommended for cloth wraps to prevent wrinkles (see Fig. 2–4A). Manually roll elastic wraps and be sure the wraps are completely dry before rolling. If multiple wraps are to be cleaned, tie the wraps together to prevent tangling .

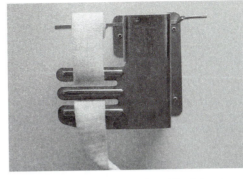

Figure 2-4 Hand-driven roller with cloth wrap.

> **Helpful Hint:** After collecting the used wraps, lay them lengthwise on a table or bench top. Using 1 inch non-elastic tape, gather one end of the bundle and tightly encircle the wraps. At 24–36 inch increments, continue to encircle the wraps with the tape. Because the wraps will most likely be different lengths, continue with taping as far as possible to include the majority of them. Wash and dry the bundle together. Near the completion of the drying cycle, cut the tape to allow the taped areas to dry.

Braces

Braces are normally kept in a storage room or cabinet and brought to the application area for use. The storage area should be ventilated and free of moisture to prevent damage to the braces. The size of many designs prohibits storage in taping tables and benches.

Pads

Soft, low-density pads can be stored in taping tables and benches in the application area. Arrange the pads in drawers by thickness and length. Hard, high-density materials of thermoplastics and cast tapes should be stored in a cool, dry area. It may be a good idea to store small pieces of thermoplastic material in tables and benches for easy access during application sessions.

the flow of traffic. The lower traffic flow also allows additional space in which to move during technique application. Construct benches with hinged tops to provide storage underneath for supplies. Use Formica or another durable, easy-to-clean material for construction of the benches or chairs.

FLOORS

The floor of the application area is both a cosmetic and sanitary concern (Fig. 2–5). High traffic and use of adherent tape spray, fiberglass casting tape, and water can quickly stain and damage floor coverings. At the same time, continuous technique application for one to two hour periods can cause back and lower body fatigue. If the facility has pre-existing carpet in the area, use non-

Critical Thinking Question 2

You have a limited storage area in your facility, and only a portion of this area is well ventilated.

▶ **Question: What taping, wrapping, bracing, and padding materials will you store in this area?**

...IF/THEN...

IF the storage space allows, **THEN** place wooden pallets directly on the floor and stack tape on the pallets to allow cool, dry air to circulate freely around the boxes/cases.

SEATING

If space is available in the application area, use benches or chairs for individuals as they wait, which should lessen

slip plastic, rubber, or carpet runners or mats to lessen soiling and damage and provide some cushion (see Fig. 2–5A). Using non-slip runners or mats over tile or vinyl is also possible (see Fig. 2–5B).

As the runners or mats become soiled or damaged, clean or replace them with new ones. Remove the runners or mats to clean the carpet, tile, or vinyl floor. Clean plastic and rubber runners and mats with a mild dish soap and warm water. Rinse completely to remove any sticky residue. A bristle brush will lift dirt from any grooves. Carpets can be cleaned by a wet or dry process with

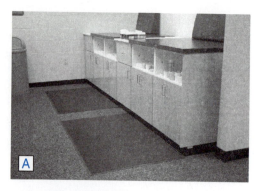

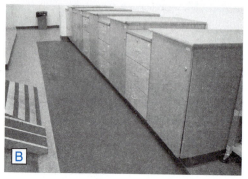

Figure 2-5 A Non-slip carpet mats placed over carpet. **B** Non-slip rubber runner placed over tile.

electric shampoo machines. Clean tile with an electric floor washer or polisher-scrubber with ¼ cup of low-suds-ing detergent in 1 gallon of water. Rinse completely. Vinyl can be cleaned with a mild dish soap and mop. Rinse with a towel. Removing tape and adhesive residue from the runners, mats, and floor often requires commercial cleans-ing products and solvents. This residue attracts additional dirt and debris, and can build up quickly. Several of these products contain harsh chemicals and can damage these surfaces. Before using a commercial product, always test a spot for damage, such as color fastness.

> **...IF/THEN...**
>
> **IF** back and lower body fatigue occurs during technique application despite the use of carpet mats/runners, **THEN** place carpet padding underneath the existing mats/runners or pur-chase off-the-shelf padded mats/runners for additional cushion.

WALLS

Walls can be constructed with a variety of materials, such as cinder block, drywall, or tile. Use paint that will resist moisture and allow for easy cleaning. Many facilities with high traffic loads attach Plexiglas or similar material to the wall directly behind taping tables and benches. When an individual is sitting on the table or bench, her/his back rests against the material on the wall. The material pro-tects the wall from dirt and may be cleaned and disinfect-ed daily without damage to the actual wall surface.

CEILING

The application area ceiling should be easy to clean and resistant to moisture. The ceiling must be at a height to provide clearance for individuals in standing positions on tables and benches. For example, a standing position is required for applying an adductor strain wrapping technique. Exposed plumbing pipes or ventilation ducts may reduce ceiling heights. Adjust the position of tables and benches in the application area to find ceiling heights that allow clearance for individuals in standing positions. The prescribed ceiling height depends on the height of the tables and benches and the individual.

ELECTRICAL

The demand for electrical outlets in the application area may be less than in other specialized areas in a health-care facility (Fig. 2–6). Outlets are required when using cast cutters, heat guns, supplemental lighting, and clean-ing equipment. Referring to the facility as a whole, Secor[3] suggested placement of electrical outlets every four feet. Outlets are normally placed approximately 3–4 feet off the floor so that they are safe in the event of accidental spills. If involved in the pre-design of new construction or renovations of a facility, plan for exact placement of out-lets between tables and benches. Equip all outlets in a health-care facility with **ground fault interrupter (GFI)** breakers (see Fig. 2–6). GFI breakers and hospital grade plugs protect individuals, health-care professionals, and equipment from electrical damage.

PLUMBING

The plumbing system is perhaps one of the most expen-sive components of a health-care facility. Attention to cur-rent and future water needs is important in the pre-design process. A supply of hot and cold water in the application area is convenient, but not required. Water is required for constructing thermoplastic materials, applying casting tapes, and hand cleansing after using adherent tape sprays and adhesive tapes. A hand-washing station with hot and cold water is ideal. Fixtures that allow control of water with foot pedals, along with soap and paper towel dis-pensers, should meet the demands of the application area.

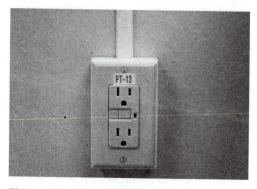

Figure 2-6 GFI breaker on wall.

VENTILATION

Because the application area often has high traffic, and because the area often serves as the storage facility for supplies, proper ventilation is a major concern. Ray[2] stated that temperature and humidity are the two most important ventilation concerns. Separate thermostat controls for the athletic training room or outpatient clinic allow for ventilation adjustments during periods of high traffic and seasonal environmental changes. Placing thermostats in each room or specialized area in a facility is optimal to control temperature and humidity. Penman and Penman[1] recommend a humidity level between 40% and 50%. High levels of humidity not only can result in uncomfortable working conditions but also may promote the growth of bacteria and fungi, and may damage supplies. Taping, wrapping, bracing, and padding supplies require storage in cool, dry places. Supplemental or portable air conditioners, heaters, or fans assist with temperature and humidity control during high traffic periods.

LIGHTING

The application area does not require the most intense illumination in a health-care facility. While the area should be lit better than storage rooms, examination and treatment areas typically require more illumination. Recessed lighting commonly found in health-care facilities is sufficient for the application area. Use mounted or floor lamps of various intensities if additional lighting is desired. Natural light from windows or skylights can enhance illumination in the application area. However, many health-care facilities are located within buildings, well away from natural lighting. Such internal locations are often chosen for individual privacy and equipment/ supply security.

...IF/THEN...

IF footwear, school textbooks or bags and athletic equipment constantly clutter the application area, **THEN** have athletes leave these items in the locker room or outside the door of the athletic training room to lessen congestion during technique application.

Critical Thinking Question 3

Each day, your application area becomes congested because several sport teams practice at the same time. The coaches are unwilling to change practice times to lessen the congestion.

▶ **Question: How can you manage this situation?**

CASE STUDY

Heather Jones, a PT/ATC, works in the town's Boone Orthopedic Clinic, which has just started an outreach program with Mogol High School. For the past three years, a teacher/ATC has been employed at the high school. Recently, the teacher/ATC left the high school to accept another position. Although Mogol High School is known for its modern facilities, the school is planning renovations. The athletic booster organization at the high school has raised substantial private funds for the project and supports the health-care services provided to the athletes. The high school administrators approach Heather in hopes that she will assist them in the renovation of their facility, specifically the athletic training room. Heather tours the building with the administrators. The athletic training room is divided into several distinct sections, one of which appears to be an application area for taping, wrapping, bracing, and padding. One individual taping table stands against the wall. Overhead, ventilation duct work is visible. The floor in the area is tile, and several pieces are cracked. A vertical support beam for the second floor is located in one corner of the area. The dimensions of the application area are as follows: 12 feet by 12 feet with an 8 foot ceiling. The high school administrators tell Heather that the room will not be expanded, but changes can be made within the existing walls. Because of the original construction of the plumbing and ventilation systems, the application area must remain in its existing space. Prior to meeting with the high school administrators to discuss her ideas for the renovations, Heather has several questions regarding the program, athlete population, and future plans of the school.

First, what current and future program needs of the high school should Heather possibly consider that may affect the renovations of the application area? Second, design an application area, within the dimensions given, that would meet the needs of a typical high school athletic program.

WRAP UP

- Design and construction of the application area should be based upon ergonomic principles.
- The design of the application area should include current and future program needs and structural considerations.
- Use taping tables and benches in varying heights with storage areas for technique application.
- Store taping, wrapping, bracing, and padding materials in a well-ventilated area.
- Use additional seating to lower the flow of traffic.
- Non-slip plastic, rubber, or carpet runners or mats protect the floor and may reduce lower body fatigue.
- Use moisture-resistant paint on the wall and ceilings.
- Ceiling heights should allow for individuals to stand on taping tables and benches.
- Place electrical outlets equipped with GFI breakers 3–4 feet off the floor.
- A hand-washing station should provide the water needs for the application area.
- Control temperature and humidity with a separate thermostat located in the application area.
- Illumination in the application area can be supplied with standard recessed lighting.
- Clean and disinfect tables, benches, and countertops with appropriate agents following use.

WEB REFERENCES

U.S. Department of Labor Occupational Safety and Health Administration. Ergonomics
http://www.osha.gov/SLTC/ergonomics/
- This Web site provides ergonomic guidelines and solutions for health-care facilities.

U.S. Department of Labor Occupational Safety and Health Administration. Bloodborne Pathogens
http://www.osha.gov/SLTC/bloodbornepathogens/index.html
- This site contains OSHA standards and safety and health topics related to bloodborne pathogens.

Athletic Business
http://www.athleticbusiness.com
- This site provides access to a monthly magazine that contains information about facility planning. The magazine is distributed free to owners, operators, and directors of sport/athletic facilities.

Bailey Manufacturing Company
http://www.baileymfg.com
- This Web site is an online catalog for the manufacturer and provides information on a variety of sports medicine equipment, including taping tables and benches.

REFERENCES

1. Penman, KA, and Penman, TM: Training rooms aren't just for colleges. Athletic Purchasing and Facilities 6:34–37, 1982.
2. Ray, R: Management Strategies in Athletic Training, ed 2. Human Kinetics, Champaign, 2000.
3. Secor, MR: Designing athletic training facilities or "Where do you want the outlets?" Athl Train J Natl Athl Train Assoc 19:19–21, 1984.
4. Taber's Cyclopedic Medical Dictionary, ed 20. FA Davis, Philadelphia, 2001.
5. U.S. Department of Labor Occupational Safety and Health Administration. Bloodborne pathogens, 2003. http://www.osha.gov/SLTC/bloodbornepathogens/index.html

Foot and Toes

LEARNING OBJECTIVES

1. Recognize common injuries and overuse conditions that occur to the foot and toes.
2. Demonstrate applying tapes, wraps, braces, and pads to the foot and toes when preventing, treating, and rehabilitating injuries.
3. Discuss and demonstrate appropriate taping, wrapping, bracing, and padding techniques for the foot and toes within a therapeutic exercise program.

INJURIES AND CONDITIONS

During athletic, work, and casual activities, the foot and toes must react to acute and chronic forces. As a result, injuries and overuse conditions often occur. Walking produces constant shearing forces between the foot and toes and ground in anteroposterior, lateral-to-medial, and vertical directions. During running, these same forces increase as speeds increase. In sports, sudden cutting, twisting, and deceleration movements further increase the stresses. A contusion, sprain, or fracture can occur when a football wide receiver decelerates and plants his right foot to make a cut or quick turn to his left, placing anteroposterior, lateral-to-medial, and rotational stresses on the foot and toes. Common injuries to the foot and toes include the following:

• Contusions
• Sprains
• Strains
• Fractures
• Overuse injuries and conditions
• Blisters

Contusions

Contusions to the foot and toes are caused by compressive forces and weight-bearing activities. A contusion is trauma to the soft tissue. Compression on the **dorsal** or **plantar** surface of the area can cause inflammation and pain. For example, activities that require jumping and sudden change of direction can lead to contusion of the calcaneus, referred to as a heel bruise (Illustration 3–1). Training errors and the use of poorly designed shoes may contribute to such injuries.

Sprains

Sprains to the toes are typically caused by contact with an unmovable object, producing abnormal joint range of motion. A sprain involves trauma to ligaments and, based on the severity of the injury, commonly categorized as Grade I, II, or III, may result in only mild pain or complete loss of function. Forced hyperextension of the **metatarsophalangeal (MTP) joint** of the great toe (turf toe) is associated with excessive flexibility of athletic shoes and sport activities on artificial grass surfaces (Illustration 3–1). Another sprain to the great toe MTP joint is caused by forced **hyperflexion** (soccer toe) and may occur with instep ball strike of a soccer ball.[1] Sprains to the MTP and **interphalangeal (IP) joints** of the toes are caused by **valgus** and **varus** stresses and result in injury to the collateral ligaments (Illustration 3–1). Midfoot sprains occur through excessive **plantar flexion, dorsiflexion,** or rotational stress that can occur with stepping on an opponent's foot or stepping into a hole.

Strains

Strains to the foot commonly affect the **longitudinal, metatarsal,** or **transverse arch** (Illustration 3–2). Strains involve trauma to a muscle and/or tendon. Injury can be caused by overloads of the musculature and ligamentous support, through activity on rigid surfaces.[29] Repetitive activity on asphalt or concrete surfaces in footwear without arch support can contribute to a strain. **Pes cavus** or high arches, may also contribute to an arch strain.

Fractures

Fractures to the foot and toes may involve the tarsals, metatarsals, or phalanges (Illustration 3–1). Mechanisms of injury commonly include excessive **inversion, eversion,** dorsiflexion, plantar flexion, rotation, and axial loading.[1,29] For example, a fracture can occur as a basketball player jumps to rebound the ball, either landing directly on the calcaneus or on an opponent's foot, causing excessive inversion or eversion. If there is a possibility of a fracture, refer the individual to a physician.

Overuse

Overuse injuries and conditions are caused by excessive, repetitive stress to the foot and toes. Pressure from the heel

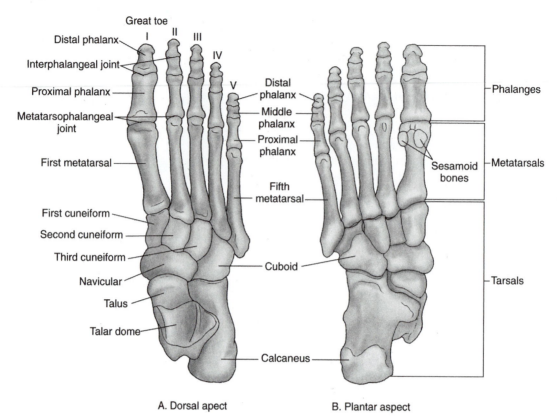

Illustration 3-1 Bones and joints of the foot and toes.

box of a shoe may lead to **retrocalcaneal bursitis**. Medial heel pain, commonly **plantar fasciitis,** may result from poor running technique and inflexible musculature. Repetitive hyperextension of the great toe may cause **sesamoiditis** (Illustration 3–1).[29] **Metatarsalgia** may follow injury to the transverse arch. Ill fitting shoes and foot pronation can lead to plantar **interdigital neuroma**. **Bunions** and **bunionettes** may be the result of ill fitting shoes.

Blisters

The foot and toes play a large role in athletic, work, and everyday activities. Because the majority of these activities require some type of footwear, blisters caused by shearing forces are common. Blisters are particularly common during the beginning of competitive sport seasons or when wearing new shoes.

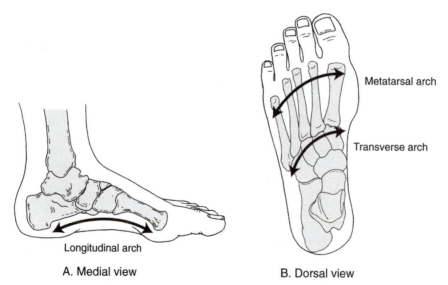

Illustration 3-2 Arches of the foot.

Taping Techniques

Provide support to the arch and forefoot areas with the use of several arch taping techniques. While one technique may provide adequate support for one individual, applying the same technique on another individual with a similar injury may be ineffective, because of the mechanism of injury, foot structure, or sport or activity. When deciding on a technique, consider the intended purposes of the technique, the injury, the individual, and the activity, then select the appropriate technique, and monitor the outcomes. Note that many of these techniques may be used for lower leg injuries and conditions as indicated.

CIRCULAR ARCH Figure 3–1

- **Purpose:** The circular arch technique provides mild support to the longitudinal arch (Fig. 3–1). Use this straightforward technique for longitudinal arch strains and pes cavus and **pes planus** conditions.

- **Materials:**
  - 1½ inch non-elastic tape
  - Options:
  - Pre-tape material or self-adherent wrap, adherent tape spray
  - ⅛ inch or ¼ inch foam or felt, taping scissors
  - 2 inch or 3 inch elastic tape

- **Position of the individual:** Sitting on a taping table or bench with the leg extended off the edge and the foot placed at a 90° angle.

- **Preparation:** Apply the technique directly to the skin.
  Options: *Apply adherent tape spray, then apply pre-tape material or self-adherent wrap around the midfoot area to provide additional adherence and lessen irritation.*
  Incorporate a felt pad with the circular arch to provide additional support. This technique is illustrated in the Padding section (see Fig. 3–26).

- **Application:**
  STEP 1: Anchor 1½ inch non-elastic tape on the **medial** aspect of the foot, just proximal to the MTP joint of the great toe (see Fig. 3–1A).
  Option: *Use 2 inch or 3 inch elastic tape instead of non-elastic tape for added comfort and conformability.*

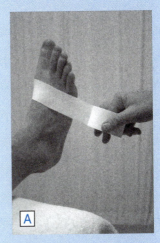

Figure 3-1

STEP 2: Pull the tape in a **lateral** direction across the dorsum of the foot and continue across the plantar surface. Anchor the strip on the dorsal aspect of the foot (Fig. 3–1B). Avoid excessive roll tension that may cause constriction of the foot upon weight-bearing.

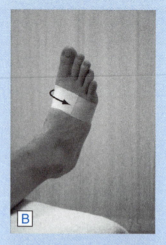

STEP 3: Continue with three to five additional strips in a proximal direction (Fig. 3–1C). Overlap each strip by ½ of the width of the tape.

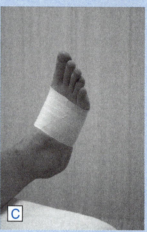

Figure 3-1 *continued*

"X" ARCH Figure 3–2

▶ **Purpose:** Use the "X" arch technique to provide mild to moderate support for the longitudinal arch and forefoot in the treatment of arch strains, plantar fasciitis, pes cavus, and pes planus (Fig. 3–2).

▶ **Materials:**
  • 1 inch and 1½ inch non-elastic tape, adherent tape spray

▶ **Position of the individual:** Sitting on a taping table or bench with the leg extended off the edge and the foot placed at a 90° angle.

▶ **Preparation:** Apply adherent tape spray on the plantar forefoot area.

▶ **Application:**
  STEP 1: Place a 1 inch non-elastic tape anchor directly on the skin over the base of the metatarsal heads (Fig. 3–2A). This anchor may encircle the foot, but this is not necessary.

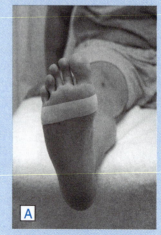

Figure 3-2

STEP 2: Anchor the first "X" strip of 1 inch non-elastic tape under the base of the fifth toe, proceed at an angle around the medial heel with moderate roll tension, and finish at the base of the great toe (see Fig. 3–2B).

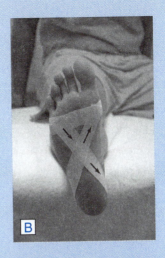

STEP 3: Anchor the next "X" strip at the base of the great toe, angle around the lateral heel with moderate roll tension, and finish at the base of the fifth toe (see Fig. 3–2C).

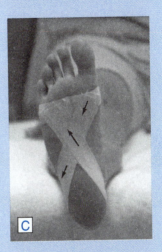

STEP 4: Continue with each strip two to three additional times, overlapping each on the plantar surface of the foot by ⅓ to ½ of the tape width (see Fig. 3–2D).

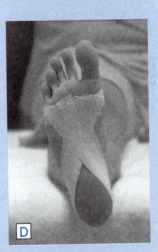

Figure 3-2 *continued*

STEP 5: Finish by applying an anchor strip over the MTP joints, covering the ends of the tape (see Fig. 3–2E).

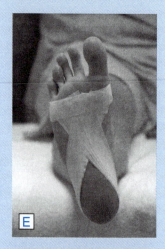

STEP 6: Apply four to five circular strips with 1½ inch non-elastic tape, as illustrated in Fig. 3–1, to cover the arch (see Fig. 3–2F).

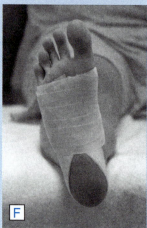

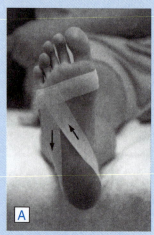

Figure 3-2 *continued*

LOOP ARCH Figure 3–3

▶ **Purpose:** The loop arch technique also provides mild to moderate support to the longitudinal arch and forefoot (see Fig. 3–3).

▶ **Materials:**
  • 1 inch and 1½ inch non-elastic tape, adherent tape spray

▶ **Position of the individual:** Sitting on a taping table or bench with the leg extended off the edge and the foot placed at a 90° angle.

▶ **Preparation:** Apply adherent tape spray to the plantar forefoot area.

▶ **Application:**
  STEP 1: Apply a 1 inch non-elastic tape anchor over the base of the metatarsal heads. Begin the first loop strip of 1 inch non-elastic tape at the base of the fifth toe, proceed around the lateral heel with moderate roll tension, and finish at the base of the fifth toe (Fig. 3–3A).

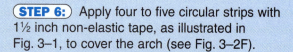

Figure 3-3

STEP 2: Anchor the next loop strip at the base of the great toe, continue around the medial heel with moderate roll tension, and finish at the great toe (Fig. 3–3B).

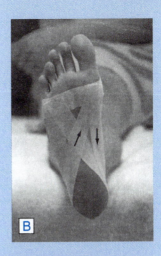

B

STEP 3: Repeat each loop strip two to three times, overlapping each by ⅓ to ½ of the tape width on the plantar foot (Fig. 3–3C).

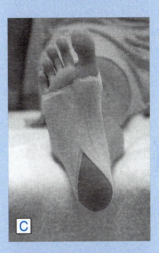

C

STEP 4: Apply a 1 inch non-elastic anchor strip over the tape ends on the plantar foot. Use 1½ inch non-elastic tape circular strips to cover the arch (Fig. 3–3D).

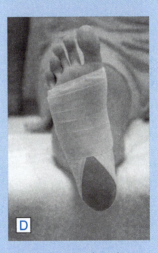

D

Figure 3-3 *continued*

○ **DETAILS**

The "X" and loop arch taping techniques are interchangeable, as both provide mild to moderate support for the longitudinal arch and forefoot. The health-care professional and individual's preference commonly determines which technique is applied.

WEAVE ARCH Figure 3–4

▶ **Purpose:** The weave arch technique is perhaps the most supportive of the arch techniques, providing moderate support to the longitudinal arch and forefoot (Fig. 3–4).

▶ **Materials:**
   • 1 inch and 1½ inch non-elastic tape, adherent tape spray

▶ **Position of the individual:** Sitting on a taping table or bench with the leg extended off the edge and the foot placed at a 90° angle.

▶ **Preparation:** Apply adherent tape spray to the plantar forefoot.

▶ **Application:**

STEP 1: Place a 1 inch non-elastic tape anchor over the metatarsal heads. Anchor a strip of 1 inch non-elastic tape over the third metatarsal head, proceed at an angle around the lateral heel, and finish just lateral to the starting point near the third metatarsal head (Fig. 3–4A).

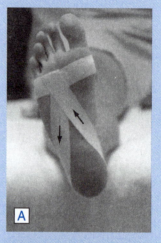

STEP 2: Anchor the next strip on the second metatarsal head, continue around the lateral heel, and finish on the fourth metatarsal head (Fig. 3–4B).

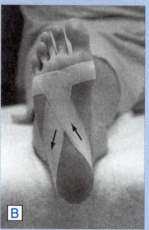

STEP 3: Begin the next strip on the fourth metatarsal head, continue around the lateral heel, and finish on the fifth metatarsal head (Fig. 3–4C).

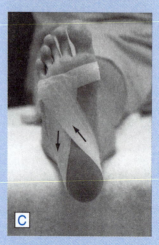

Figure 3-4

STEP 4: Begin the last strip on the great toe metatarsal head, continue around the lateral heel, and finish on the great toe metatarsal head (Fig. 3–4D). Apply the strips with a moderate amount of roll tension. The strips should resemble a weave pattern on the plantar surface of the foot.

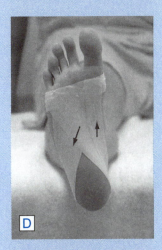

STEP 5: Apply supportive 1½ inch non-elastic tape anchor strips over the pattern, as illustrated in the circular arch technique (see Fig. 3–4E).

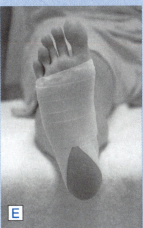

Anchor Variation to the "X," Loop, and Weave Arch Techniques

▶ **Purpose:** A variation to anchor the "X," loop, or weave arch techniques entails applying a series of tape strips across the plantar foot. Consider using these strips to provide additional support to the plantar foot when treating arch strains, plantar fasciitis, pes cavus, and pes planus.

▶ **Materials:**
  • 1 inch non-elastic tape

▶ **Position of the individual:** Sitting on a taping table or bench with the leg extended off the edge and the foot placed at a 90° angle.

▶ **Preparation:** Application of "X," loop, or weave arch technique, excluding the circular strips.

▶ **Application:**
  STEP 1: Tear individual strips of 1 inch non-elastic tape and apply with equal tension inwards toward the plantar foot. Anchor each strip on the medial and lateral borders of the foot. Begin on the proximal foot and continue with additional strips in a distal direction, overlapping by ½ of the tape width to cover the entire arch (Fig. 3–4F).

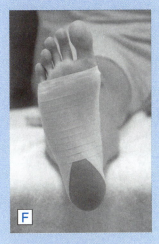

Figure 3-4 *continued*

STEP 2: Four to five circular strips may be applied to cover the arch.

DETAILS

For the circular, "X," loop, and weave techniques, elastic tape of 1 inch width may be used in place of non-elastic tape for comfort and conformability, but elastic tape provides less support to the arch and forefoot. Non-elastic tape of 1 inch width is most commonly used for the techniques, but 1½ inch may be required for large feet. If one of these techniques is applied daily, monitor the heel area for skin irritation. Thin foam pads or adhesive gauze material placed directly on the heel prior to applying the tape should lessen irritation.

LOW-DYE Figures 3–5, 3–6

▶ **Purpose:** The Low-Dye technique is commonly used in treating arch strains, plantar fasciitis, and lower leg conditions to provide moderate support and correct structural abnormalities. Anecdotally, researchers have suggested that this technique may reduce the symptoms of many conditions, such as tendinitis and stress syndromes, caused by excessive pronation.[2,8,33,34,38] Two methods that are interchangeable are illustrated in applying the Low-Dye technique (Fig. 3–5).

Low-Dye Technique One

▶ **Materials:**
  • 1 inch and 2 inch non-elastic and 2 inch elastic tape, adherent tape spray

▶ **Position of the individual:** Sitting on a taping table or bench with the leg extended off the edge and the foot in a **neutral** position.

▶ **Preparation:** Apply adherent tape spray to the lateral and medial surfaces of the foot.

▶ **Application:**
  STEP 1: Anchor 1 inch non-elastic tape directly to the skin over the lateral surface of the fifth MTP joint, continue around the heel, and finish on the medial surface of the first MTP joint (Fig. 3–5A).

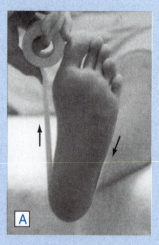

Figure 3-5

STEP 2: Repeat this step twice, overlapping by ½ of the tape width (Fig. 3–5B). Apply the tape with moderate roll tension **inferior** to the medial and lateral malleoli.

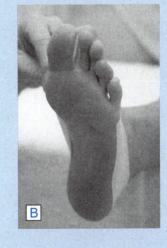

STEP 3: Anchor a strip of 2 inch non-elastic tape on the lateral dorsum of the proximal foot, continue across the plantar aspect, and finish on the medial dorsum (Fig. 3–5C).

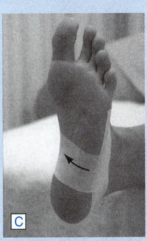

STEP 4: Apply two additional strips in the same manner, overlapping each by ½ of the tape width with moderate roll tension (Fig. 3–5D). These strips, C and D, should cover the 1 inch tape strips (see Figs. 3–5A and B), but not encircle the foot. Next, apply a 1 inch non-elastic strip as illustrated in Fig. 3–5A.

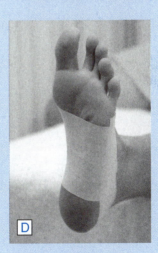

Figure 3-5 *continued*

STEP 5: Finish by applying an anchor strip of 2 inch elastic tape on the lateral dorsum, continue across the plantar surface, and finish on the lateral dorsum to encircle the arch with mild to moderate roll tension (see Fig. 3–5E).

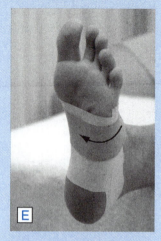

E

Figure 3-5 *continued*

Low-Dye Technique Two

▶ **Materials:**
- 1 inch and 2 inch non-elastic and 2 inch elastic tape, adherent tape spray, 3 inch heavyweight moleskin, taping scissors

▶ **Position of the individual:** Sitting on a taping table or bench with the leg extended off the edge and the foot in a neutral position with the great toe and medial foot in plantar flexion.

▶ **Preparation:** Apply adherent tape spray to the plantar foot.

▶ **Application:**

STEP 1: Using 3 inch width heavyweight moleskin, cut a piece in a pattern to cover the foot from the metatarsal heads to the calcaneus (Fig. 3–6A).

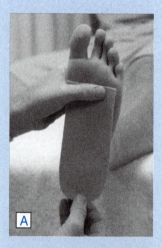

A

STEP 2: Anchor the moleskin to the metatarsal heads (Fig. 3–6B). Ensure the plantar flexed position of the great toe and medial foot, and reposition if necessary.

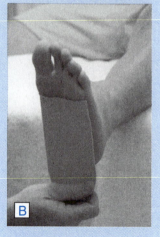

B

Figure 3-6

STEP 3: Apply slight tension to the moleskin and anchor on the calcaneus (Fig. 3–6C).

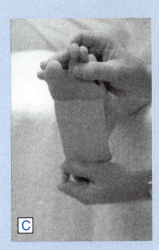

STEP 4: Anchor a 1 inch strip of non-elastic tape over the lateral surface of the fifth MTP joint, continue around the heel, and finish over the medial aspect of the first MTP joint (Fig. 3–6D).

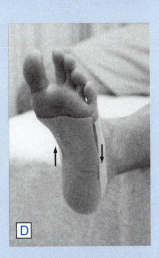

STEP 5: Apply two to three additional 1 inch strips with moderate roll tension, overlapping each by ½ of the tape width (Fig. 3–6E). Place these strips inferior to the medial and lateral malleoli.

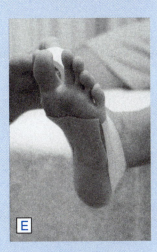

Figure 3-6 *continued*

STEP 6: Anchor a strip of 2 inch non-elastic tape on the lateral dorsum proximally, continue across the plantar surface, and anchor on the medial dorsum (Fig. 3–6F).

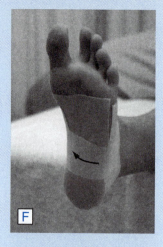

STEP 7: Repeat this step with three additional strips, overlapping each with moderate roll tension (Fig. 3–6G). Do not encircle the foot with these strips.

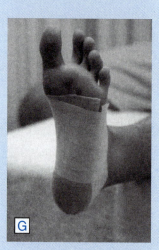

STEP 8: Apply 2 inch elastic tape from the lateral dorsum, across the plantar surface, and finish on the lateral dorsum to encircle the arch (Fig. 3–6H).

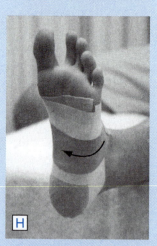

Figure 3-6 *continued*

STEP 9: Apply two to three additional overlapping strips with mild to moderate roll tension to anchor the moleskin and non-elastic tape (Fig. 3–6I).

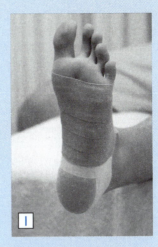

Figure 3-6 *continued*

PLANTAR FASCIA STRAP Figure 3–7

▶ **Purpose:** Use the plantar fascia strap technique to provide moderate support to the longitudinal arch and lessen the symptoms associated with plantar fasciitis (Fig. 3–7). This technique requires fewer supplies than the Low-Dye techniques in treating plantar fasciitis.

▶ **Materials:**
  • 2 inch or 3 inch width heavyweight moleskin (pre-cut straps or from roll), taping scissors
  Options:
  • Adherent tape spray
  • 2 inch elastic tape

▶ **Position of the individual:** Sitting on a taping table or bench with the leg extended off the edge and the foot placed in a neutral position.

▶ **Preparation:** To make a strap, cut a piece of 2 inch or 3 inch width moleskin in a 9–11 inch length strip. Determine the length of the strap by the size of the foot. Measure approximately 1–1½ inches from one end and draw a line. From this line, measure another 1–1½ inches and draw a second line.
  Option: *Apply adherent tape spray to the plantar forefoot to provide additional adherence.*

▶ **Application:**
  STEP 1: On each side of the strip beginning at the second line, make an angled cut toward the first line, leaving about 1 inch between the cuts at the first line (Fig. 3–7A).

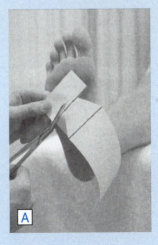

Figure 3-7

STEP 2: Anchor the cross bar end of the strap directly to the skin over the posterior heel (Fig. 3–7B). Position the cut in the strap just **superior** to the plantar surface of the foot.

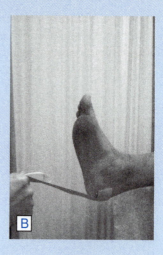

B

STEP 3: Pull the strap with slight tension toward the metatarsal heads and anchor (Fig. 3–7C). Check the tension of the strap by allowing the individual to step down and take a few steps. Appropriate tension should support the longitudinal arch and lessen pain with weight-bearing movements. If necessary, reposition the strap by removing the end at the metatarsal heads and reanchor.

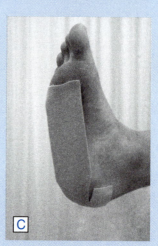

C

STEP 4: Smooth the strap directly to the skin with your hands and cut any excess moleskin from the metatarsal heads (Fig. 3–7D).
Option: *An anchor of 2 inch elastic tape may be applied around the metatarsal heads to anchor the strap, but this is not required.*

...IF/THEN...

IF application of the circular, "X," and/or loop arch taping technique does not provide adequate support for a longitudinal arch strain, **THEN** consider using the weave, Low-Dye, or plantar fascia strap taping or orthotic technique, which may provide greater support to the longitudinal arch.

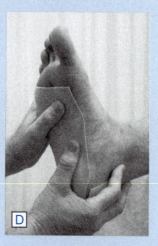

D

Figure 3-7 *continued*

Critical Thinking Question 1

Late in the season, an intercollegiate softball outfielder begins to demonstrate pain over the medial heel. You suspect plantar fasciitis and are proficient in applying several taping techniques to treat the injury. However, your supply inventory is low, leaving only non-elastic tape available for use.

▶ **Question: What taping techniques can you use to treat plantar fasciitis?**

HEEL BOX Figure 3–8

▶ **Purpose:** Use the heel box technique to provide mild support to the calcaneus when treating a heel contusion and to attach pads to the heel (Fig. 3–8).

▶ **Materials:**
  • ½ inch or 1 inch non-elastic tape, adherent tape spray

▶ **Position of the individual:** Sitting on a taping table or bench with the leg extended off the edge and the foot in a dorsiflexed position.

▶ **Preparation:** Apply adherent tape spray to the heel area.

▶ **Application:**
  STEP 1: Place an anchor with ½ inch or 1 inch non-elastic tape directly to the skin from the inferior medial malleolus, across the distal Achilles tendon, finishing inferior to the lateral malleolus (Fig. 3–8A).

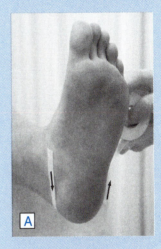

  STEP 2: Next, apply a strip from the inferior medial malleolus, across the plantar foot, and anchor inferior to the lateral malleolus (Fig. 3–8B).

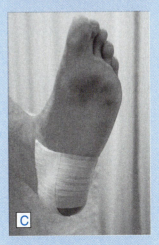

  STEP 3: Continue to apply strips in this alternating pattern to the anchors with moderate roll tension, overlapping by ½ of the tape width until the majority of the heel is covered (Fig. 3–8C).

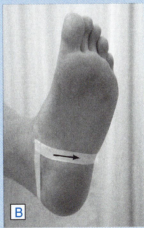

Figure 3-8

BUDDY TAPE Figure 3–9

▸ **Purpose:** Use the buddy tape technique following sprains, dislocations, and fractures of the toes to provide mild to moderate stability for the collateral ligaments. The injured toe is taped together with the largest adjacent toe (Fig. 3–9).

▸ **Materials:**
- ½ inch non-elastic tape, ⅛ inch foam or felt, adherent tape spray, taping scissors
  Options:
- 1 inch non-elastic or elastic tape or self-adherent wrap

▸ **Position of the individual:** Sitting on a taping table or bench with the leg extended off the edge and the foot placed in a neutral position.

▸ **Preparation:** Apply adherent tape spray to the involved toes. To maintain anatomical alignment, cut a piece of ⅛ inch foam or felt the length of the shortest toe to be taped. Do not apply tape directly over the joints. When applying tape to the toes, monitor for skin irritation of adjacent toes ✂.

 Helpful Hint: Apply a skin lubricant such as petroleum jelly over the tape and to adjacent toes. The lubricant will reduce friction between the tape and skin to prevent blisters and abrasions.

▸ **Application:**

STEP 1: Apply a strip of ½ inch non-elastic tape around the proximal end of the foam or felt and place between the toes (Fig. 3–9A).

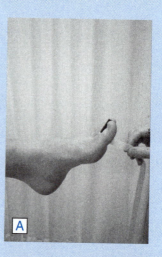

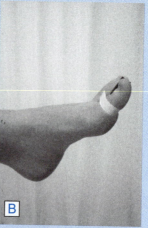

STEP 2: Encircle the toes between the MTP and PIP joints with the tape lock-in strip ✂ (Fig. 3–9B). The direction of the tape does not matter (hereinafter symbolized by ◀▶).

Figure 3-9

 Helpful Hint: The lock-in strip will prevent the foam or felt from dislodging and loosening during activity as perspiration and moisture begin to affect the tape adhesive.

STEP 3: Maintain alignment of the toes and apply three to five circular strips of ½ inch non-elastic tape with mild to moderate roll tension between the MTP and PIP and the PIP and DIP joints ◄► (Fig. 3–9C).
Option: *Use 1 inch non-elastic or elastic tape or self-adherent wrap on large toes to provide adequate support.*

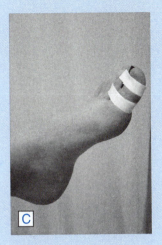

Figure 3-9 *continued*

TOE SPICA Figure 3–10

▶ **Purpose:** The toe spica technique provides mild support to the MTP joint of the great toe in the treatment of great toe sprains (Fig. 3–10).

▶ **Materials:**
  • 1 inch non-elastic or elastic tape, 2 inch elastic tape, adherent tape spray

▶ **Position of the individual:** Sitting on a taping table or bench with the leg extended off the edge and the foot placed in a neutral position.

▶ **Preparation:** Apply adherent tape spray to the involved toe.

▶ **Application:**
  STEP 1: Anchor a strip of 1 inch non-elastic or elastic tape directly to the skin at an angle on the medial plantar surface of the foot (Fig. 3–10A).

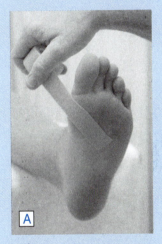

STEP 2: Proceed up and around the medial aspect of the great toe, down and between the great and second toe, across the plantar surface, and anchor on the dorsum of the foot near the third metatarsal (Fig. 3–10B).

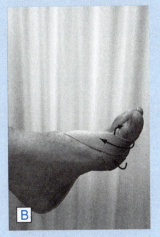

Figure 3-10

STEP 3: Apply slight roll tension to **adduct** the great toe as the dorsal anchor is placed to provide additional support to the MTP joint. Repeat this step with two to three additional strips, overlapping by ⅓ to ½ of the tape width (Fig. 3–10C).

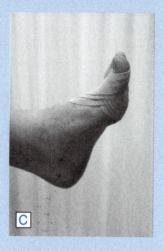

STEP 4: Anchor the strips with mild roll tension around the distal foot with 2 inch elastic tape ⬅ (Fig. 3–10D).

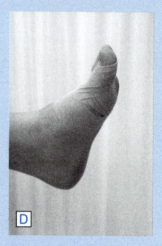

Figure 3-10 *continued*

TOE STRIPS Figure 3–11

▶ **Purpose:** Use the toe strip technique following a hyperextension (turf toe) or hyperflexion (soccer toe) sprain to provide mild to moderate support and reduce range of motion at the MTP joint (Fig. 3–11). Depending on the specific injury (turf or soccer toe) hyperextension, hyperflexion, or multidirectional range of motion can be reduced.

▶ **Materials:**
  • 1 inch non-elastic or elastic tape, 2 inch elastic tape or self-adherent wrap, adherent tape spray

▶ **Position of the individual:** Sitting on a taping table or bench with the leg extended off the edge and the foot placed in a neutral position. Determine painful range(s) of motion by stabilizing the midfoot, proximal to the metatarsal heads. To determine painful flexion, place a finger on the proximal dorsal phalanx of the great toe and slowly move the toe into flexion until pain occurs. Place a finger on the proximal plantar phalanx and slowly move the toe into extension to determine painful extension. Once painful range of motion is determined, place the great toe in a pain-free range and maintain this position during application.

▶ **Preparation:** Apply adherent tape spray to the midfoot and great toe.

▶ **Application:**

STEP 1: Place a 1 inch non-elastic or elastic tape anchor directly to the skin around the distal great toe and a 2 inch elastic tape or self-adherent wrap anchor around the midfoot with mild roll tension ◀▬▶ (Fig. 3–11A).

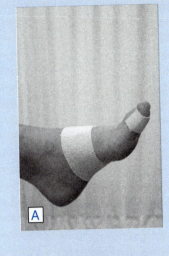

STEP 2: To limit hyperextension, anchor a 1 inch non-elastic tape strip on the lateral plantar surface of the toe and continue to the midfoot anchor (Fig. 3–11B).

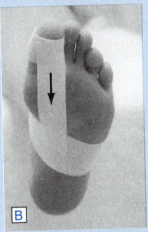

STEP 3: Apply three to four additional strips, overlapping by ½ of the tape width (Fig. 3–11C).

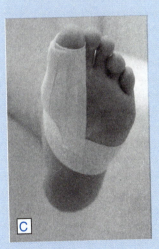

Figure 3-11

STEP 4: To limit hyperflexion, anchor a 1 inch non-elastic strip on the lateral dorsal surface of the toe and continue to the midfoot anchor (Fig. 3–11D).

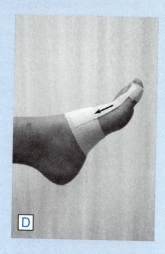

STEP 5: Apply three to four additional strips, overlapping each one (Fig. 3–11E).

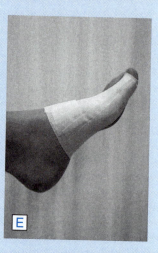

STEP 6: To limit multidirectional motion, anchor a 1 inch non-elastic tape strip on the lateral plantar toe, proceed at an angle over the medial foot, and finish on the dorsal midfoot anchor (Fig. 3–11F).

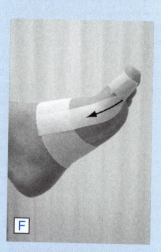

Figure 3-11 *continued*

STEP 7: Next, anchor a strip on the lateral dorsal toe, proceed at an angle over the medial foot, and finish on the plantar midfoot anchor (Fig. 3–11G).

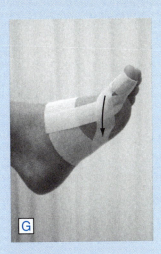

STEP 8: Place three to four additional strips, alternating anchor points, to produce a weave-type pattern (Fig. 3–11H).

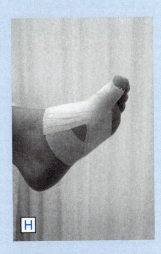

STEP 9: Place a 1 inch non-elastic or elastic tape anchor around the distal great toe and a 2 inch elastic tape anchor around the midfoot with mild roll tension ◀▶ (Fig. 3–11I).

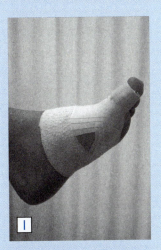

Figure 3-11 *continued*

Toe Strip Variation

▶ **Purpose:** A variation to the toe strips technique to limit multidirectional motion involves applying tape strips that enclose the great toe. Use this technique with painful hyperflexion and hyperextension associated with an MTP joint sprain.

▶ **Materials:**
• 1 inch non-elastic or elastic tape, 2 inch elastic tape or self-adherent wrap, adherent tape spray

▶ **Position of the individual:** Sitting on a taping table or bench with the leg extended off the edge and the foot placed in a neutral position. Determine painful range(s) of motion. Once determined, place the great toe in a pain-free range and maintain this position during application.

▶ **Preparation:** Apply adherent tape spray to the midfoot and great toe.

▶ **Application:**

STEP 1: Place a 1 inch non-elastic or elastic tape anchor directly to the skin around the distal great toe and a 2 inch elastic tape or self-adherent wrap anchor around the midfoot with mild roll tension ◀▶ . Beginning on the lateral plantar toe, apply individual 1 inch non-elastic tape strips, anchoring on the midfoot. Continue to place individual strips in the same manner around the toe, overlapping by ½ of the tape width (Fig. 3–11J).

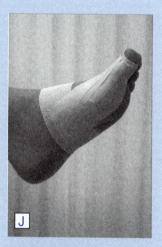

STEP 2: Place the last strip on the lateral dorsal surface of the great toe (Fig. 3–11K).

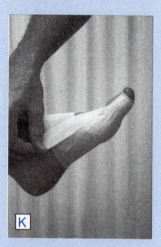

Figure 3-11 *continued*

STEP 3: Place a 1 inch non-elastic or elastic tape anchor around the distal great toe and a 2 inch elastic tape anchor around the midfoot (Fig. 3–11L).

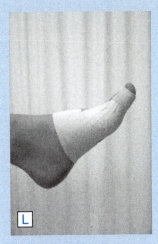

L

Figure 3-11 *continued*

TURF TOE STRAP   Figure 3–12

▶ **Purpose:** The turf toe strap technique provides moderate support to the great toe and limits excessive range of motion, typically hyperextension (Fig. 3–12). This technique requires fewer supplies than the toe strips technique in treating MTP joint sprains.

▶ **Materials:**
  • 2 inch or 3 inch width heavyweight moleskin (pre-cut straps or from roll), 1 inch non-elastic or elastic tape, taping scissors
  Options:
  • Adherent tape spray
  • 2 inch elastic tape

▶ **Position of the individual:** Sitting on a taping table or bench with the leg extended off the edge and the foot placed in a neutral position. Determine painful range(s) of motion. Once determined, place the great toe in a pain-free range and maintain this position during application.

▶ **Preparation:** Cut individual straps in the shape of an uppercase "T" from a roll of 2 inch or 3 inch heavy-weight moleskin by following the technique illustrated in Fig. 3-7, but leaving only ½–¾ inches for the cross bar.
  Option: *Apply adherent tape spray to the toe and plantar forefoot to provide additional adherence.*

▶ **Application:**
  STEP 1: Anchor the strap directly to the skin on the plantar surface of the distal great toe (Fig. 3–12A).

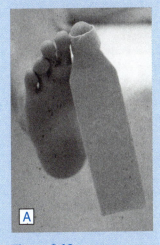

A

Figure 3-12

STEP 2: Check the position of the toe and apply slight tension to the strap and anchor on the plantar surface of the foot near or over the calcaneus (Fig. 3–12B). Check for appropriate strap tension by allowing the individual to step down and walk. Appropriate tension should limit excessive hyperextension and reduce pain with weight-bearing movements. Reposition the plantar foot anchor if necessary. Smooth the moleskin to the skin.

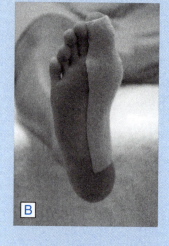

STEP 3: Apply a 1 inch non-elastic or elastic tape anchor with mild roll tension around the strap on the distal toe ◄► (Fig. 3–12C).
Option: An anchor of 2 inch elastic tape can be applied around the midfoot to anchor the strap, but this is not required. ◄►

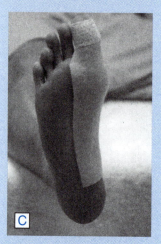

Figure 3-12 *continued*

ELASTIC MATERIAL Figures 3–13, 3–14

▶ **Purpose:** Use elastic materials to cover wound dressings and attach pads to the foot (Fig. 3–13) and toes (Fig. 3–14) in treating wounds, contusions, and blisters. The material should be lightweight and not restrict range of motion. Because of the elastic material's thin profile and great adhesive strength, use the material in place of tape.

▶ **Materials:**
• Adhesive gauze material, ½ inch non-elastic tape, taping scissors
Option:
• 2 inch or 3 inch lightweight elastic tape

▶ **Position of the individual:** Sitting, prone, or supine on a taping table or bench with the leg extended off the edge and the foot in a neutral position.

▶ **Preparation:** Apply adhesive gauze material directly to the skin and use without adherent tape spray.

Application:

STEP 1: After applying a sterile wound dressing or pad, cut a piece of the material. The piece of adhesive gauze material should extend from ½–1 inch beyond the dressing or pad to adhere properly to the skin (Fig. 3–13). Smooth the material to the foot.

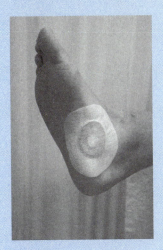

Figure 3-13

Helpful Hint: Round all corners of the material to prevent the edges from rolling upon contact with clothing.

STEP 2: For the toes, cut a piece of the elastic material to cover an area from the tip of the toe to just proximal to the DIP or PIP joint. Place the center of the material over the toe (Fig. 3–14A). *Option: If adhesive gauze material is not available, use 2 inch or 3 inch lightweight elastic tape.*

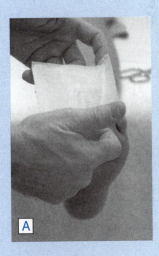

STEP 3: Fold the sides over the toe, avoiding wrinkles. Press the sides of the material together against the toe (Fig. 3–14B).

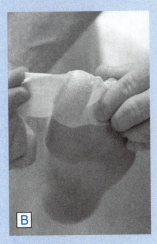

Figure 3-14

STEP 4: Cut the excess material away from the sides, leaving enough of the material to maintain adherence (Fig. 3–14C). If the toe is large enough, place anchors with ½ inch non-elastic tape around the distal, middle, or proximal phalanx ◀▬▶ .

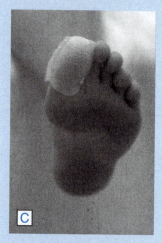

C

Figure 3-14 *continued*

Critical Thinking Question 2

You are treating a recreational runner for a distal third phalanx fracture with the buddy tape technique. After applying the technique several times, the adjacent toes become abraded.

▶ **Question: How can you treat the abrasion and prevent future blisters and abrasions from occurring?**

Wrapping Techniques

By applying mechanical pressure around the injured site, compression wraps assist in reducing the amount of space available for swelling.[30] Use elastic and self-adherent wraps and elastic tape on the foot and toes to treat inflammation that accompanies contusions, sprains, strains, and overuse injuries and conditions (Fig. 3-15).

COMPRESSION WRAP Figure 3–15

▶ **Purpose:** The compression wrap technique for the foot or toe aids in reducing mild, moderate, or severe swelling.

▶ **Materials:**
  • 2 inch, 3 inch, or 4 inch width by 5 yard length elastic wrap determined by the size of the foot, metal clips, 1½ inch non-elastic or 2 inch elastic tape, taping scissors
  • 1 inch elastic tape or self-adherent wrap for the toes
  Options:
  • ⅛ inch or ¼ inch foam or felt
  • 2 inch, 3 inch, or 4 inch width self-adherent wrap or elastic tape, pre-tape material, thin foam pads

▶ **Position of the individual:** Sitting on a taping table or bench with the leg extended off the edge and the foot in a dorsiflexed position.

▶ **Preparation:** Apply the technique directly to the skin.
  Option: Cut a ⅛ inch or ¼ inch foam or felt pad and place it over the inflamed area directly to the skin to assist in venous return.
  Using tape, apply one layer of pre-tape material directly to the skin and use thin foam pads over the heel and lace areas to prevent irritation.

▶ **Application:**

STEP 1: Holding the elastic wrap, anchor the extended end on the distal plantar surface of the foot and proceed around to encircle the anchor 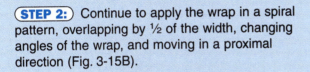 (Fig. 3–15A).

Option: 2 inch, 3 inch, or 4 inch width self-adherent wrap or elastic tape can also be used when an elastic wrap is not available.

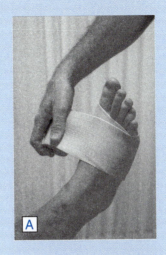

STEP 2: Continue to apply the wrap in a spiral pattern, overlapping by ½ of the width, changing angles of the wrap, and moving in a proximal direction (Fig. 3-15B).

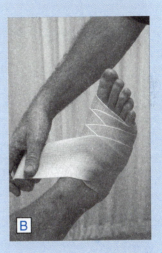

STEP 3: Incorporate the heel lock technique (see Fig. 4-2) with the spiral pattern to enclose the heel (Fig. 3-15C). Avoid gaps, wrinkles, or inconsistent roll tension in the distal-to-proximal application.

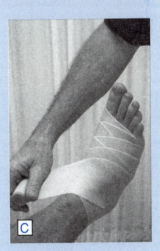

Figure 3-15

STEP 4: Continue with the spiral pattern and anchor over the distal lower leg with Velcro, metal clips, or loosely applied 1½ inch non-elastic or 2 inch elastic tape ◀▶ (Fig. 3–15D). With practice, apply the greatest amount of roll tension distally and lessen tension as the wrap continues proximally.

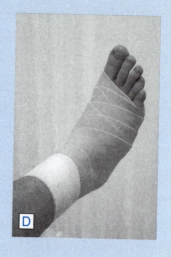

STEP 5: For the toes, apply 1 inch elastic tape or self-adherent wrap in a distal-to-proximal circular pattern over the toe ◀▶ (Fig. 3–15E). Apply pressure greatest at the distal end and less toward the proximal end. The tip of the toe should remain exposed to monitor circulation. No additional anchor is required.

...IF/THEN...

IF an elastic wrap compression technique does not provide adequate pressure around the foot, allowing swelling to migrate distally following a dorsal midfoot contusion, **THEN** consider using self-adherent wrap or pre-tape material and elastic tape, which possess greater ability to conform to the contours of the foot, to provide adequate pressure.

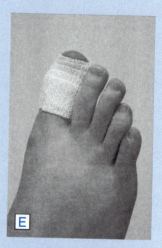

Figure 3-15 *continued*

Bracing Techniques

Bracing techniques provide immobilization or support, or correct structural abnormalities in preventing and treating injuries and conditions of the foot and toes. Many of these techniques also work for other lower extremity injuries and conditions.

Orthotics

The use and construction of orthotics have been and continue to be a common practice in the health-care setting. Orthotics are designed to correct and support structural abnormalities of the foot, such as excessive supination and pronation, and pes cavus, and can be purchased off-the-shelf or individually fabricated in a variety of shapes with many different types of materials. Generally, orthotics can be categorized as three types: soft, semirigid, and rigid. Research determining the effectiveness of orthotics in preventing and treating injuries and conditions both supports and questions their use.

Soft Orthotics

Soft orthotics are designed to absorb shock and reduce friction and stress of the foot. They are constructed of a variety of materials such as felt, foam, plastic, rubber, silicone, and viscoelastic polymers (Fig. 3–16). Many of these orthotics can be purchased off-the-shelf and do not require cast molds or fabrication.

Felt and foam are frequently used to construct soft orthotics. For our purposes, the construction and application of felt and foam orthotics in treating sesamoiditis, metatarsalgia, interdigital neuroma, heel contusions, and bunions are discussed in the Padding section of this chapter. The types of soft orthotics are discussed next.

HEEL CUPS Figure 3–16A

▸ **Purpose:** Use heel cups for heel pain associated with contusions, spurs, plantar fasciitis, and lower leg, knee, and back injuries and conditions.

▸ **Design**:
  • Hard heel cups are made from plastic to provide support; soft cups are constructed of latex rubber, silicone, and viscoelastic polymers to provide support and shock absorption.
  • Heel cups come according to the foot size or weight of the individual.
  • To prevent adaptive changes with the use of one heel cup, place a cup in each shoe. Clean heel cups with soap and water and reuse them.

▸ **Application:**
  (STEP 1:) Insert the cups into the heel box of each shoe over the insole. Additional adhesive to prevent migration is normally not required (Fig. 3–16A).

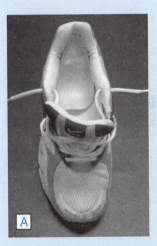

SOFT INSOLES Figure 3–16B

▸ **Purpose:** Full-length neoprene, silicone, and viscoelastic polymer insoles provide shock absorption for the entire plantar surface of the foot.

▸ **Design**:
  • Purchase the insoles off-the-shelf in specific shoe sizes or cut them from a large roll of the soft material.
  • Use the insoles over the existing insoles or as replacements.

▸ **Application:**
  (STEP 1:) Trimming the insole with taping scissors may help in finding the best fit. Additional adhesive is typically not required to hold the insole in place. Loosen the shoe laces and slide the soft insole toward the toe box (Fig. 3-16B).

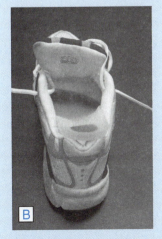

Figure 3-16 Soft insole partially inserted into a shoe.

Semirigid Orthotics

Semirigid orthotics are constructed from thermoplastic, cork, leather, and foam materials and are designed to absorb shock, reduce friction and stress, and support and correct structural abnormalities of the forefoot and/or rearfoot (Fig. 3-17).[20] Because of the adaptability, support, control, and flexible construction, semirigid orthotics are perhaps the most widely used type with the athletic population.[30] Purchase the orthotics in off-the-shelf designs or have them custom-made in a health-care facility or orthotic laboratory.

▶ **Purpose:** Use semirigid orthotics in preventing and treating many rearfoot and forefoot injuries and conditions such as MTP sprains, arch strains, interdigital neuroma, sesamoid fractures, metatarsalgia, bunions, and plantar fasciitis.

▶ **Design:**
- These orthotics typically consist of a semirigid outer shell with a soft, durable covering.
- Off-the-shelf designs are manufactured according to shoe size to provide cushion and support to the longitudinal and metatarsal arches (Fig. 3–17A).
- Other off-the-shelf designs consist of a steel, graphite, or thermoplastic material insert to restrict forefoot and toe range of motion, such as hyperextension with turf toe injuries (Fig. 3–17B).
- Custom-made designs are fabricated after foot impressions or casts are taken (Fig. 3–17C).

○ DETAILS

With custom-made semirigid designs, posts are used to correct structural abnormalities and are either intrinsic or extrinsic.[20] Intrinsic posts are built into the orthotic mold, and extrinsic posts are applied on the orthotic shell. Extrinsic posts, constructed of foam or cork material, are used more often with semirigid orthotics and can be modified easily by adding or removing the material.

Rigid Orthotics

Rigid orthotics are used when the injury or condition warrants absolute biomechanical control of structural abnormalities (Fig. 3–18).[20] The rigid properties of the materials make fabrication time consuming and do not allow for errors. Many health-care professionals send casts or molds to orthotic laboratories for construction. Intrinsic posts are commonly used with rigid designs.

Important facts to be familiar with regarding the use of rigid orthotics include the following:

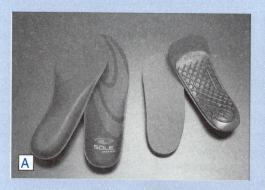
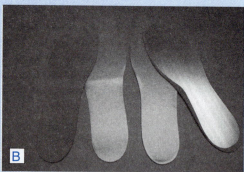
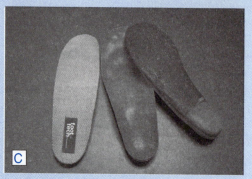

Figure 3-17 A Off-the-shelf semirigid orthotics. (Left) Full length. (Right) ¾ length. **B** Off-the-shelf steel semirigid orthotics. (Left) ½ length. (Right) Full length. **C** Custom-made semirigid orthotics.

- Because of the inflexibility of the materials, fewer athletes use rigid orthotics.[30]
- The designs have frequently been used with limited success in treating structural abnormalities in adolescents.[27]
- Use rigid orthotics in preventing and treating MTP sprains, arch strains, and excessive pronation or supination.
- The orthotics are constructed from a foot cast and made of rigid acrylic plastic or graphite materials (Fig. 3-18).

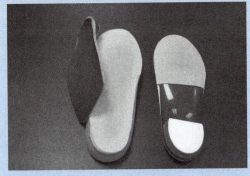

Figure 3-18   Custom-made rigid orthotics.

RESEARCH BRIEF

Examining active subjects with knee, shin, and ankle pain,[13,21] plantar fasciitis,[18] and excessive foot eversion,[5,18] between 70% and 80% reported relief of pain and a return to preinjury activity levels with the use of semirigid or rigid orthotics. Other researchers have shown that among military recruits with low arches, the use of semirigid or cushioned orthotics reduced the incidence of metatarsal stress fractures.[36] Viscoelastic polymer orthotics have been reported to decrease back, leg, and foot pain following prolonged standing,[4] and reduce impact forces from ambulation as much as 42%.[12,39] Many different types of injuries and conditions can be prevented and treated with the same orthotic technique.[26]

These same orthotic techniques have also been questioned. Several researchers have found that among active individuals, the use of orthotics did not affect pes cavus[10,11] or pronation,[32] reduce the incidence of metatarsal stress fractures,[23,35] or reduce impact forces greater than 10%–20%.[9,14,22,25] Nigg, Nurse, and Stefanyshyn[26] have stated that the idea of orthotics aligning the skeleton is based on a substantial amount of uncertainty. Questions regarding the cost versus the effectiveness[16] and concern about overprescribing orthotics[37] for individuals leave many variables for the health-care professional to consider. The use of any orthotic technique should fit the needs of the individual and be part of the overall prevention and treatment program.

Critical Thinking Question 3

A construction worker is experiencing general pain along the entire plantar surface of both feet during work. His boots have a steel shank sole.

▶ **Question: What bracing technique would you use to treat his condition?**

Orthotics Fabrication Process

The fabrication of custom-made soft, semirigid, and rigid orthotics typically takes place either in health-care facilities or orthotic laboratories. Fabrication techniques require skill and expertise obtained through experience with foot biomechanics, pathological conditions, and orthotic materials and fabrication equipment. This experience has resulted in the development of many different types of fabrication techniques that are currently used by health-care professionals. Several advantages of in-house fabrication include a shorter time from construction to use and the ability to make modifications to the designs. The following discussion provides an overview of a general fabrication process of soft, semirigid, and rigid designs.

Foot Impressions and Molds

With many designs, the fabrication process begins with the health-care professional taking an impression of the foot to obtain a neutral subtalar joint position (Fig. 3–19).[20] Impressions are commonly taken with boxes of impression foam or with plaster casting, as detailed below.

FOAM IMPRESSION BOX Figure 3–19A,B

▶ **Purpose:** Use a foam impression box when the orthotic design does not require an exact fit. This method is often used with soft and semirigid designs. The foam impression box may be packaged and sent to an orthotic laboratory for fabrication.

▶ **Procedure:**

STEP 1: Place the individual in a seated position with the hip and knee at 90° and insert the foot into the foam box (Fig. 3–19A).

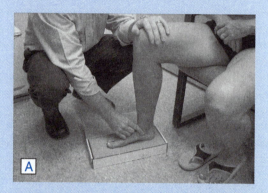

STEP 2: Push the foot well into the foam while maintaining a neutral position at the subtalar joint (Fig. 3–19B).

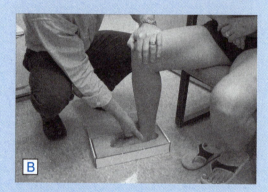

Figure 3-19

NEGATIVE CASTS AND POSITIVE MOLDS Figure 3–19C,D,E

▶ **Purpose:** Use negative casts and positive molds when exact fit of the orthotic is required.

▶ **Design:**

- Use plaster to make a negative cast, then a positive mold, while the individual is in a prone or supine non–weight-bearing position maintaining the subtalar joint neutral.[20]
- A negative cast is constructed with two plaster splints placed on the plantar surface of the foot. The plaster splints form an impression of the subtalar neutral foot position and resemble a slipper.
- Using the negative cast, a positive mold can be constructed with a plaster mixture. Another option is to send the negative cast to an orthotic laboratory to make a positive mold. The orthotic is then fabricated from the positive mold.

▶ **Procedure:**

STEP 1: Apply one splint from the posterior heel to the metatarsal heads (Fig. 3–19C) and apply the second splint extending from the toes to the posterior heel (Fig. 3–19D). Smooth the cast with your hands and allow the plaster to dry.

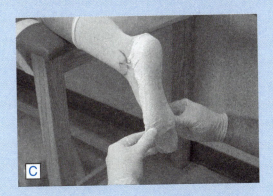

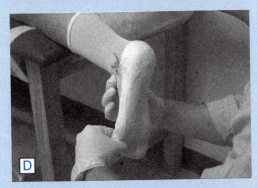

STEP 2: Pour a plaster mixture into the negative cast, allow to dry, and then remove, producing a positive mold for in-house or laboratory orthotic fabrication (Fig. 3-19E).

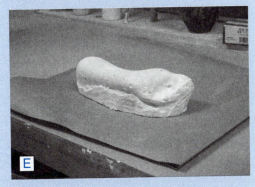

Figure 3-19 E Positive mold produced from a negative cast.

Fabrication from a Positive Mold

Fabrication of semirigid and rigid orthotics from a positive mold requires additional time and equipment (Fig. 3–20).[20] Experienced fabricators modify the mold with grinding, sanding, and shaping to correct structural abnormalities that are evident in the mold prior to fabrication of the orthotic. Plaster can also be added to the mold to correct structural abnormalities. Once the mold is completed, rigid acrylic or graphite materials are heated and pressed onto the mold with the hands or vacuum press (Fig. 3–20).

The modifications to the mold made prior to fabrication represent intrinsic posting and further changes to the orthotic are difficult. Off-the-shelf orthotic shells also come in shoe sizes, which are heated and molded over the positive mold. These shells are modified with additional heating.

Fabrication to the Foot

Other semirigid orthotic designs do not require a cast or mold, but are molded directly to the foot of the individual and fabricated in-house (Fig. 3–21). Place the individual

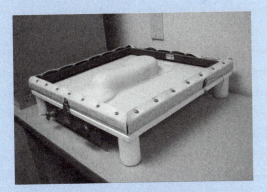

Figure 3-20 Positive mold and orthotic materials in a vacuum press.

in a prone or seated position, knee flexed at 90°, and with the foot in subtalar neutral, and follow this step-by-step procedure.

▶ **Fabrication Procedure:**

STEP 1: First, cut the thermoplastic materials larger than the foot and heat (Fig. 3–21A). When the materials are pliable, remove from the heating source and apply to the plantar surface of the foot.

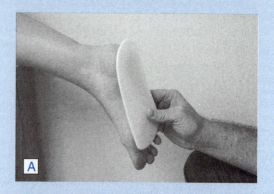

STEP 2: Mold the materials with your hands to the contours of the foot. After cooling, trim the materials to match the size of the foot (Fig. 3–21B).

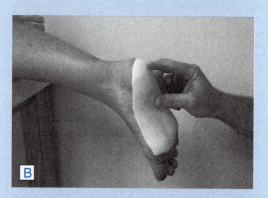

STEP 3: The general orthotic fabrication process continues with the use of an electric grinder to bevel the outside edge of the soft, semirigid, or rigid orthotic to assist with proper fit in the shoe (Fig. 3–21C). Use eye, nose, mouth, and hand protection when operating the equipment. Many grinders are available with vacuums attached to decrease the amount of debris in the air and clean-up time.

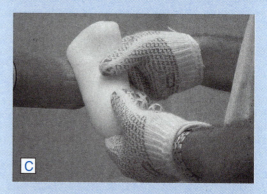

STEP 4: Grind the orthotic to produce a flat bottom with tapering toward the distal foot under the metatarsals or toes (Fig. 3-21D) .

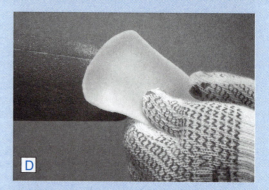

Figure 3-21

Helpful Hint: Many health-care professionals incorporate additional support through extrinsic posting at this stage of fabrication. Support and cushioning for the longitudinal and metatarsal arch, heel, or sesamoids are accomplished by molding thermoplastic wedges, and horse-shoe, tear drop, or half-circle shapes to the dorsal or plantar surface of the orthotic.

STEP 5: After determining alignment, attach the thermoplastic pieces with cement and ground to produce a beveled edge and flattened bottom (Fig. 3–21E). Modifications can be performed through additional grinding.

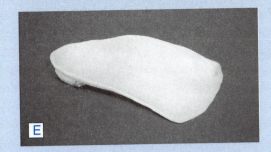

E

STEP 6: Attach a covering of soft, durable material with cement on the top for cushioning and to lessen migration of the orthotic in the shoe (Fig. 3–21F).

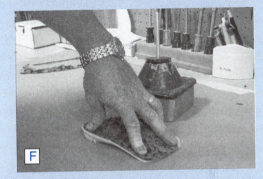

F

Figure 3-21 *continued*

Fabrication Systems

Orthotic fabrication systems that include all the materials necessary for in-house construction may be purchased from several manufacturers. The materials are constructed in various designs and sizes according to purpose and can be cut and ground to achieve proper fit.

One system utilizes a water-activated material placed between the top and bottom sections of the orthotic. Insert water into the material, and molding occurs in the shoe while the individual is weight-bearing.

Another system uses a stand to align the individual in a standing subtalar neutral position. Heat a pre-sized shell and place it on the cushioned surface of the stand. The individual then stands on the shell. Cement the bottom portion of the orthotic onto the shell, trim, and ground to fit.

Aside from orthotics, other bracing techniques for the foot and toes provide immobilization or support, or absorb shock in the treatment of sprains, strains, stable acute and stress fractures, overuse injuries and conditions, and postoperative procedures.

OFF-THE-SHELF NIGHT SPLINTS Figure 3–22A

▸ **Purpose:** Night splints are designed to keep the ankle and foot in 5° of dorsiflexion and the toes in slight dorsiflexion to provide a static stretch of the plantar fascia and Achilles tendon while the individual is sleeping to reduce pain in treating plantar fasciitis (Fig. 3–22).

▸ **Design:**
  • Off-the-shelf splints are designed in predetermined sizes that correspond to shoe size.
  • These splints are contoured to the lower leg and foot and made of rigid plastic, covered with soft foam material.
  • Many designs include a removable foam wedge used to place the foot and toes into additional dorsiflexion.
  • Velcro straps are typically used to attach the splint to the lower leg and foot.

RESEARCH BRIEF

A review of the literature reveals that night splints are effective in the treatment of plantar fasciitis when used alone,[7,28] early in the treatment protocol,[3] or in combination with heel cups or pads,[6,17,40] lower leg stretching,[6,31,40] anti-inflammatory medication,[6,17,31,42] and orthotics.[17,24,42]

▶ **Position of the individual:** Sitting on a taping table or bench with the leg extended off the edge and the foot in a dorsiflexed position.

▶ **Application:**

STEP 1: To apply most designs, release the straps, place on the lower leg and foot, and fasten the straps (Fig. 3–22A).

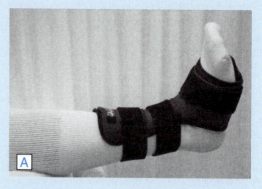

Figure 3-22

CUSTOM-MADE NIGHT SPLINTS Figure 3–22B

▶ **Purpose:** Thermoplastic material also is useful for the construction of a night splint when an off-the-shelf design is unavailable. The splint covers the posterior aspect of the lower leg and foot, including the gastrocnemius-soleus, calcaneus, plantar surface of the foot, and distal toes.

▶ **Materials:**
- Paper, felt tip pen, thermoplastic material, ¼ inch soft foam, taping scissors, a heating source, 4 inch or 6 inch width elastic wrap or 3 inch or 4 inch self-adherent wrap

Options:
- Glue, plastic rivets, Velcro straps

▶ **Position of the individual:** Sitting, prone, or supine on a taping table or bench with the leg extended off the edge and the foot in a dorsiflexed position.

▶ **Application:**

STEP 1: Construct a custom-made splint using thermoplastic material. See Fig. 1–15 for thermoplastic material construction guidelines .

 Helpful Hint: Depending on the resistance and thickness of the thermoplastic material used, reinforcements at the heel angle or double-layering of the material may be required to provide adequate rigidity of the splint.

STEP 2: Place soft foam of at least ¼ inch thickness on the inside of the splint to lessen skin irritation. If foam is not available, have the individual wear a knee-high sock under the splint.

STEP 3: Apply a 4 inch or 6 inch width elastic wrap in a circular pattern or self-adherent wrap in a circular pattern at several intervals with mild roll tension to attach the splint ◀▶ (Fig. 3–22B). *Option: Velcro straps may be attached to the splint with glue or plastic rivets to hold the splint in place.*

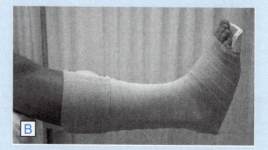

Figure 3-22

DETAILS

Although not as effective as off-the-shelf and thermoplastic night splints, lace-up ankle braces provide some static stretch to the plantar fascia and Achilles tendon (see Fig. 4–14). Properly fitted ankle braces do not incorporate the toes, which is a disadvantage of using this technique as a night splint. However, lace-up ankle braces are commonly found in health-care settings and may be used if other splints are not available. A complete discussion of lace-up ankle braces is found in Chapter 4.

WALKING BOOT Figure 3–23

▸ **Purpose:** Walking boots or walkers provide complete support and immobilization in treating sprains, strains, and stable acute and stress fractures, and in postoperative procedures involving the foot and toes (Fig. 3–23). Boots can replace a traditional plaster or fiberglass cast. The advantages of boots over traditional casting include lightweight design, lower cost, removal to allow for treatment and rehabilitation, adjustable range of motion, and lower adverse effects on gait kinematic and kinetic patterns.[15]

▸ **Design:**
- The boots are manufactured in predetermined sizes according to shoe size.
- The shell and medial and lateral upper arms and struts of the boots are constructed of aluminum, molded plastic, or lightweight steel materials.
- The soles consist of soft or hard rubber with a flat or rocker-shaped bottom.
- Inside the shell, a nylon foam liner wraps around the lower leg and foot to provide cushioning.
- Velcro straps incorporated through the shell secure the boot to the lower leg and foot.
- Boots come in a tall design that extends to the upper portion of the lower leg and a short design that extends to the middle portion of the lower leg (Fig. 3–23A).
- Several boot designs contain dials that allow for adjustments in range of motion (Fig. 3–23B).

▸ **Position of the individual:** Sitting on a taping table or bench with the leg extended off the edge and the foot in a dorsiflexed position.

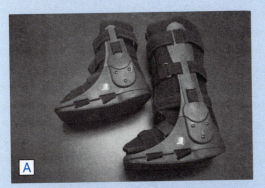 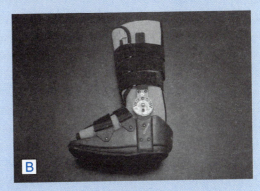

Figure 3-23 A Walking boots. (Left) Short. (Right) Tall. **B** Walking boot with an adjustable range of motion dial.

▶ **Application:**

STEP 1: Application begins with loosening the straps and separating the liner. Place the foot into the boot, moving the heel against the heel box (Fig. 3–23C).

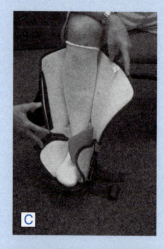

STEP 2: Wrap the liner around the foot and lower leg and fasten each strap (Fig. 3–23D). Adjust the fit by tightening or loosening the straps.

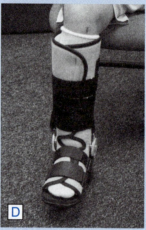

Figure 3–23 *continued*

CAST BOOT Figure 3–24

▶ **Purpose:** Cast boots are used as a sandal with lower leg casting or alone with postoperative procedures to absorb shock and provide mild support, allowing for a normal gait (Fig. 3–24).

▶ **Design:**
- The boots are constructed of a canvas upper and ethylene vinyl acetate (EVA) rocker-bottom with fore-foot and heel Velcro straps. EVA is a thermoplastic material used in the construction of orthotics and soles of running shoes.
- The boots may be purchased in predetermined sizes according to shoe size.

▶ **Position of the individual:** Sitting on a taping table or bench with the leg extended off the edge and the foot in a dorsiflexed position.

▶ **Application:**

STEP 1: To use, simply loosen the straps, place on the plantar surface of the cast or foot, then fasten the straps (Fig. 3–24).

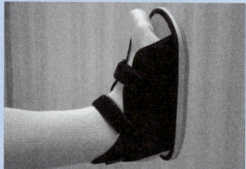

Figure 3-24

POST-OPERATIVE SHOE Figure 3–25

▶ **Purpose:** The post-operative shoe is similar in design to the cast boot but has a wooden rocker-bottom (Fig. 3–25). The stiffness of the sole reduces range of motion in the foot and toes. The shoe is used to treat metatarsal, calcaneus, and sesamoid stress fractures, foot and toe sprains, and post-operative conditions.

▶ **Position of the individual:** Sitting on a taping table or bench with the leg extended off the edge and the foot in a dorsiflexed position.

▶ **Application:**

STEP 1: Apply the shoe in the same manner as the cast boot (Fig. 3–25).

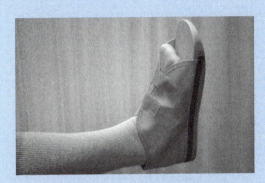

Figure 3-25

Critical Thinking Question 4

A police officer returns to work in the communications center after a surgical procedure to the left foot. The surgeon allows weight-bearing activities with an emphasis on a normal preoperative gait if support is provided to his foot.

▶ **Question: What type of brace could you apply to treat his foot while allowing for a normal gait?**

...IF/THEN...

IF off-the-shelf semirigid orthotics are effective in correcting a rear or forefoot abnormality, but lose their structure and support after a short period of use, **THEN** consider a custom-made design, which will likely retain structure and support for a longer period of time because of the more durable materials used in the construction process.

Padding Techniques

A variety of felt, foam, viscoelastic polymers, and thermoplastic materials provide support, shock absorption, and protection, and lessen stress for foot and toe injuries and conditions. Because felt and foam are readily available, many health-care professionals use these materials to construct soft orthotic designs in the treatment of sesamoiditis, metatarsalgia, interdigital neuroma, heel contusions, and bunions.

LONGITUDINAL ARCH Figure 3–26

▶ **Purpose:** Use the longitudinal arch pad technique to provide mild to moderate support of the longitudinal arch in the treatment of arch strains, plantar fasciitis, and pes planus and cavus conditions (Fig. 3–26).

▶ **Materials:**
- ⅛ inch or ¼ inch foam or felt (pre-cut or from roll), taping scissors

▶ **Position of the individual:** Sitting on a taping table or bench with the leg extended off the edge and the foot in a dorsiflexed position.

▶ **Preparation:** Construct the pad from ⅛ inch or ¼ inch foam or felt or purchase pre-cut with an adhesive backing.

▶ **Application:**

STEP 1: Cut the pad to fit from the base of the first metatarsal head to the third metatarsal head, extending to the distal calcaneus, and along the medial aspect of the foot (Fig. 3–26A).

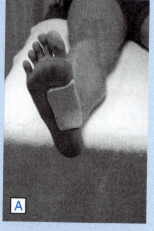

A

Helpful Hint: To obtain proper fit, outline the longitudinal arch on the individual with a felt tip marker (Fig. 3–26B). Apply adherent tape spray over the outline. Press the selected foam or felt against the outline and hold for 5–10 seconds. The outline will transfer to the foam/felt (Fig. 3-26C). Remove the foam/felt and cut as outlined (Fig. 3–26D). This procedure is helpful with many of the techniques in this section.

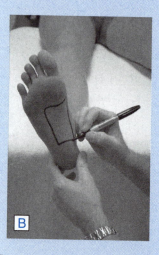

B

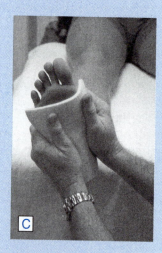

C

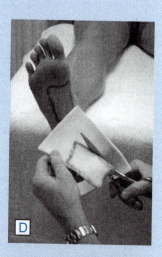

D

STEP 2: Attach the pad to the foot using the circular arch technique (see Figs. 3–1 and 3–26E).

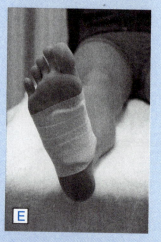

E

Figure 3-26

DONUT PADS Figure 3–27

▶ **Purpose:** Use a donut pad to lessen the amount of stress and impact over a painful area by dispersing the stress/impact outward in the treatment of foot and toe blisters, retrocalcaneal bursitis, bunions, and heel contusions (Fig. 3–27).

▶ **Materials:**
 • ⅛ inch or ¼ inch foam or felt (pre-cut or from roll), taping scissors
 • Pre-cut viscoelastic donuts also come in a variety of sizes

▶ **Position of the individual:** Sitting, prone, or supine on a taping table or bench with the leg extended off the edge and the foot in a dorsiflexed position.

▶ **Preparation:** Either make the pads from ⅛ inch or ¼ inch foam or felt or purchase pre-cut with adhesive backing. Construction of the pad begins with determining the painful area. If the area of the foot or toes allows, cut the pad to extend in all directions ½ inch to 1 inch beyond the painful area. Apply adherent tape spray if necessary.

▶ **Application:**

(STEP 1:) Cut a piece of foam/felt to the appropriate size. Mark the painful area on the piece of foam/felt and cut out the area with taping scissors, creating a hole (Fig. 3–27A). This hole protects the painful area from stress/impact.

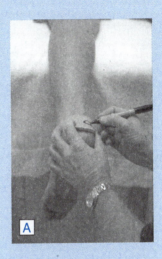

(STEP 2:) Folding the foam/felt over into one piece and cutting in a semicircle pattern is helpful (Fig. 3–27B).

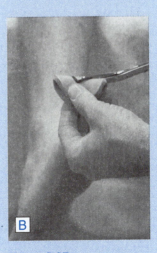

Figure 3-27

STEP 3: Place the pad on the foot or toe with the hole over the painful area, such as the retro-calcaneal bursa, bunion, or heel and attach with adhesive gauze material, or ½ inch or 1 inch non-elastic tape with the heel box technique, or 2 inch self-adherent wrap or elastic tape with the heel lock technique (see Figs. 4–2 and 3–27C).

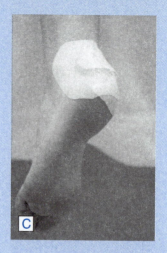

Two additional techniques, along with donut pads, also lessen stress and impact over painful areas. In treating a bunion or hallux valgus deformity, cut an "X" into the shoe over the MTP joint and bursa of the great toe or apply isopropyl alcohol to the shoe.

▶ **Materials:**
  • Felt tip pen, scalpel or sharp instrument
  • 70% isopropyl alcohol

▶ **Application:**
  STEP 1: With the individual wearing the shoe, mark the area over the inflamed MTP joint with a felt tip pen (Fig. 3–27D).

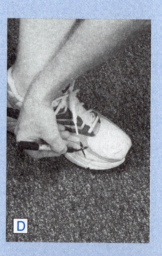

STEP 2: Remove the shoe and cut an "X" into the shoe with a scalpel or sharp instrument (Fig. 3–27E). The "X" provides additional space for the MTP joint, bursa, and/or donut pad.

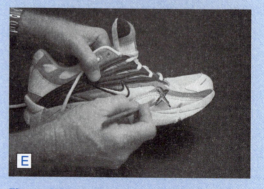

Figure 3-27 *continued*

STEP 3: The second technique involves apply-ing 70% isopropyl alcohol on the leather of a shoe .

Helpful Hint: Determine the shoe area that is causing stress and impact such as the medial or lateral toe box. Soak a cotton ball or gauze pad with 70% isopropyl alcohol and apply liberally over the outer and inner shoe leather (Fig. 3–27F). Place a shoe horn, weight, or other firm object tightly into the shoe directly against the soaked area (Fig. 3-27G). Leave the object in the shoe overnight to stretch the leather. Reapply and restretch if necessary.

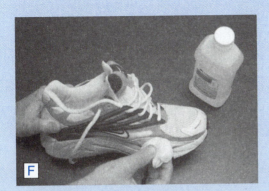

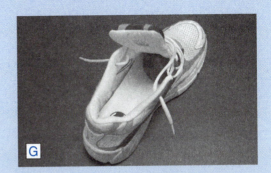

Figure 3-27 **G** Weight positioned against the toe box.

HEEL PADS Figure 3–28

▶ **Purpose:** Use heel pads in treating plantar fasciitis to provide shock absorption and relief of pain by compressing the fat pad under the calcaneus (Fig. 3-28).[29] Also use heel pads or lifts to lessen stress on the Achilles tendon in treating retrocalcaneal bursitis. The pads are commonly used when soft heel cups are not available.

▶ **Materials:**
• ¼ inch or ½ inch soft, closed-cell foam (pre-cut or from roll) or ¼ inch or ½ inch felt (pre-cut or from roll), taping scissors
Option:
• Rubber cement

▶ **Position of the individual:** Sitting on a taping table or bench with the leg extended off the edge and the foot in a dorsiflexed position.

▶ **Preparation:** Construct the pads from ¼ inch or ½ inch soft, closed-cell foam or ¼ inch or ½ inch felt or purchase in pre-cut designs with adhesive backing. Place a pad on each heel or in each shoe to prevent adaptive changes. Apply adherent tape spray if necessary.

▶ **Application:**
STEP 1: Cut the pad to cover the entire heel area or to the dimensions of the shoe liner (see Fig. 3–28A). Taper the distal end of the pad with taping scissors ✂.

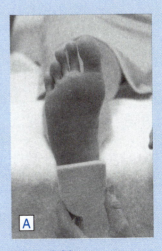

Figure 3-28

Helpful Hint: Taper a foam heel pad by cutting the distal edge at an angle toward the toes (Fig. 3-28B). Taper a felt pad by separating the distal edge into sections. With your hands, pull apart the felt into three equal sections (Fig. 3–28C). Separate the sections approximately ¾–1 inch toward the curved end of the pad. Cut the middle section out (Fig. 3-28D). Press the upper and lower sections together, producing a tapered edge (Fig. 3–28E).

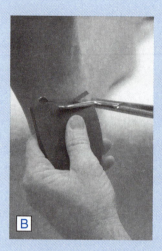

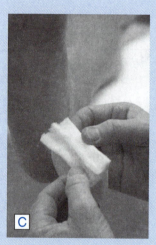

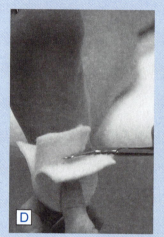

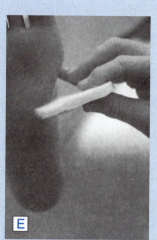

STEP 2: Either attach the pad to the heel with adhesive gauze material or with ½ inch or 1 inch non-elastic tape with the heel box technique or with 2 inch self-adherent wrap or elastic tape with the heel lock technique (see Figs. 4–2 and 3–28F).

Option: Rubber cement may be used to permanently anchor the pad to the shoe liner. Additional anchors are not required.

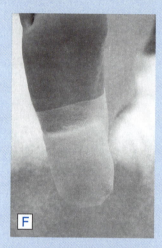

Figure 3-28 *continued*

METATARSAL BAR   Figure 3–29

▶ **Purpose:** Metatarsal bar pads reduce stress and load on the metatarsal heads in treating sesamoiditis and metatarsalgia (Fig. 3–29).

▶ **Materials:**
  • ⅛ inch or ¼ inch felt (from roll), 1 inch non-elastic tape, 2 inch self-adherent wrap or elastic tape, pre-tape material, taping scissors

▶ **Position of the individual:** Sitting on a taping table or bench with the leg extended off the edge and the foot in a dorsiflexed position.

▶ **Preparation:** Cut the bar from ⅛ inch or ¼ inch felt. The length of the bar measures across the plantar surface of the metatarsal heads and is approximately ¾ inch to 1 inch wide.

◆ **Application:**

 STEP 1: Temporarily attach the bar just proximal to the metatarsal heads with 1 inch non-elastic tape and allow the individual to walk to ensure proper alignment, indicated by a reduction in pain (Fig. 3–29A). Reposition the pad if necessary.

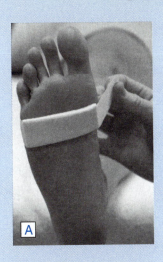

A

 STEP 2: Apply the pad with adhesive gauze material or with one to two strips of 2 inch self-adherent wrap or elastic tape directly to the skin or over pre-tape material. Anchor a strip of self-adherent wrap or elastic tape over the pad on the plantar surface of the foot. Proceed around the dorsal foot and anchor on the plantar or dorsal surface, encircling the foot ◀▬▶ (Fig. 3–29B).

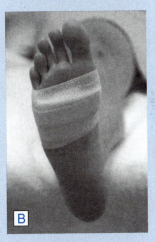

B

Figure 3-29

TEAR DROP Figure 3–30

◆ **Purpose:** The tear drop pad technique provides mild to moderate support to the metatarsal arch in treating interdigital neuroma (Fig. 3–30). The most common location is between the third and fourth metatarsals and is referred to as Morton's neuroma.[29,41] With alignment of the metatarsal arch, a decrease in inflammation and pain should occur with the use of the pad.

◆ **Materials:**
  • ⅛ inch or ¼ inch felt (pre-cut or from roll), 1 inch non-elastic tape, taping scissors

◆ **Position of the individual:** Sitting on a taping table or bench with the leg extended off the edge and the foot in a dorsiflexed position.

◆ **Preparation:** Either cut tear drop pads from ⅛ inch or ¼ inch felt or purchase pre-cut with adhesive backing.

▶ **Application:**

STEP 1: Cut the pad in a tear drop shape and apply between the heads of the third and fourth metatarsals on the plantar surface of the foot (Fig. 3–30A). Temporarily apply the pad with 1 inch non-elastic tape and have the individual walk.

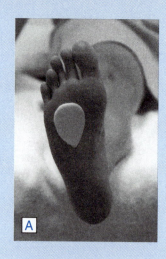

STEP 2: After ensuring proper placement, indicated by a reduction in pain, apply the pad with adhesive gauze material or one to two strips of 2 inch self-adherent wrap or elastic tape directly to the skin or over pre-tape material (Fig. 3–30B).

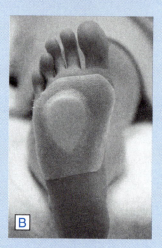

Figure 3-30

OVAL Figure 3–31

▶ **Purpose:** The oval metatarsal pad is similar to the tear drop pad in design and function (Fig. 3–31). Use the pad in treating metatarsalgia and pain caused by inflexibility of the Achilles tendon, pes cavus, Morton's toe, and metatarsal arch strains. The most common site of pain is under the second or third metatarsal head. The oval pad functions to lessen stress by aligning the metatarsal heads into a correct structural position.

▶ **Materials:**
- ⅛ inch or ¼ inch felt (pre-cut or from roll), 1 inch non-elastic tape, taping scissors

▶ **Position of the individual:** Sitting on a taping table or bench with the leg extended off the edge and the foot in a dorsiflexed position.

▶ **Preparation:** Construct the pad in an oval shape from ⅛ inch or ¼ inch felt or purchase pre-cut.

Application:

STEP 1: Place the pad just proximal to the metatarsal head on the plantar surface of the foot (Fig. 3-31A). Temporarily apply the pad with 1 inch non-elastic tape and have the individual walk.

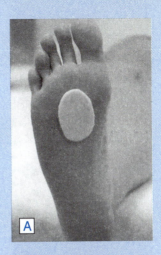

STEP 2: After proper placement and a reduction in pain, attach the pad with adhesive gauze material or one to two strips of 2 inch self-adherent wrap or elastic tape directly to the skin or over pre-tape material (Fig. 3–31B).

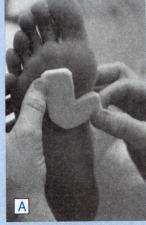

Figure 3-31

"J" Figure 3–32

▶ **Purpose:** Use the "J" pad technique in treating sesamoiditis and sesamoid fractures to unload or lessen stress to the area (Fig. 3–32).[19,20]

▶ **Materials:**
• ⅛ inch or ¼ inch felt (pre-cut or from roll), taping scissors

▶ **Position of the individual:** Sitting on a taping table or bench with the leg extended off the edge and the foot in a dorsiflexed position.

▶ **Preparation:** Make the pad from ⅛ inch or ¼ inch felt in the shape of an uppercase "J." Pre-cut designs are also available. Extend the pad from the second and third metatarsals, continue proximal, and turn in a medial direction proximal to the sesamoids. The pad is approximately 1–1½ inches wide (Fig. 3–32A).

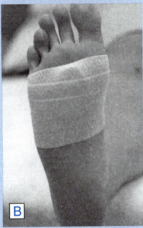

Figure 3-32

▶ **Application:**

(**STEP 1:**) Apply the pad with adhesive gauze material or two to three strips of 2 inch self-adherent wrap or elastic tape directly to the skin or over pre-tape material (Fig. 3–32B).

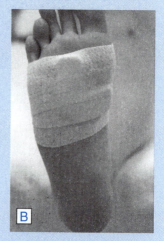

Figure 3-32 *continued*

TOE WEDGE Figure 3–33

▶ **Purpose:** Use the toe wedge technique in the treatment of bunions or hallux valgus as a spacer to lessen medial deviation of the great toe at the MTP joint (Fig. 3–33). This technique is similar to the buddy tape technique, but adequate spacing between the toes is critical.

▶ **Materials:**
- ⅛ inch, ¼ inch, or ½ inch foam, felt, or viscoelastic polymer (pre-cut or from roll), taping scissors

▶ **Position of the individual:** Sitting on a taping table or bench with the leg extended off the edge and the foot in a dorsiflexed position.

▶ **Preparation:** Choose the appropriate width of foam, felt, or viscoelastic polymer to correct structural misalignment. Apply adherent tape spray to the involved toes.

▶ **Application:**

(**STEP 1:**) Place the foam, felt, or viscoelastic polymer between the great and second toes to correct medial deviation (Fig. 3–33A).

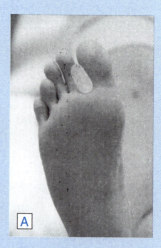

Figure 3-33

STEP 2: The buddy tape technique is useful to anchor the toe wedge (Fig. 3–33B).

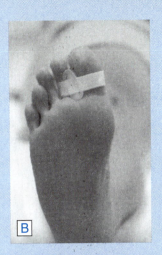

B

Figure 3-33 *continued*

VISCOELASTIC POLYMERS Figure 3–34

▶ **Purpose:** Pad the foot and toes with viscoelastic polymers to provide shock absorption and lessen friction and pressure in preventing and treating contusions, corns, calluses, wounds, and overuse conditions (Fig. 3–34). Wash and reuse the sleeves multiple times.

▶ **Materials:**
  • Off-the-shelf elastic toe sleeves lined with a padded disc, elastic toe sleeves fully lined with padding, elastic toe caps lined with padding, elastic foot sleeves lined with padding, and pads (Fig. 3–34A)

▶ **Position of the individual:** Sitting on a taping table or bench with the leg extended off the edge and the foot in a dorsiflexed position.

▶ **Preparation:** Cut the appropriate size of the material to overlap the injured area.

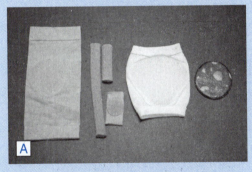

A

Figure 3-34 A Viscoelastic polymers. (Left to right) Foot and ankle sleeve, toe sleeves and cap, foot sleeve, and pad.

▶ **Application:**
  STEP 1: Slide the sleeve or cap onto the foot or toes (Fig. 3–34B). Additional anchor strips of tape or wrap are not required.

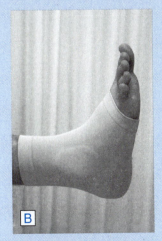

B

Figure 3-34

STEP 2: Place the pads directly onto the skin and anchor with elastic material or one to two strips of 2 inch self-adherent wrap or elastic tape directly to the skin or over pre-tape material. Clean and reuse the sleeves, caps, and pads.

OUTER TOE BOX Figure 3–35

▸ **Purpose:** Mold thermoplastic materials and attach over shoes to form a cap to provide protection in preventing and treating contusions, wounds, and fractures of the distal forefoot and toes (Fig. 3–35).

▸ **Materials:**
- Paper, felt tip pen, thermoplastic material, ⅛ inch or ¼ inch foam or felt, taping scissors, a heating source, 2 inch or 3 inch elastic tape, an elastic wrap, ½ inch high density, closed-cell foam, rubber cement

▸ **Position of the individual:** Standing in a weight-bearing position in shoes.

▸ **Preparation:** Heat the thermoplastic material.

▸ **Application:**
STEP 1: While the individual is weight-bearing in the shoe, mold the material around the dorsal, medial, and lateral surfaces (Fig. 3–35A). Fig. 1–15 illustrates the molding of thermoplastic material. Extend the pad in medial and/or lateral directions if necessary.

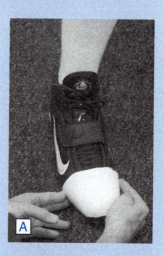

STEP 2: With some athletic shoes, the pad can encircle the distal forefoot and toe area. During molding, cut holes in the plantar surface of the pad to allow for full exposure of cleats (Fig. 3–35B).

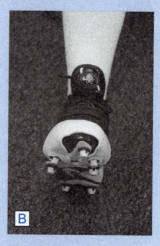

Figure 3-35

STEP 3: Drill or cut holes in the pad for incorporation of shoe lacing (Fig. 3–35C). Incorporation of shoe lacing in the pad serves as the attachment; no additional anchoring is required. The pad may be cemented to the medial and lateral sides of the shoe.

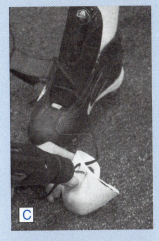

STEP 4: After cooling, line the pad with ⅛ inch or ¼ inch foam or felt for cushioning (Fig. 3–35D).

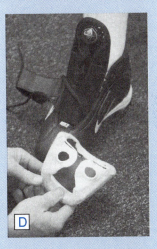

STEP 5: Cover the toe box pad with high density, closed-cell foam of at least ½ inch thickness as mandated by NCAA and NFHS rules (Fig. 3–35E).

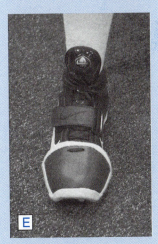

Figure 3-35 *continued*

Critical Thinking Question 5

After practice, a high school football tight end removes his cleats and walks to the locker room with bare feet. He steps on a rock and suffers a contusion to the right calcaneus. The next day, he experiences moderate pain with weight-bearing activities.

▶ **Question: What bracing or padding techniques can you use to treat his heel?**

> **...IF/THEN...**
>
> **IF** a foam or felt donut padding technique anchored to the great toe with adhesive gauze material, non-elastic or elastic tape, and/or self-adherent wrap is too bulky and uncomfortable in the attempt to lessen friction, **THEN** consider using a low-profile viscoelastic polymer elastic toe sleeve or cap.

CASE STUDY

The end of the second week of basketball practice has not brought any relief for Tony White. Tony is a forward on the team, and he has bilateral heel pain. He first reported the pain during preseason conditioning three weeks ago. Jason Heideman, the PT/ATC at Leigh University, has been treating Tony for the past three weeks with ice, massage, electrical muscle stimulation, ultrasound, over-the-counter NSAIDs for anti-inflammatory effects, lower leg stretching, and strengthening exercises.

The treatments have allowed Tony to continue with full participation in conditioning and practice sessions but have not eliminated the pain. Tony complains of pain over the anterior/medial aspect of each calcaneus and reports that the greatest pain is present during initial weight-bearing in the morning and following team film meetings. Through his evaluation, Jason elicits pain in both feet with palpation of the anterior/medial calcaneus and passive dorsiflexion of the distal foot and toes. Jason refers Tony to the team physician for an evaluation of suspected plantar fasciitis. During the evaluation, the physician finds that point tenderness is present over the calcaneus, but no crepitus, deformity, or neurological symptoms. Radiographs demonstrate no bony pathology, and the physician recommends that Jason continue with symptomatic treatment of bilateral plantar fasciitis.

Jason will continue the symptomatic treatment described and implement taping, bracing, and padding techniques in the management of this case. First, what taping techniques could you apply to support the longitudinal arch in reducing pain during basketball practices and competitions? Next, how could night splints and orthotics be used in the overall treatment plan for Tony? Lastly, what padding techniques could be used to provide support and shock absorption in treating plantar fasciitis?

WRAP UP

- Acute and chronic injuries to the foot and toes can be the result of compressive forces, abnormal ranges of motion, and excessive and repetitive stresses.
- The circular, "X," loop, weave, Low-Dye, and plantar fascia strap taping techniques support the longitudinal arch and forefoot.
- The buddy tape, toe spica, toe strip, and turf toe taping techniques provide support and reduce range of motion of the toes.
- Compression wrap techniques applied in a distal-to-proximal spiral pattern assist in reducing swelling and inflammation.
- Orthotics can be categorized into three types: soft, semirigid, and rigid.
- Soft, semirigid, and rigid orthotics can be used in preventing and treating acute and chronic injuries and conditions.
- Orthotics are fabricated in-house or in a laboratory from foot impressions or directly to the foot.

- Night splints, post-operative shoes, and walking and cast boots provide support and restrict range of motion.
- The longitudinal arch, metatarsal bar, tear drop, oval, "J," and toe wedge pad techniques provide support in correcting structural abnormalities.
- Donut, heel, viscoelastic, and thermoplastic padding techniques serve as shock absorbers and reduce stress and friction.

■ WEB REFERENCES

American Academy of Orthotists and Prosthetists
http://www.oandp.org/
- This site provides access to the Journal of Prosthetics and Orthotics, which contains clinical and educational manuscripts.

American College of Foot and Ankle Surgeons
http://www.acfas.org/
- This Web site allows you to search for information on the causes and treatment of foot and ankle injuries and conditions.

American Podiatric Medical Association
http://www.apma.org/s_apma/index.asp/
- This site provides general foot health information on a variety of injuries and conditions.

FURTHER READING

Foot Orthotics in Therapy and Sport. 1995. S. Hunter, MG Dolan, and JM Davis. Champaign, IL. Human Kinetics. Detailed examination of the indications for orthotics and step-by-step fabrication techniques.

REFERENCES

1. Anderson, MK, Hall, SJ, and Martin, M: Sports Injury Management, ed 2. Lippincott Williams & Wilkins, Philadelphia, 2000.
2. Ator, R, Gunn, K, McPoil, TG, and Knecht, HG: The effect of adhesive strapping on medial longitudinal arch support before and after exercise. J Orthop Sports Phys Ther 14:18–23, 1991.
3. Barry, LD, Barry, AN, and Chen Y: A retrospective study of standing gastrocnemius-soleus stretching versus night splinting in the treatment of plantar fasciitis. J Foot Ankle Surg 41:221–227, 2002.
4. Basford, JR, and Smith, MA: Shoe insoles in the workplace. Orthopedics 11:285–288, 1988.
5. Bates, BT, Ostering, LR, Mason, B, and James, LS: Foot orthotic devices to modify selected aspects of lower extremity mechanics. Am J Sports Med 7:338–342, 1979.
6. Batt, ME, Tanji, JL, and Skattum, N: Plantar fasciitis: A prospective randomized clinical trial of the tension night splint. Clin J Sports Med 6:158–162, 1996.
7. Berlet, GC, Anderson, RB, Davis, H, and Kiebzak, G: A prospective trial of night splinting in the treatment of recalcitrant plantar fasciitis: The Ankle Dorsiflexion Dynasplint. Orthopedics 25:1273–1275, 2002.
8. Brukner, P, and Khan, K: Clinical Sports Medicine. McGraw-Hill, Sidney, 1997.
9. Clarke, TE, Frederick, EC, and Hamill, CL: Effects of shoe cushioning upon ground reaction forces in running. Int J Sports Med 4:247–251, 1983.
10. D'Ambrosia, RD: Orthotic devices in running injuries. Clin Sports Med 4:611–618, 1985.
11. D'Ambrosia, RD, and Douglas, R: Orthotics. In D'Ambrosia, RD, and Drez, Jr, D (eds): Prevention and Treatment of Running Injuries. Slack, Thorofare, 1982, pp 155–164.
12. DeMaio, M, Paine, R, Mangine, R, and Drez, D: Plantar fasciitis. Orthopedics 16:1153–1163, 1993.
13. Donatelli, R, Hurlbert, C, Conaway, D, and St. Pierre, R: Biomechanical foot orthotics: A retrospective study. J Orthop Sports Phys Ther 10:205–212, 1988.
14. Dufek, JS, Bates, BT, Davis, HP, and Malone, LA: Dynamic performance assessment of selected sport shoes on impact forces. Med Sci Sports Exerc 23:1062-1067, 1991.
15. Fabian, EP, Gowling, TL, and Jackson, RW: Walking boot design: A gait analysis study. Orthopedics 22:503–508, 1999.
16. Gill, E: Orthotics. Runners's World February:55–57, 1985.
17. Gill, LH: Plantar fasciitis: Diagnosis and conservative management. J Am Acad Orthop Surg 5:109–117, 1997.
18. Gross, ML, Davlin, LB, and Evanski, PM: Effectiveness of orthotic shoe inserts in the long-distance runner. Am J Sports Med 19:409–412, 1991.
19. Hockenbury, RT: Forefoot problems in athletes. Med Sci Sports Exerc 31:S448–S458, 1999.
20. Hunter, S, Dolan, MG, and Davis, JM: Foot Orthotics in Therapy and Sport. Human Kinetics, Champaign, 1995.
21. James, SL, Bates, BT, and Ostering, LR: Injuries to runners. Am J Sports Med 6:40–50, 1978.
22. McNair, PJ, and Marshall, RN: Kinematic and kinetic parameters associated with running in different shoes. Br J Sports Med 28:256–260, 1994.
23. Milgrom, C, Giladi, M, Kashtan, H, Simkin, A, Chisin, R, Marguiles, J, Steinberg, R, Aharonson, Z, and Stein, M: A prospective study of the effect of a shock absorbing orthotic device on the incidence of stress fractures in military recruits. Foot Ankle 6:101–104, 1985.
24. Mizel, MS, Marymont, JV, and Trepman, E: Treatment of plantar fasciitis with a night splint and shoe modification consisting of a steel shank and anterior rocker bottom. Foot Ankle Int 17:732–735, 1996.
25. Nigg, BM, Luethi, SM, Denoth, J, and Stacoff, A: Methodological aspects of sport shoe and sport surfaces analysis. In Matsui, H, and Kobayashi, K (eds): Biomechanics VIII-B. Human Kinetics, Champaign, 1983, pp 1041–1052.
26. Nigg, BM, Nurse, MA, and Stefanyshyn, DJ: Shoe inserts and orthotics for sport and physical activities. Med Sci Sports Exerc 31:S421–S428, 1999.
27. Penneau, K, Lutter, LD, and Winter, RD: Pes planus: Radiographic changes with foot orthoses and shoes. Foot Ankle 2:299–302, 1982.
28. Powell, M, Post, WR, Keener, J, and Wearden, S: Effective treatment of chronic plantar fasciitis with dorsiflexion night splints: A crossover prospective randomized outcome study. Foot Ankle Int 19:10–18, 1998.
29. Prentice, WE: Arnheim's Principles of Athletic Training, ed 11. McGraw-Hill, Boston, 2003.
30. Prentice, WE: Rehabilitation Techniques, ed 3. McGraw-Hill, Boston, 1999.
31. Probe, RA, Baca, M, Adams, R, and Preece, C: Night splint treatment for plantar fasciitis. A prospective randomized study. Clin Orthop 368:190–195, 1999.
32. Rodgers, M, and LeVeau, B: Effectiveness of foot orthotic devices used to modify pronation in runners. J Orthop Sports Phys Ther 4:86–90, 1982.
33. Russo, SJ, and Chipchase, LS: The effect of low-Dye taping on peak plantar pressures of normal feet during gait. Austr J Physiotherapy 47:239–244, 2001.
34. Saxelby, J, Betts, RP, and Bygrave, CJ: Low-Dye taping on the foot in the management of plantar fasciitis. The Foot: Int J Clin Foot Sci 7:205–209, 1997.
35. Schwellnus, MP, Jordaan, G, and Noakes, TD: Prevention of common overuse injuries by the use of shock absorbing insoles: A prospective study. Am J Sports Med 18:636–641, 1990.
36. Simkin, A, Leichter, I, Giladi, M, Stein, M, and Milgrom, C: Combined effect of foot structure and an orthotic device on stress fractures. Foot Ankle 10:25–29, 1989.
37. Subotnick, S: Foot orthoses: An update. Phys Sportsmed 11:103–109, 1983.
38. Vicenzino, B, Feilding, J, Howard, R, Moore, R, and Smith, S: An investigation of the anti-pronation effect of two taping methods after application and exercise. Gait and Posture 5:1–5, 1997.
39. Voloshin, A, and Wosk, J: Influence of artificial shock absorbers on human gait. Clin Orthop Rel Res 160:52–56, 1981.
40. Wapner, KL, and Sharkey, PF: The use of night splints for treatment of recalcitrant plantar fasciitis. Foot Ankle 12:135–138, 1991.
41. Wu, KK: Morton's interdigital neuroma: A clinical review of its etiology, treatment, and results. J Foot Ankle Surg 35:112–119, 1996.
42. Young, CC, Rutherford, DS, and Niedfeldt, MW: Treatment of plantar fasciitis. Am Fam Physician 64:467–474, 477–478, 2001.

Ankle

1. Discuss common injuries that occur to the ankle.
2. Demonstrate taping, wrapping, bracing, and padding techniques for the ankle when preventing, treating, and rehabilitating injuries.
3. Explain and demonstrate the application of taping, wrapping, bracing, and padding techniques for the ankle within a therapeutic exercise program.

INJURIES AND CONDITIONS

Injury to the ankle can occur during any weight-bearing activity, due to excessive range of motion and repetitive stress. Injury to the bony and ligamentous structures of the ankle can occur from excessive range of motion caused by stepping off a curb while walking and sudden changes of direction during athletic activities. Casual and athletic activities on uneven or poorly maintained surfaces may also contribute to injury. Common injuries to the ankle include:

- Sprains
- Fractures
- Blisters

Sprains

Ankle sprains are one of the most common sport-related injuries.[3,54] Injuries are caused by excessive, sudden inversion or eversion at the **subtalar joint** and can be associated with plantar flexion or dorsiflexion at the **talocrural joint** (Illustration 4-1). **Rotation** of the foot, either **internal** or **external,** can also contribute to injury. An inversion or eversion sprain can result, for instance, when a baseball batter steps on the corner of first base while running straight ahead to beat a throw from the second baseman, causing excessive inversion, eversion, rotation, and/or dorsiflexion. Inversion sprains are more common and can lead to damage of the **anterior talofibular, calcaneofibular,** and/or **posterior talofibular ligaments. Eversion sprains** can result in injury to the **deltoid ligament** and are often accompanied by an **avulsion fracture** of the distal tibia with severe eversion force. Excessive dorsiflexion and external rotation can cause a **syndesmosis sprain** involving the **anterior** and **posterior tibiofibular ligaments.** A syndesmosis sprain can occur, for example, during a fumble recovery in football, as the ankle of a player on the ground is forced into dorsiflexion and external rotation by others diving for the ball.

Fractures

Fractures of the distal tibia or fibula can occur in combination with ankle sprains. A severe inversion mechanism can cause an avulsion fracture of the **lateral (fibular) malleolus** and sometimes an accompanying fracture of the **medial (tibial) malleolus,** known as a **bimalleolar fracture.** With eversion sprains, the longer fibular malleolus can be fractured as the talus is forced into the distal end. If the eversion mechanism continues, an avulsion fracture of the tibial malleolus can occur, resulting in a bimalleolar fracture. Mechanisms of injury for distal tibia and fibula fractures include forcible inversion, eversion, dorsiflexion, and internal rotation.

Blisters

Athletic, work, and casual footwear can cause irritation of the skin. Application of taping, wrapping, and bracing techniques themselves can cause blisters from shearing forces over the heel, lace, and bony prominence areas such as the medial and lateral malleoli.

Taping Techniques

Several taping techniques reduce inversion and eversion at the subtalar joint, and reduce plantar flexion and dorsiflexion at the talocrural joint, protecting against excessive range of motion. Some techniques are used in preventing sprains to support and limit excessive range of motion, while others provide support to the ankle during a return to activities. Several techniques are used specifically in the acute treatment of sprains and fractures to support or immobilize the ankle. The appropriate technique to use should be based on the intended purpose, the injury, the individual, and the activity.

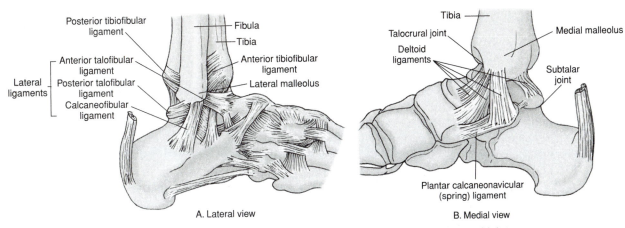

Posterior tibiofibular ligament — Fibula — Tibia — Anterior tibiofibular ligament — Lateral malleolus

Anterior talofibular ligament
Posterior talofibular ligament
Calcaneofibular ligament

Lateral ligaments

A. Lateral view

Tibia — Medial malleolus
Talocrural joint
Deltoid ligaments
Subtalar joint

Plantar calcaneonavicular (spring) ligament

B. Medial view

Illustration 4-1 Ligaments of the subtalar and talocrural joints.

CLOSED BASKETWEAVE Figures 4–1, 4–2, 4–3

▶ **Purpose:** The closed basketweave technique is used both to prevent and treat inversion and eversion sprains (Fig. 4–1). It provides moderate support to the subtalar and talocrural joints and reduces range of motion. For our purposes, we review a basic closed basketweave first, and then illustrate several variations used to provide additional support.

⊙ **DETAILS**

There may be as many different basketweave techniques as there are health-care professionals applying them, but the majority of the techniques contain some of the procedures described by Gibney[15] over 100 years ago.

▶ **Materials:**
   • 1½ inch or 2 inch non-elastic tape, taping scissors

   Options:
   • Pre-tape material or self-adherent wrap, adherent tape spray, thin foam pads, skin lubricant

▶ **Position of the individual:** Sitting on a taping table or bench with the leg extended off the edge with the foot in 90° of dorsiflexion.

▶ **Preparation:** Apply the basketweave technique directly to the skin.

   Option: Apply pre-tape material or self-adherent wrap, adherent tape spray, thin foam pads, and skin lubricant over the heel and lace areas to provide additional adherence and lessen irritation. Using pre-tape material appears to provide some additional support to the ankle.[40]

▶ **Application:**
   STEP 1: In this example, apply one layer of pre-tape material ◀▶ (Fig. 4–1A).

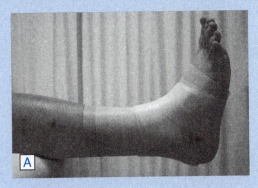

Figure 4-1

STEP 2: Using 1½ inch or 2 inch non-elastic tape, apply two anchor strips at a slight angle around the distal lower leg, just inferior to the gastrocnemius belly with moderate roll tension ◀▶ (Fig. 4–1B). An anchor strip can be placed around the midfoot ◀▶, proximal to the fifth metatarsal head, but this is not required. If this anchor strip is applied, monitor roll tension to prevent constriction as the foot expands upon weight-bearing.

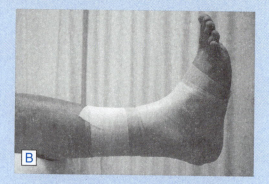

Option: *Use self-adherent wrap of 2 inch width for these anchors to prevent constriction.*

STEP 3: When preventing and treating inversion sprains, start the first stirrup on the medial lower leg anchor. Proceed down over the posterior medial malleolus (Fig. 4–1C), across the plantar surface of the foot, and continue up and over the posterior lateral malleolus with moderate roll tension (Fig. 4–1D).

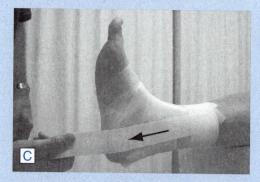

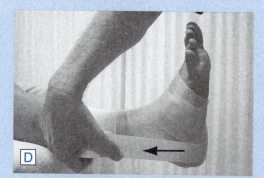

STEP 4: Finish on the lateral lower leg anchor (Fig. 4–1E).

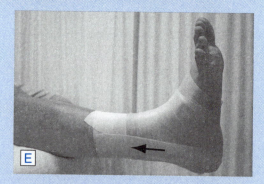

STEP 5: When preventing and treating eversion sprains, apply the stirrups on the lateral lower leg anchor and follow the same steps, finishing on the medial lower leg anchor (Fig. 4–1F).

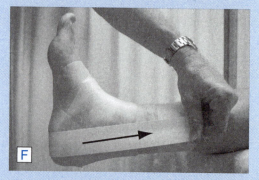

Figure 4-1 *continued*

STEP 6: Begin the first horseshoe strip on the medial aspect of the midfoot (Fig. 4–1G), continue around the distal Achilles tendon, across the distal lateral malleolus, and finish on the lateral midfoot with moderate roll tension, proximal to the fifth metatarsal head (Fig. 4–1H).

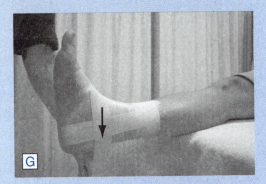

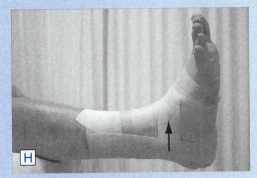

STEP 7: Start the second stirrup on the medial lower leg by overlapping the first by ½ of the tape width, continue down over the medial malleolus (Fig. 4–1I), across the plantar foot, up and over the lateral malleolus, and anchor on the lateral lower leg (Fig. 4–1J).

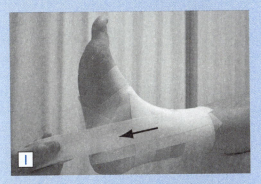

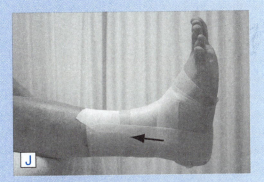

STEP 8: The second horseshoe begins on the medial forefoot and overlaps the first by ½ of the tape width (Fig. 4–1K).

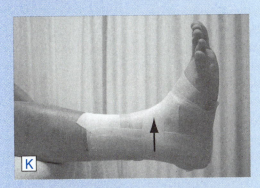

STEP 9: The third stirrup, beginning on the medial lower leg, overlaps the second and covers the anterior medial and lateral malleoli (Fig. 4–1L).

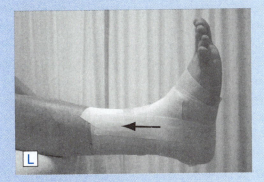

Figure 4-1 *continued*

STEP 10: Starting on the medial forefoot, apply the third horseshoe, overlapping the second (Fig. 4–1M).

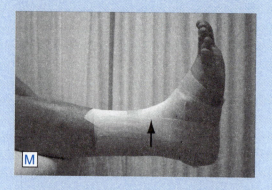

STEP 11: Beginning at the third horseshoe, apply closure strips in a proximal direction with moderate roll tension, overlapping each ◄► (Fig. 4–1N). Apply the last closure strip over the distal lower leg anchors. Progress proximally, and angle the tape to prevent gaps or wrinkles.

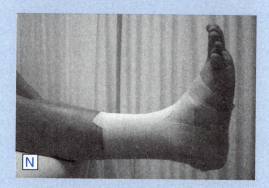

STEP 12: Apply 2–3 closure strips around the midfoot in a medial-to-lateral direction with mild to moderate roll tension, remaining proximal to the fifth metatarsal head (Fig. 4–1O).

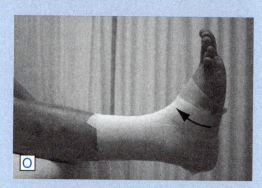

Figure 4-1 *continued*

Heel Locks

▸ **Purpose:** Use heel locks to provide additional support to the subtalar and talocrural joints and secure the closed basketweave technique (Fig. 4–2). Based on individual preferences, apply heel locks in either an individual or continuous pattern. Many apply the continuous heel lock to conserve time when applying the basketweave technique.

▸ **Materials:**
  • 1½ inch or 2 inch non-elastic tape

▸ **Position of the individual:** Sitting on a taping table or bench with the leg extended off the edge with the foot in 90° of dorsiflexion.

▸ **Preparation:** Application of the closed basketweave taping technique.

Individual Heel Locks

▶ **Application:**

STEP 1: Using the individual technique, anchor the lateral heel lock with 1½ inch or 2 inch non-elastic tape across the lateral lace area at an angle toward the longitudinal arch (Fig. 4–2A).

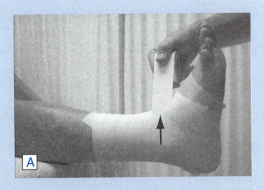

STEP 2: Continue across the arch, then angle the tape upward and pull across the lateral calcaneus with moderate roll tension (Fig. 4–2B), around the posterior heel, and finish on the lateral lace area (Fig. 4–2C).

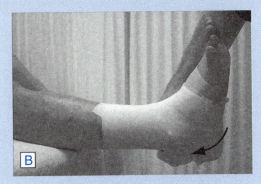
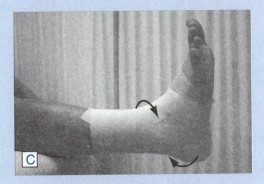

STEP 3: The medial heel lock begins over the medial lace area at an angle toward the lateral malleolus (Fig. 4–2D) and continues across the posterior heel.

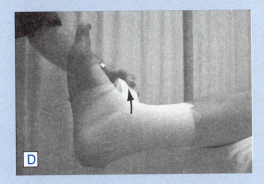

STEP 4: Then, angle the tape downward and pull across the medial calcaneus with moderate roll tension (Fig. 4–2E), under the heel, and finish on the medial lace area (Fig. 4–2F). Typically, the lateral and medial heel locks are repeated.

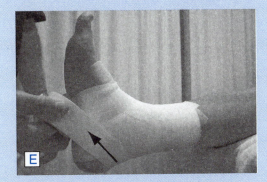
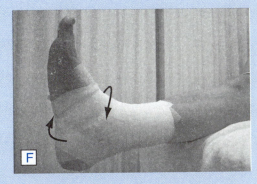

Figure 4-2

Continuous Heel Locks

▶ **Application:**

STEP 1: The continuous heel lock technique combines the individual locks and is applied within a figure-of-eight pattern with moderate roll tension. Apply a lateral heel lock as shown in Figure 4-2A–C.

STEP 2: Instead of tearing the tape when finished, continue around the distal Achilles tendon (Fig. 4–2G).

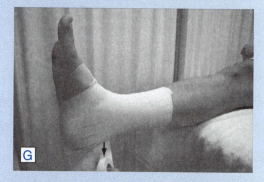

STEP 3: Angle downward and pull the tape across the medial calcaneus (Fig. 4–2H).

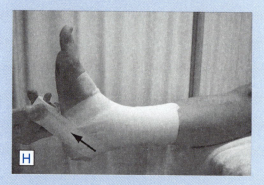

STEP 4: Continue across the plantar foot, then up and over the dorsum of the foot toward the superior medial malleolus (Fig. 4–2I), around the posterior lower leg, and finish on the anterior lower leg (Fig. 4–2J). The continuous technique is also often repeated.

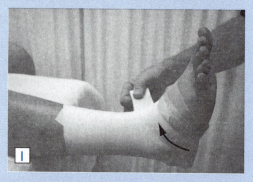
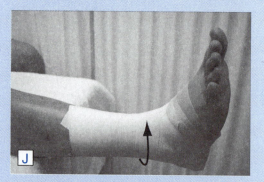

Figure 4-2 *continued*

Because non-elastic tape does not possess elastic properties, starting with and maintaining the proper angles of the body contours is important .

Helpful Hint: Proper angles will be created if the center of the tape width covers the lateral and medial malleoli. Begin the continuous technique by anchoring the center of the tape directly over the lateral malleolus, at an angle toward the longitudinal arch. Center tape placement over the lateral malleolus guides toward a correct lateral heel lock and medial malleolus center placement toward a correct medial heel lock.

Basketweave Variation One

‣ **Purpose:** Several variations to the basic closed basketweave technique provide additional support to the subtalar and talocrural joints and reduce range of motion (Fig. 4-3). These variations are used when individuals are returning to activity or work while treating inversion, eversion, and syndesmosis sprains, and fractures.

‣ **Materials:**
- 2 inch or 3 inch elastic tape, taping scissors
- 2 inch or 3 inch semirigid cast tape, gloves, water, taping scissors

‣ **Position of the individual:** Sitting on a taping table or bench with the leg extended off the edge with the foot in 90° of dorsiflexion.

‣ **Preparation:** Application of the closed basketweave taping technique.

‣ **Application:**

STEP 1: After applying the closed basketweave, use elastic tape in 2 inch or 3 inch widths for heel locks (Fig. 4–3A). Apply the elastic tape with the individual or continuous technique. Non-elastic tape heel locks can be applied over the elastic tape to provide additional support.

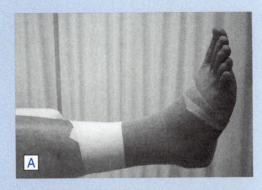

STEP 2: If greater support is required, use semirigid cast tape in 2 inch or 3 inch widths for heel locks (Fig. 4–3B). Apply the basketweave technique with heel locks of non-elastic or elastic tape. Anchor the cast tape around the distal lower leg and continue with the continuous heel lock technique with mild to moderate roll tension. Smooth, mold, and shape the cast tape to the ankle. Allow 10–15 minutes for the tape to cure. Additional anchors over the cast tape are not required.

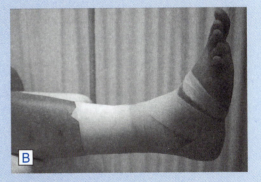

Figure 4-3

Basketweave Variation Two

‣ **Purpose:** Another variation is the application of moleskin or thermoplastic material stirrups with the closed basketweave technique. This variation, using semirigid materials, provides maximal support to the subtalar and talocrural joints, specifically inversion and eversion.

‣ **Materials:**
- 2 inch or 3 inch moleskin, taping scissors
- Paper, felt tip pen, ⅛ inch thermoplastic material, taping scissors, a heating source, an elastic wrap, 2 inch or 3 inch moleskin

‣ **Position of the individual:** Sitting on a taping table or bench with the leg extended off the edge with the foot in 90° of dorsiflexion.

‣ **Preparation:** Application of the closed basketweave taping technique.

▶ **Application:**

STEP 1: Cut moleskin stirrups from 2 inch or 3 inch width material into 25–30 inch length straps (Fig. 4–3C).

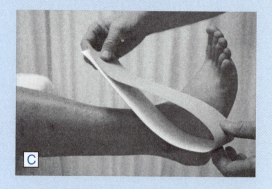

STEP 2: Fold and cut the middle of the strap at an angle to achieve better fit over the plantar calcaneus (Fig. 4–3D).

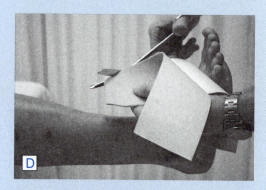

STEP 3: After applying tape anchors, grasp the ends of the strap and anchor the stirrup on the plantar surface of the calcaneus (Fig. 4–3E).

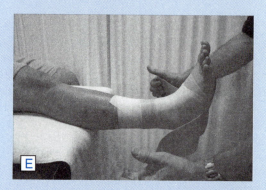

STEP 4: Pull the ends toward the lower leg anchors with equal tension (Fig. 4–3F). The center of the stirrup should be located over the medial and lateral malleoli. The stirrup may also be anchored directly to the skin. Continue applying the closed basketweave and heel lock techniques.

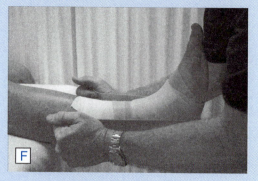

Figure 4-3 *continued*

STEP 5: Thermoplastic material of ⅛ inch thickness may also be cut into a 3–4 inch width stirrup and fitted to the individual. Design, cut, heat, and mold the material (see Figs. 1–14 and 1–15C–G) over the area from the lateral lower leg anchor, over the lateral malleolus, under the calcaneus, across the medial malleolus, and finish at the medial lower leg anchor. The stirrup can be lined with moleskin (Fig. 4–3G). Apply the closed basketweave and heel lock techniques.

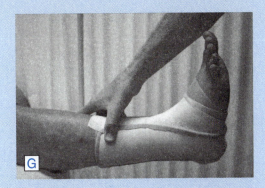

STEP 6: Place the thermoplastic stirrup on the ankle and apply 2 inch or 3 inch elastic tape heel locks and elastic anchor strips around the distal lower leg with moderate roll tension to attach the stirrup ◀▬▶ (Fig. 4–3H).

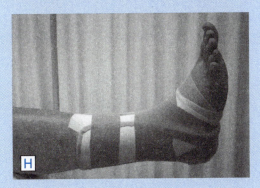

Figure 4-3 *continued*

Critical Thinking Question 1

A center on the basketball team is currently in phase III of a rehabilitation program for a second degree eversion ankle sprain. This phase includes position-specific shooting, rebounding, and agility exercises. A closed basketweave technique was applied for support and protection. During the exercises, the center asks whether additional support can be provided. The entire inventory of ankle braces is being used by other members of the team, leaving only taping supplies available for use.

▶ **Question: What can be done in this situation?**

ELASTIC Figure 4–4

▶ **Purpose:** The elastic technique is an alternative to the closed basketweave and can be applied quickly (Fig. 4–4). Because this technique offers mild support to the subtalar and talocrural joints, the elastic technique is typically used only when preventing inversion and eversion sprains for noninjured individuals.

▶ **Materials:**
- 1½ inch or 2 inch non-elastic tape, 2 inch or 3 inch elastic tape, pre-tape material or self-adherent wrap, thin foam pads, skin lubricant, taping scissors

  Option:
  - Adherent tape spray

▶ **Position of the individual:** Sitting on a taping table or bench with the leg extended off the edge with the foot in 90° of dorsiflexion.

▶ **Preparation:** Apply pre-tape material or self-adherent wrap, and thin foam pads and skin lubricant over the heel and lace areas.

  Option: *Apply adherent tape spray under the pre-tape material or self-adherent wrap for additional adherence.*

Ankle

• Application:

STEP 1: Begin by placing 1½ inch or 2 inch non-elastic tape distal lower leg anchors directly to the skin or over pre-tape material or self-adherent wrap.

STEP 2: Apply three consecutive stirrups with 1½ inch or 2 inch non-elastic tape in a medial-to-lateral direction, beginning the first over the posterior medial and lateral malleolus (Fig. 4–4A), overlapping each by ½ of the tape width (Fig. 4–4B).

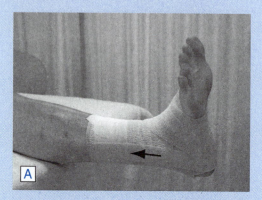
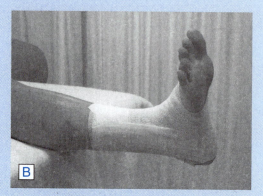

STEP 3: Using 2 inch or 3 inch elastic tape, anchor on the lateral lace area and apply two continuous heel locks (Fig. 4–4C).

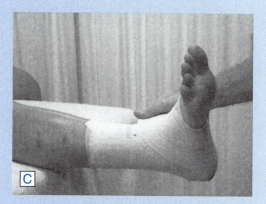

STEP 4: From the anterior lower leg, continue to apply the elastic tape in a circular or spiral pattern with moderate roll tension (Fig. 4–4D), overlapping by ½ of the tape width, and finish on the lower leg anchor (Fig. 4–4E).

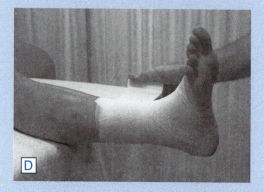
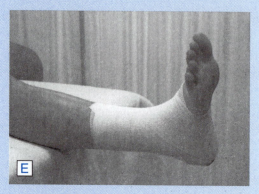

Figure 4-4

STEP 5: Apply a heel lock with 1½ inch or
2 inch non-elastic tape with moderate roll tension
(Fig. 4–4F).

*Option: Anchor the elastic tape at the distal lower
leg with 1½ inch or 2 inch non-elastic tape* ◀.

> **...IF/THEN...**
>
> **IF** choosing a taping technique to support the
> subtalar and talocrural joints of a noninjured
> individual and time is limited, **THEN** consider
> using the elastic technique, which involves
> fewer steps and can be applied more quickly
> than the closed basketweave.

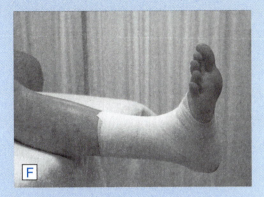

Figure 4-4 *continued*

OPEN BASKETWEAVE Figure 4–5

▶ **Purpose:** The open basketweave technique is used in the acute treatment of inversion, eversion, and syndesmosis sprains to provide mild support and compression (Fig. 4–5). This technique differs from the closed
basketweave in that the anterior lower leg, ankle, and dorsal aspect of the foot are not enclosed by horseshoes or closure strips. The anterior opening is designed to accommodate swelling and effusion, which may
be present following a sprain. However, this technique uses the same sequence of stirrups and horseshoes.

▶ **Materials:**
• 1½ inch or 2 inch non-elastic tape, adherent tape spray, 3 inch or 4 inch by 5 yard length elastic wrap

▶ **Position of the individual:** Sitting on a taping table or bench with the leg extended off the edge. If pain
and swelling allow, place the foot in 90° of dorsiflexion.

▶ **Preparation:** Apply adherent tape spray.

▶ **Application:**
STEP 1: Apply lower leg anchors, stirrups, and
horseshoes directly to the skin with 1½ inch or
2 inch non-elastic tape, as described in Figures
4–1B–M, leaving the anterior lower leg, ankle,
and dorsal aspect of the foot open (Fig. 4–5A).

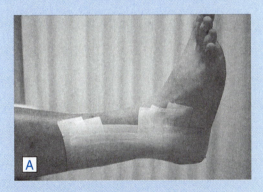

STEP 2: Apply closure strips in a proximal direction to the lower leg anchor (Fig. 4–5B) and in a distal
direction to the forefoot (Fig. 4–5C), covering the calcaneus and plantar foot ◀.

Option: Apply individual heel locks, but do not encircle the ankle.

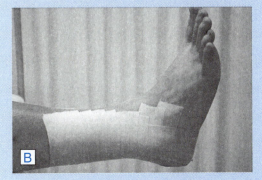

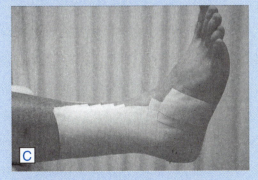

Figure 4-5

STEP 3: Anchor the ends of the horseshoes and closure strips with 1½ inch or 2 inch non-elastic tape ◀▬▶ (Fig. 4–5D).

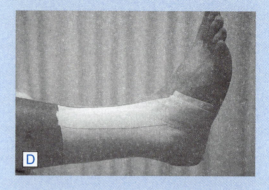

STEP 4: Apply a compression wrap (see Fig. 4-10A) over the open basketweave for further compression (Fig. 4–5E).

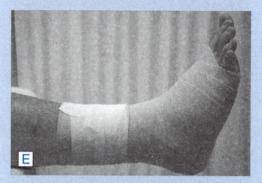

Figure 4-5 *continued*

SPARTAN SLIPPER Figure 4–6

▸ **Purpose:** The Spartan Slipper technique is used in combination with the closed basketweave in treating inversion, eversion, and syndesmosis sprains to provide additional support during return to activity and/or work (Fig. 4–6).

▸ **Materials:**
  • 1½ inch, 2 inch, and 3 inch non-elastic tape
  Options:
  • Pre-tape material or self-adherent wrap, adherent tape spray, thin foam pads, skin lubricant

▸ **Position of the individual:** Sitting on a taping table or bench with the leg extended off the edge with the foot in 90° of dorsiflexion.

▸ **Preparation:** Apply directly to the skin.

  Option: *Apply pre-tape material or self-adherent wrap, adherent tape spray, and thin foam pads and skin lubricant over the heel and lace areas to provide adherence and to lessen irritation.*

▸ **Application:**
  STEP 1: Start the technique by placing anchors on the distal lower leg with 1½ inch or 2 inch non-elastic tape.

  STEP 2: With 3 inch non-elastic tape, measure and tear a strip to serve as a stirrup. Holding the ends of the stirrup, anchor on the plantar surface of the calcaneus (Fig. 4–6A).

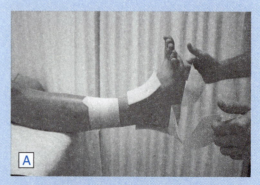

Figure 4-6

STEP 3: Pull, with equal tension, the ends of the stirrup toward the distal lower leg, and anchor (Fig. 4–6B). The center of the stirrup should cover the medial and lateral malleoli.

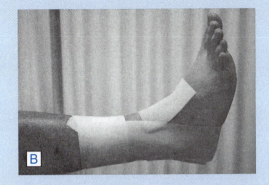

STEP 4: Tear another stirrup strip of 3 inch non-elastic tape slightly longer than the first one. Anchor the strip on the plantar surface of the calcaneus over the previous stirrup. Starting at the ends, tear or cut lengthwise down the middle of the stirrup to the inferior medial and lateral malleoli (Fig. 4–6C).

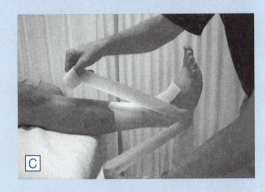

STEP 5: Wrap the lateral stirrup ends individually around the lower leg in a spiral pattern with moderate tension (Fig. 4–6D), finishing on the distal lower leg anchor.

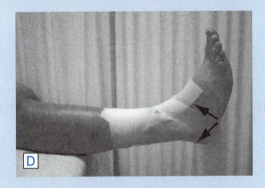

 Helpful Hint: As the stirrup ends progress from the plantar foot, crease or pinch the tape, if needed, to allow for smooth contact on the foot.

STEP 6: Wrap the medial stirrup ends around the lower leg with moderate tension in a spiral pattern, finishing on the distal lower leg anchor, to form a slipper (Fig. 4–6E).

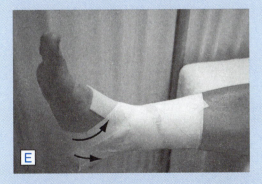

Figure 4-6 *continued*

STEP 7: Continue the Spartan Slipper technique by applying a closed basketweave, with heel locks of non-elastic, elastic, or semirigid cast tape. Another option is to use additional stirrups of moleskin or thermoplastic materials.

SUBTALAR SLING Figure 4–7

▸ **Purpose:** The subtalar sling technique is also used in combination with the closed basketweave to provide additional support to the subtalar joint in treating inversion, eversion, and syndesmosis sprains (Fig. 4–7).[20,26,61,64]

▸ **Materials:**
 • 2 inch heavyweight elastic tape, taping scissors

▸ **Position of the individual:** Sitting on a taping table or bench with the leg extended off the edge with the foot in 90° of dorsiflexion.

▸ **Preparation:** Application of the closed basketweave taping technique.

▸ **Application:**
  STEP 1: Apply the anchors, stirrups, and horseshoes of the closed basketweave technique with 1½ inch or 2 inch non-elastic tape.

  STEP 2: To prevent subtalar inversion, use a lateral sling. Anchor 2 inch heavyweight elastic tape on the medial plantar forefoot at an angle toward the distal fifth metatarsal (Fig. 4–7A).

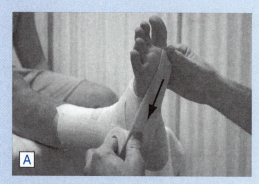

  STEP 3: Continue with moderate roll tension up and over the lateral foot toward the lateral malleolus (Fig. 4–7B), around the posterior lower leg, and anchor on the lateral lower leg (Fig. 4–7C). Monitor roll tension to prevent irritation of the forefoot lateral border.

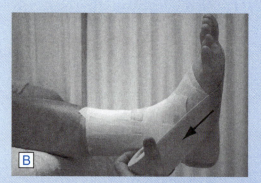 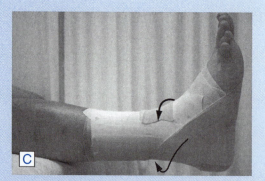

  STEP 4: A medial sling is used to prevent subtalar eversion. The medial sling also can be used when treating syndesmosis sprains. Anchor 2 inch heavyweight elastic tape on the lateral plantar forefoot at an angle toward the longitudinal arch (Fig. 4–7D).

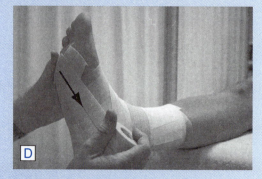

Figure 4-7

STEP 5: Proceed up and across the arch, with moderate roll tension toward the medial malleolus (Fig. 4–7E), around the posterior lower leg, and anchor on the medial lower leg (Fig. 4–7F).

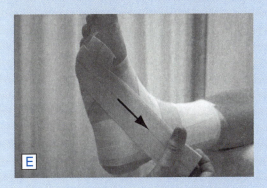

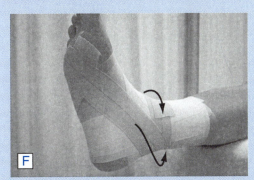

STEP 6: An additional lateral and/or medial sling may be applied, anchoring in a more distal position on the medial or lateral forefoot (Fig. 4–7G).

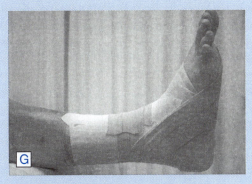

Figure 4-7 *continued*

STEP 7: After applying the subtalar sling(s), continue with closed basketweave closure strips and heel locks with 1½ inch or 2 inch non-elastic tape. Additional anchors over the distal forefoot are not required.

○ **DETAILS**

Because of the high incidence of inversion sprains, apply a lateral sling when using the medial sling technique to compensate for the inversion tension of the medial sling.[63]

...IF/THEN...

IF application of the basic closed basketweave taping technique is not effective in supporting the ankle during the return to activity following a sprain, **THEN** consider using elastic or cast tape heel locks, moleskin or thermoplastic stirrups, the Spartan Slipper, and/or the subtalar sling in combination with the closed basketweave to provide greater support to the subtalar and talocrural joints.

SPATTING Figure 4–8

▸ **Purpose:** The spatting technique entails applying tape over athletic shoes (Fig. 4–8). Spatting is commonly performed in the sport of American football, perhaps more for cosmetic than supportive purposes. While spatting does provide minimal support, this technique should not be used alone for preventing and treating inversion, eversion, and syndesmosis sprains.[54] Tapes in team or shoe colors are often used for the technique.

▸ **Materials:**
  • Pre-tape material or self-adherent wrap, 1½ inch or 2 inch non-elastic tape, 2 inch or 3 inch elastic tape, taping scissors

▸ **Position of the individual:** Sitting on a taping table or bench with the leg extended off the edge with the foot in 90° of dorsiflexion.

▸ **Preparation:** When spatting is used to provide additional support, the closed basketweave and heel lock techniques are commonly applied first. Then apply socks and shoes.

▶ **Application:**

STEP 1: Apply pre-tape material or self-adherent wrap from the midsole area of the shoe to the distal lower leg (Fig. 4–8A). The application of the material or wrap will allow for easy removal of the tape following use.

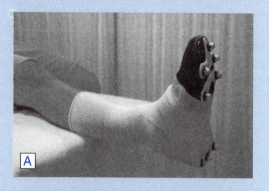

A

STEP 2: One method of spatting is applying the closed basketweave and heel lock techniques with 1½ inch or 2 inch non-elastic tape over the shoe (Fig. 4–8B). Because of the unusual contours of the shoe, do not be concerned by wrinkles in the tape.

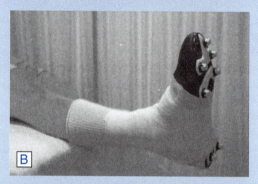

B

STEP 3: Another method is applying the elastic technique with 1½ inch or 2 inch non-elastic and 2 inch or 3 inch elastic tape (Fig. 4–8C) 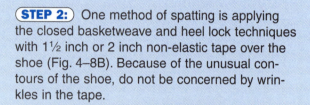 .

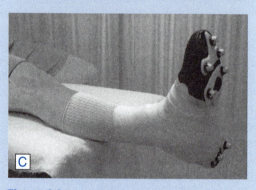

C

Figure 4-8

 Helpful Hint: Spatting may lessen contact of the plantar surface of the shoe with the ground. Therefore, cut tape away from cleats and contact areas such as the heel and forefoot.

POSTERIOR SPLINT Figure 4–9

▶ **Purpose:** The posterior splint technique is used to immobilize the subtalar and talocrural joints in the acute treatment of fractures and severe inversion, eversion, and syndesmosis sprains (Fig. 4–9). Use the splint as temporary immobilization prior to further evaluation by a physician. Temporary immobilization may be required while waiting overnight for a physician appointment or returning home with an athletic team from an away competition. Two methods that are interchangeable are illustrated in the application of this technique.

◯ **DETAILS**

Periods of immobilization are normally determined by a physician following evaluation of the individual. To provide complete immobilization, rigid cast tape is applied over stockinet and cast padding by cast technicians and physicians.

▶ **Design:**
  • Rigid splints available off-the-shelf in pre-cut and padded designs provide temporary immobilization in the treatment of fractures and sprains. The splints are constructed of several layers of rigid fiberglass material, covered with fabric and foam padding in 2, 3, 4, and 5 inch widths by 10, 12, 15, 30, 35, and 45 inch lengths.

Posterior Splint Technique One

▶ **Materials:**
  • Off-the-shelf rigid, padded splint, gloves, water, towel, two 4 inch width by 10 yard length elastic wraps, metal clips, 1½ inch non-elastic tape

▶ **Position of the individual:** Prone on a taping table or bench with the leg extended off the edge. If pain and swelling allow, place the ankle in subtalar neutral.

▶ **Preparation:** Mold and apply the padded splint directly to the skin.

▶ **Application:**
  (**STEP 1:**) Remove the splint from the package and immerse in water of 70° to 75°F to begin the chemical reaction. Remove the splint and place lengthwise on a towel.

  (**STEP 2:**) Quickly roll the splint and towel together to remove excess water (Fig. 4–9A).

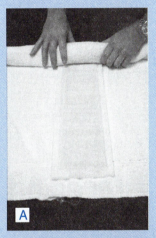

  (**STEP 3:**) Apply the splint from just inferior to the posterior knee, across the plantar foot, to the distal toes (Fig. 4–9B).

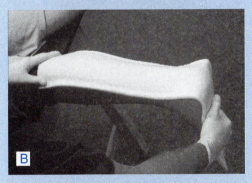

  (**STEP 4:**) Mold the splint to the body contours with the application of a 4 inch width by 10 yard length elastic wrap in a spiral pattern with moderate roll tension ◀▶ (Fig. 4–9C). Continue to mold and shape the splint with the hands. Monitor the pain-free position of the ankle. After 10–15 minutes, the fiberglass should be cured; remove the elastic wrap.

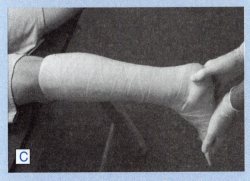

Figure 4-9

STEP 5: Using another 4 inch width by 10 yard length elastic wrap, attach the splint with moderate roll tension to the posterior lower leg, ankle, and foot in a spiral, distal-to-proximal pattern 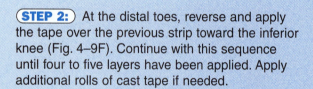 (Fig. 4–9D). Anchor the wrap with metal clips or loosely applied 1½ inch non-elastic tape. The individual will require crutches for non–weight-bearing ambulation.

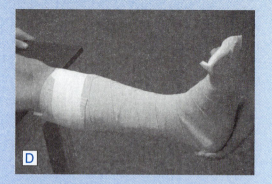

Posterior Splint Technique Two

▶ **Materials:**
  • 4 inch or 5 inch width rigid cast tape, stockinet, gloves, 4 inch width by 10 yard length elastic wrap, metal clips, 1½ inch non-elastic tape, taping scissors

▶ **Position of the individual:** Prone on a taping table or bench with the leg extended off the edge. If pain and swelling allow, place the ankle in subtalar neutral.

▶ **Preparation:** Apply one layer of stockinet from the knee to the distal toes.

▶ **Application:**
STEP 1: Remove the cast tape from the pouch and immerse in water of 70° to 75°F. Start just inferior to the knee. Apply the tape on the posterior lower leg, proceed over the heel and plantar foot, and finish at the distal toes (Fig. 4–9E).

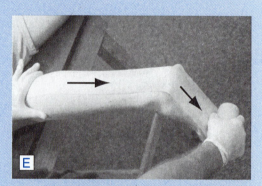

STEP 2: At the distal toes, reverse and apply the tape over the previous strip toward the inferior knee (Fig. 4–9F). Continue with this sequence until four to five layers have been applied. Apply additional rolls of cast tape if needed.

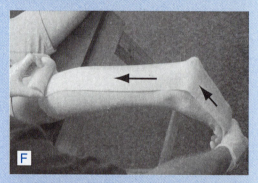

STEP 3: Mold the tape with gloved hands. Monitor the pain-free position of the ankle. Curing should be complete in 10–15 minutes. Cut the stockinet lengthwise down the anterior lower leg and fold the stockinet over the splint to protect against skin irritation (Fig. 4–9G).

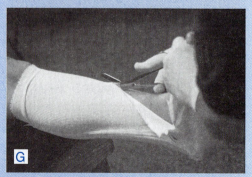

Figure 4-9 *continued*

STEP 4: Attach the splint with a 4 inch width by 10 yard length elastic wrap with moderate roll tension in a spiral, distal-to-proximal pattern ◄— (Fig. 4–9H). Anchor the wrap with metal clips or loosely applied 1½ inch non-elastic tape. Place the individual on crutches.

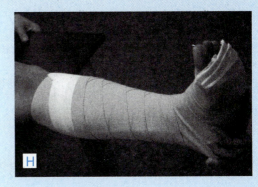

Figure 4-9 *continued*

Critical Thinking Question 2

Through the outpatient orthopedic clinic, you perform outreach services with an amateur rugby team. A flanker on the team suffers a syndesmosis sprain of his left ankle. Following rehabilitation, a physician allows the flanker to return to practice and competition with appropriate ankle support.

▶ **Question: What taping techniques can be used in this situation?**

...IF/THEN...

IF applying the continuous heel lock taping technique and the correct angles remain problematic, **THEN** apply pre-tape material in the same pattern at the start of a taping technique for additional practice.

Wrapping Techniques

Wrapping techniques are used to provide compression to control swelling and effusion, to provide support, and to reduce range of motion.

COMPRESSION WRAPS   Figures 4–10, 4–11

▶ **Purpose:** The compression wrap technique is used in the acute treatment of inversion, eversion, and syndesmosis sprains to control mild, moderate, or severe swelling and effusion (Fig. 4–10).

▶ **Materials:**
  • 2 inch, 3 inch, or 4 inch width by 5 yard length elastic wrap, metal clips, 1½ inch non-elastic or 2 inch elastic tape, taping scissors
  Options:
  • ¼ inch or ½ inch foam or felt
  • 2 inch, 3 inch, or 4 inch self-adherent wrap or elastic tape, pre-tape material, thin foam pads

▶ **Position of the individual:** Sitting on a taping table or bench with the leg extended off the edge and the foot in pain-free dorsiflexion.

▶ **Preparation:** Apply the technique directly to the skin.

  Option: *Cut a ¼ inch or ½ inch foam or felt horseshoe pad (see Fig. 4–19A–E). With the use of elastic tape, apply one layer of pre-tape material directly to the skin and use thin foam pads over the heel and lace areas.*

▶ **Application:**

STEP 1: The wrap technique for the ankle is identical to the compression technique for the foot illustrated in Chapter 3, Fig. 3–15 (Fig. 4–10A). Apply the greatest amount of roll tension distally and lessen tension as the wrap continues proximally.

Option: Apply the ¼ inch or ½ inch foam or felt horseshoe pad to the medial and/or lateral aspect of the ankle to provide additional compression to assist in the control of swelling and effusion (Fig. 4–10B). Two inch, 3 inch, or 4 inch self-adherent wrap or elastic tape may be used if an elastic wrap is not available.

> **...IF/THEN...**
>
> **IF** the elastic compression wrap migrates or slides over or off the calcaneus during ambulation and movement of footwear, **THEN** loosely apply a 1½ inch non-elastic or 2 inch elastic tape or self-adherent wrap circular strip from the lace area, across the plantar calcaneus, and finish over the lace area to anchor the elastic wrap ◀▬▶.

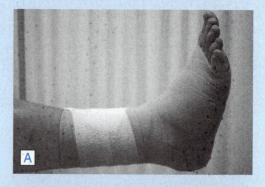

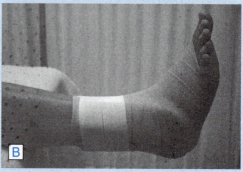

Figure 4-10

Elastic Sleeve

▶ **Purpose:** Use an elastic sleeve over the ankle to provide compression when controlling mild, moderate, or severe swelling and effusion when treating sprains (Fig. 4–11). Unlike elastic wraps, this compression wrap, with proper instruction, can be applied and removed by the individual without assistance.

▶ **Materials:**
  • 3 inch elastic sleeve, taping scissors

  Options:
  • ¼ inch or ½ inch foam or felt

▶ **Position of the individual:** Sitting on a taping table or bench with the leg extended off the edge, or sitting in a chair.

▶ **Preparation:** Cut a sleeve from a roll to extend from the proximal toes to the distal lower leg. Cut and use a double length sleeve to provide additional compression.

▶ **Application:**

STEP 1: Pull the sleeve onto the foot and ankle directly to the skin in a distal-to-proximal direction (Fig. 4–11). If using a double length sleeve, pull the distal end over the first layer to provide an additional layer. No anchors are required; the sleeve can be cleaned and reused.

Option: Apply the ¼ inch or ½ inch foam or felt horseshoe pad to the medial and/or lateral aspect of the ankle to provide additional compression.

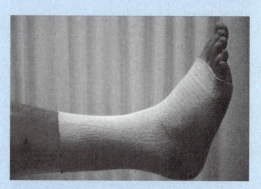

Figure 4-11

SOFT CAST Figure 4–12

▶ **Purpose:** Compression and mild support can be provided with the soft cast technique in the acute treatment of sprains (Fig. 4–12). Because of the materials used, this technique is perhaps the most comfortable for the individual with moderate or severe swelling and can be left in place for several days.

▶ **Materials:**
• 2 inch, 3 inch, or 4 inch width cast padding, 2 inch, 3 inch, or 4 inch width by 5 yard length elastic or self-adherent wrap

▶ **Position of the individual:** Sitting on a taping table or bench with the leg extended off the edge and the foot in pain-free dorsiflexion.

▶ **Preparation:** Apply the soft cast directly to the skin.

▶ **Application:**
STEP 1: Apply 2 inch, 3 inch, or 4 inch width cast padding from the proximal toes to the distal lower leg in a spiral, distal-to-proximal pattern with moderate roll tension ◀▬▶ (Fig. 4–12A). Applying three layers of the material should provide adequate compression around the ankle.

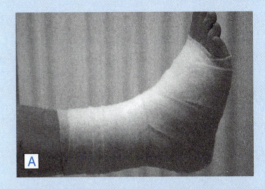

STEP 2: Next, apply a compression wrap technique over the cast padding with a 2 inch, 3 inch, or 4 inch width by 5 yard length elastic wrap or self-adherent wrap (Fig. 4–12B).

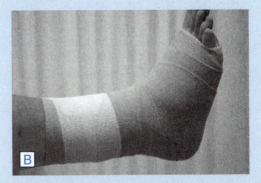

Figure 4-12

CLOTH WRAP Figure 4–13

▶ **Purpose:** Use the cloth wrap technique to provide mild support in preventing inversion and eversion sprains during athletic activities (Fig. 4–13).

▶ **Materials:**
• 2 inch width by 72–96 inch length cloth wrap, thin foam pads, 1½ inch or 2 inch non-elastic tape

▶ **Position of the individual:** Sitting on a taping table or bench with the leg extended off the edge with the foot in 90° of dorsiflexion.

▶ **Preparation:** Apply over a sock and use thin foam pads over the heel and lace areas to lessen irritation.

▶ **Application:**

STEP 1: Place the end of a 72–96 inch length cloth wrap on the distal lateral lower leg superior to the lateral malleolus and anchor around the leg in a lateral-to-medial direction (Fig. 4–13A).

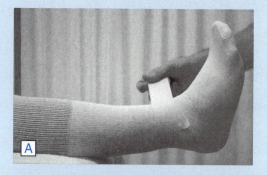

STEP 2: Continue applying the wrap with the continuous heel lock technique with moderate roll tension (Fig. 4–13B). The length of the cloth wrap should allow for the application of at least two sets of heel locks.

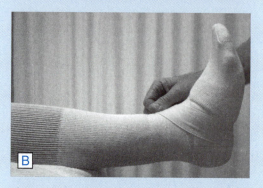

STEP 3: Finish the wrap around the distal lower leg and anchor with 1½ inch or 2 inch non-elastic tape ◀▬▶ (Fig. 4–13C).

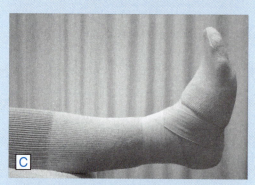

STEP 4: Heel locks may be applied with 1½ inch or 2 inch non-elastic tape with moderate roll tension over the cloth wrap for additional support (Fig. 4–13D).

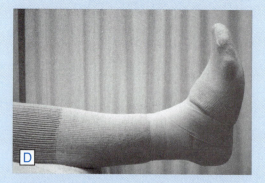

Figure 4-13

Critical Thinking Question 3

While working on a job site, an electrician steps off the unfinished stairs that lead to an outside door. His right foot lands on several pieces of scrap wood, causing a moderate inversion ankle sprain. A physician applies an air/gel bladder brace on the ankle for support and compression. The electrician is also placed on crutches for ambulation.

▶ **Question:** What type of compression wrap technique can you use with the brace?

...IF/THEN...

IF an individual has swelling following an ankle sprain, but will not be seen for treatment for an extended period of time because of work commitments, **THEN** consider using an elastic sleeve to provide compression; after receiving application instruction, the individual can apply and remove the sleeve herself or himself.

Bracing Techniques

Bracing techniques for preventing and treating ankle sprains generally can be classified into four categories: lace-up, semirigid, air/gel bladder, and wrap. Bracing offers several advantages over taping in preventing and treating injuries. With fitting instructions, braces can be applied and removed by the individual, and can be reused. During activity, straps and/or laces can be adjusted to maintain proper fit, comfort, and support. Several braces are designed to assist in venous return in the treatment of swelling and effusion. Using braces also has been proven cost effective for reducing the incidence of ankle sprains.[14,29,58]

LACE-UP Figure 4–14

‣ **Purpose:** Lace-up braces are designed to provide moderate support and limit inversion, eversion, plantar flexion, and dorsiflexion in preventing and treating inversion and eversion ankle sprains (Fig. 4–14).

DETAILS

Lace-up braces are commonly used when preventing and treating inversion and eversion sprains of athletes in sports such as baseball, basketball, field hockey, football, gymnastics, ice hockey, lacrosse, soccer, softball, track and field, volleyball, and wrestling. The braces can also be used with work and casual footwear. Lace-up ankle braces may be used in combination with the closed basketweave, elastic, Spartan Slipper, and subtalar sling taping techniques to provide maximal support during activities.

‣ **Design:**
- The braces are available off-the-shelf in predetermined sizes, corresponding either to ankle circumference or to shoe size.
- Some designs are universal and can be used on either ankle, while others are purchased in a right or left style.
- The brace is applied directly over a sock and is constructed of a variety of strong, breathable materials, such as ballistic nylon, neoprene, nylon/polyester fabric, vinyl laminate, or mesh fabric.
- Eyelets for lacing are located on the anterior aspect of the brace in a longitudinal pattern. The tongue, located beneath the laces, is constructed of a durable, padded material to lessen irritation. This padded material is also found over the posterior heel area.
- To provide additional support, outer straps or flaps are incorporated into the designs. Nylon straps with Velcro closures are applied in a figure-of-eight and/or heel lock pattern over the brace. Flaps are used to secure the laces and prevent loosening.

- Many of the designs that have straps contain an elastic Velcro closure strip to anchor the strap and lace ends at the proximal end of the brace on the distal lower leg.
- From the basic lace-up design, many braces include various plastic materials or use additional straps to provide support.
- Insert plastic stays to serve as stirrups with some designs. Others are manufactured with a thermoplastic stirrup that forms to the contour of the ankle during use.
- Some designs have forefoot and calcaneal straps to restrict range of motion in those areas.
- Several other design features found in lace-up braces include buttress pads, to prevent migration and lessen swelling; tabs, to speed lacing and assist with application; elastic materials, to prevent irritation; and contoured arches, to provide support.

▶ **Position of the individual:** Sitting on a taping table or bench or chair.

▶ **Preparation:** Apply a sock over the foot and ankle. Loosen the laces and straps of the brace.

Specific instructions for fitting and applying the brace are included with each design. For proper fit and support, carefully follow the step-by-step procedures from the manufacturer. The following application guidelines pertain to most braces.

▶ **Application:**

(STEP 1:) Over a sock, hold each side of the brace and pull it over the foot until the heel is firmly positioned in the brace (Fig. 4–14A).

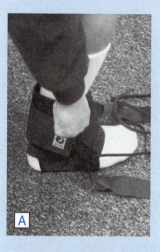

(STEP 2:) Put the laces through the eyelets in a distal-to-proximal pattern and tie at the proximal end (Fig. 4–14B). With many designs, the distance between the left and right eyelets should be less than 2 inches. If greater, use the next larger brace size. If the brace does not utilize straps, application is complete.

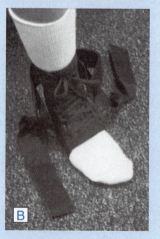

Figure 4-14

STEP 3: Applying straps will depend on the specific brace design. Figure-of-eight and heel lock straps commonly begin with application over the dorsum of the foot, continuing under the longitudinal arch, around the heel, and anchoring on the lateral or medial lower leg (Fig. 4–14C).

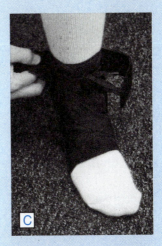

C

STEP 4: Pull these straps tight and secure to the brace with Velcro. Anchor the strap and lace ends with the elastic closure strip (Fig. 4–14D).

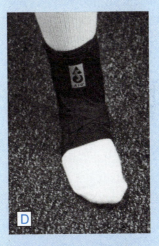

D

...IF/THEN...

IF lace-up braces gradually stretch after days or weeks of use, **THEN** wash and dry the braces and laces to shrink the materials to near original size to achieve proper fit.

Figure 4-14 *continued*

SEMIRIGID Figure 4–15

▶ **Purpose:** Semirigid braces provide moderate support and are used when preventing and treating inversion, eversion, and syndesmosis ankle sprains. These braces limit inversion, eversion, and rotation, allowing normal plantar flexion and dorsiflexion (Fig. 4–15).

DETAILS

Semirigid designs are very popular with basketball and volleyball players because these designs do not restrict plantar flexion and dorsiflexion range of motion. However, athletes participating in baseball, field hockey, football, gymnastics, ice hockey, lacrosse, soccer, softball, track and field, and wrestling can also wear the braces. The braces can also be used in casual and work footwear. Use semirigid designs in combination with the closed basketweave, elastic, Spartan Slipper, and subtalar sling taping techniques to provide maximal support during activities.

Ankle

- **Design:**
  - The braces are manufactured in universal or individual fit designs in predetermined sizes.
  - Most semirigid designs consist of a medial and lateral stirrup, attached through a hinge to either a heel or foot plate. The stirrups and plates are constructed from semirigid plastics and carbon composites.
  - Several designs allow for custom molding and fitting.
  - Another semirigid design uses a plastic heel cup attached to a longitudinal spring-loaded post, anchored at the distal posterior lower leg through a padded cuff. The cuff translates up and down during activity.
  - Semirigid braces are lined with EVA, neoprene, or air cell padding to provide compression, support, and comfort during activity.
  - Various nylon straps with Velcro attachments incorporated into the stirrups anchor the brace to the distal lower leg.
  - Many of the semirigid braces are available with extra design features to assist with support and comfort.
  - The foot plates of some designs are molded similarly to an orthotic to support the longitudinal arch. Other foot plates have small cleats on the plantar surface to prevent migration during activity.
  - In several designs, the lining of the stirrups can be changed to accommodate abnormal body contours and to vary the amount of compression.
  - In several designs, the anchor strap can be adjusted according to the type of footwear worn, such as low or high top athletic styles.

- **Position of the individual:** Sitting on a taping table or bench or chair.

- **Preparation:** Apply a sock over the foot and ankle.

Application of semirigid designs should follow manufacturers' instructions, which are included with the braces when purchased. The following general application guidelines apply to most semirigid designs.

- **Application:**

STEP 1: Begin by examining the insole of the shoe. If the insole is not attached, or if an orthotic is being used, remove and place the heel or foot plate underneath (Fig. 4–15A). Reposition the insole or orthotic in the shoe. Push the heel or foot plate of the brace against the heel box of the shoe.

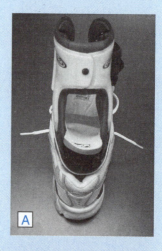

A

STEP 2: Loosen the shoe laces and place the foot inside the shoe, sliding the heel against the heel box (Fig. 4–15B).

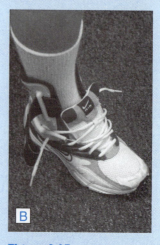

B

Figure 4-15

STEP 3: Position the stirrups over the lateral and medial malleoli and anchor the brace around the distal lower leg with the strap (Fig. 4–15C). Finish by tying the shoe laces.

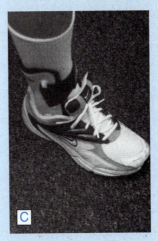

C

Figure 4-15 *continued*

AIR/GEL BLADDER Figure 4–16

▶ **Purpose:** Air/gel bladder braces are designed only to limit inversion and eversion in preventing and treating inversion and eversion ankle sprains (Fig. 4–16). The braces are used most often during the acute phase of treatment to provide compression and moderate support.

> **DETAILS**
>
> The braces are used to prevent and treat sprains for athletes participating in baseball, basketball, field hockey, football, gymnastics, ice hockey, lacrosse, soccer, softball, track and field, volleyball, and wrestling. While somewhat larger than lace-up, semirigid, and wrap designs, air/gel bladder braces can be used with work and casual footwear. Air/gel bladder braces may be used in combination with the closed basketweave, elastic, Spartan Slipper, and subtalar sling taping techniques to provide maximal support during activities, and with the open basket weave taping technique and compression, elastic sleeve, and soft cast wrapping techniques to provide moderate support during the acute phase of treatment.

▶ **Design:**
  • The braces are available in universal or individual fit designs of various widths and lengths in predetermined sizes.
  • Air/gel bladder designs consist of medial and lateral thermoplastic stirrups or shells, pre-molded to the contours of the lower leg and ankle.
  • The stirrups/shells are lined with various combinations of air and/or gel bladders. Many pre-inflated air bladder liners contain a proximal valve that allows for adjustments in compression. Some of the air/gel and gel liners may be removed and placed in a freezer to cool. After the liners are cooled, reattach the liners to the stirrups/shells to provide compression and cryotherapy. Several liner designs are covered with soft foam material for additional comfort.
  • The stirrups/shells are connected with an adjustable nylon strap that is worn across the plantar calcaneus.
  • The braces are anchored to the lower leg and ankle with two vinyl straps with Velcro closures.

▶ **Position of the individual:** Sitting on a taping table or bench or chair.

▶ **Preparation:** Apply a sock over the foot and ankle.

  Instructions for application are included with each brace. The following guidelines pertain to most designs.

▶ **Application:**

STEP 1: Begin by loosening the lower leg straps and distal air/gel bladders from the stirrups/shells to expose the plantar calcaneus strap (Fig. 4–16A). Adjust the calcaneus strap to allow the stirrups/shells to fit snugly around the lower leg and ankle.

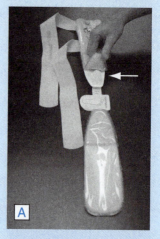

A

Figure 4-16A Plantar calcaneus strap.

STEP 2: Over a sock, place the heel onto the calcaneus strap and position the stirrups/shells over the ankle and lower leg (Fig. 4–16B).

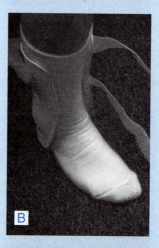

B

STEP 3: Anchor the brace with the lower leg straps.

STEP 4: Place the foot and brace into the shoe and adjust the straps if needed to achieve a snug fit (Fig. 4–16C).

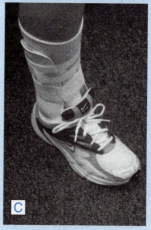

C

Figure 4-16

Critical Thinking Question 4

Near the conclusion of the spring semester, an intercollegiate soccer midfielder who sustained a right ankle syndesmosis sprain during spring practice comes into the athletic training room. She plans to participate in a summer league at home and asks about what type of protection she can use for her right ankle during practices and competitions. The Spartan Slipper and subtalar sling taping techniques were applied upon her return in the spring. These techniques allowed a return, but limited her ability to dribble and shoot the ball on goal.

▶ **Question: What technique(s) can you use in this situation?**

WRAP Figure 4–17

▸ **Purpose:** Wrap braces are used in the prevention and treatment of inversion and eversion ankle sprains and provide mild support (Fig. 4–17). These off-the-shelf braces can be categorized into two basic designs based on their function: support or treatment.

◯ **DETAILS**

Support braces can be used with work and casual footwear, and for athletes participating in baseball, basketball, field hockey, football, gymnastics, ice hockey, lacrosse, soccer, softball, track and field, volleyball, and wrestling. The support design may be used in combination with the closed basketweave, elastic, Spartan Slipper, and subtalar sling taping techniques to provide moderate support. The treatment brace, on the other hand, is designed to be used for non–weight-bearing therapeutic activities to provide compression.

▸ **Design:**
- Support designs are available in universal or individual fit in predetermined sizes. The braces are constructed of ballistic nylon, nylon/lycra, or neoprene. Support to the ankle is provided through various nylon straps with Velcro closures that are applied in figure-of-eight and/or heel lock patterns.
- Treatment designs are available in universal fit and are made of neoprene with removable gel packs attached in the inner liner of the brace. Many packs can be removed and heated and/or cooled, then reattached to provide treatment to the ankle. Anchor the treatment designs with Velcro closures.

▸ **Position of the individual:** Sitting on a taping table or bench or chair.

▸ **Preparation:** Apply support design braces over a sock. Apply treatment designs directly to the skin.

Follow the manufacturer's instructions when applying the braces.

▸ **Application:**
(STEP 1:) Apply some of the support designs by loosening the closures, positioning the foot onto the brace, wrapping the brace around the foot and ankle, and anchoring with Velcro closures (Fig. 4–17A).

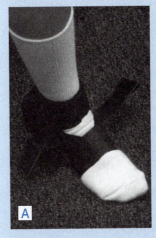

A

Figure 4-17

STEP 2: Apply the nylon straps in a figure-of-eight, heel lock, and/or stirrup pattern as indicated by the manufacturer (Fig. 4–17B). Pull other designs onto the foot and ankle in a distal-to-proximal pattern.

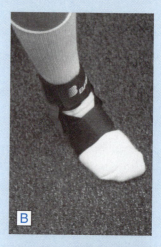

STEP 3: Apply the treatment designs by positioning the foot onto the brace, wrapping around the foot and ankle, and anchoring with the Velcro closures (Fig. 4–17C).

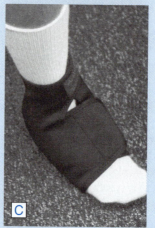

Figure 4-17 *continued*

Critical Thinking Question 5

This season, you decide to purchase and use lace-up ankle braces in place of taping techniques to prevent ankle sprains in the basketball athletes. During the first few practices, several athletes complain about the fit of the braces and the lack of support provided.

▶ **Question: What can you do to accommodate the basketball athletes?**

...IF/THEN...

IF choosing a brace design for an athlete returning to practice following a syndesmosis ankle sprain, **THEN** consider a semirigid design, which will limit external rotation. Also consider using the brace in combination with several taping techniques to provide maximal support.

...IF/THEN...

IF support is needed in the acute treatment of a first degree eversion sprain with mild to moderate swelling, **THEN** consider the use of an air/gel bladder brace design, which limits inversion and eversion and can be applied over a compression wrap technique in the control of swelling.

RESEARCH BRIEF

Health-care professionals use a variety of taping, and lace-up, semirigid, air/gel bladder, and wrap bracing techniques in preventing and treating inversion, eversion, and syndesmosis sprains. The high incidence of ankle sprains has led to the development of these multiple tape techniques and brace designs.[36,57] Determining the appropriate technique/design to utilize for a particular individual and injury can be confusing. However, investigations to determine the effectiveness of taping and bracing can assist in matching the appropriate technique/design to the individual.

The majority of the research has examined the influence of ankle taping and bracing on ankle range of motion, proprioception, postural control, muscle response, and overall functional performance. Past investigations examined passive ankle range of motion in pre-exercise and postexercise conditions with a variety of tape and brace designs. In pre-exercise conditions, tape and softshell and semirigid braces have been found to reduce inversion and eversion.[19,21,24] Following 10 minutes of exercise, semirigid braces provided the greatest reduction in range of motion, but tape did restrict inversion.[21] Other researchers have demonstrated that tape and semirigid braces had a greater restriction on inversion than softshell and lace-up braces.[24] With tape and lace-up and semirigid braces,[17,19,24] eversion range of motion increased after exercise, perhaps as a result of the design and application emphasis on preventing inversion sprains.[9] Examining passive range of motion measures following exercise of longer durations, lace-up and semirigid braces appeared to restrict range of motion more than tape.[17,18,47] Investigations of ankle range of motion with dynamic movements, such as walking and running, revealed that tape did not restrict inversion, but lace-up and semirigid braces were effective in limiting inversion.[42,45]

Many have suggested that tape quickly loses its restrictive qualities during exercise.[40,41,53] While it is true that tape loosens, it does restrict extreme ranges of motion, even after prolonged activity.[1,8,32,34,51,60] Some studies have noted that ideal tape and brace techniques and designs should not restrict normal range of motion, but rather provide support at anatomical limits of motion.[14,44]

Many researchers agree that taping and bracing provides mechanical stability to the ankle,[1,8,32,51] and others suggest that the techniques/designs may also influence proprioceptive input of the surrounding musculature.[12,37,48] Findings from several studies[10,11,25,28,56] indicated that tape and lace-up and semirigid braces improved stimulation of cutaneous mechanoreceptors located around the ankle. Adequate levels of coordination and balance have been shown to be important in preventing and treating ankle sprains.[59] Likewise, adequate postural control may lessen the risk of injury and/or re-injury.[16,59] Some researchers have suggested that semirigid braces[10]

assist in maintaining postural control while others reported that tape[56] and lace-up braces[49] had no influence. The reaction time of the peroneus longus during a simulated ankle sprain has been shown to increase following application of tape[32] and lace-up and semirigid braces.[7,48] However, other researchers demonstrated that tape[1,37] and lace-up[6] and semirigid braces[6] had no effect on reaction time. Researchers have revealed that the response of the peroneus longus plays a large role in preventing inversion injury to the ankle.[27,33] The long-term use of lace-up and semirigid braces was shown to have no effect on peroneus longus reaction time, possibly dispelling the myth that long-term use weakens the musculature.[6,7,9] Although the main function of taping and bracing is perhaps mechanical stability, the positive influence on proprioceptive input, postural sway, and peroneal muscle activity warrants further investigation.[9,63]

Investigators have demonstrated that taping and bracing techniques/designs can reduce ankle injury[55,58,59] and injury rates.[2,13,55,58,59] However, if individuals believe the techniques/designs will hamper their performances in the athletic and/or work setting, their compliance may be spotty. Nevertheless, the majority of the research has demonstrated that taping and bracing does not decrease running performance, specifically sprint times.[4,23,38,39,43,62] Examining agility performance, some researchers[4,23,30,39,50,52,62] have found that taping and bracing had no effect on drills consisting of rapidly changing direction, sprinting, and accelerating and decelerating; others[5,46] found a decrease in performance. Several studies revealed that taping and bracing had no effect on vertical jump height[4,17,22,35,39,62] while others found a decrease in height.[5,31,43,46,50] In these studies, the design and application of tape and lace-up braces may have contributed to the decrease in vertical jump height as a result of restriction in plantar flexion range of motion.[9] Overall, the research findings suggest that taping and bracing techniques/designs have a minimal negative effect on sprint, agility, and vertical jump performance.

Health-care professionals have used ankle taping and bracing techniques/designs for years and, because of the high incidence of sprains, will continue to use them. Current research has assisted in determining which technique/design may offer the optimal protection, support, and treatment for the individual. You should base decisions regarding the use of the techniques/designs on the individual, injury, sport and/or occupation, and stage of healing, as well as available resources such as budget, availability, and skill of the health-care professional.

WALKING BOOT

▶ **Purpose:** Walking boots or walkers (see Fig. 3–23) are used in treating inversion, eversion, and syndesmosis ankle sprains, as well as with stable acute and stress fractures.
  • Use the boots in the postacute treatment and rehabilitation period when limited range of motion and weight-bearing are allowed to provide support.
  • The ability to remove the boot for treatment, adjust the range of motion, and proceed with gait training provides an effective bracing technique at a lower cost than traditional casting.

Padding Techniques

Use padding techniques to lessen shear forces and provide compression with various injuries and conditions of the ankle. Applying taping, wrapping, and bracing techniques can cause trauma to the skin and result in irritation, blisters, and lacerations. Several padding techniques can be used to prevent and treat these injuries and conditions.

VISCOELASTIC POLYMERS Figure 4–18

▶ **Purpose:** Use viscoelastic polymers in preventing and treating skin irritations to the ankle (Fig. 4–18). Blisters are common over the heel, lace, and medial and lateral malleoli, and are caused by footwear and the application of tapes, wraps, and braces.

▶ **Design:**
  • Several designs come in predetermined sizes, with viscoelastic pads or discs attached to the inside of neoprene material sleeves over the high shear areas (Fig. 4–18A).

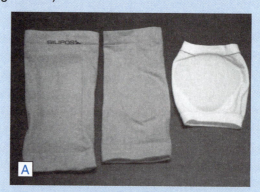

Figure 4-18A Viscoelastic polymers. Foot and ankle sleeves.

▶ **Materials:**
  • Viscoelastic pad or disc sleeves

▶ **Position of the individual:** Sitting on a taping table or bench or chair.

▶ **Preparation:** Apply the sleeves directly to the skin.

▶ **Application:**
  (**STEP 1:**) Pull the sleeves onto the foot and ankle in a distal-to-proximal pattern (Fig. 4–18B). The individual can wear socks, ankle braces, and athletic, work, and casual footwear over the sleeves.

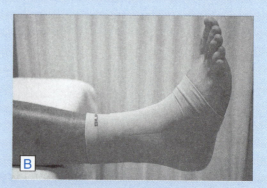

Figure 4-18

HORSESHOE PAD   Figure 4–19

▶ **Purpose:** Use the horseshoe pad technique in the acute treatment of ankle sprains to provide additional compression to assist with reducing swelling and effusion (Fig. 4–19).

▶ **Materials:**
  • ¼ inch or ½ inch foam or felt, taping scissors

▶ **Position of the individual:** Sitting on a taping table or bench with the leg extended off the edge and the foot in pain-free dorsiflexion.

▶ **Preparation:** Cut the horseshoe pad from ¼ inch or ½ inch foam or felt to fit over the medial and/or lateral aspect of the ankle. Off-the-shelf pre-cut designs are also available.

▶ **Application:**
  STEP 1: Cut a piece of foam or felt approximately 4–5 inches in width and 6–8 inches in length (Fig. 4–19A).

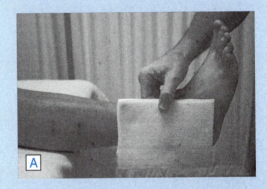

STEP 2: Cut a narrow "U" shape pattern, 5–7 inches lengthwise into the foam or felt (Fig. 4–19B).

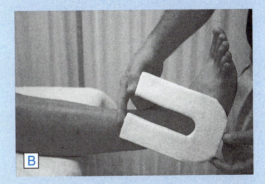

STEP 3: Another horseshoe technique is to cut a hole in the middle of the foam or felt 5–7 inches from the proximal end (Fig. 4–19C).

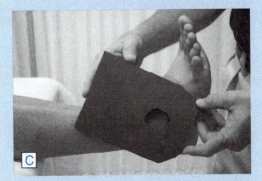

Figure 4-19

Ankle

STEP 4: Position the horseshoe pad over the medial and/or lateral ankle with the malleoli placed at the bottom of the "U" or in the hole of the pad (Fig. 4–19D).

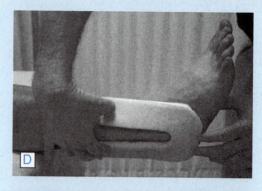

STEP 5: Apply the compression or elastic sleeve wrapping techniques over the horseshoe pad to anchor (Fig. 4–19E).

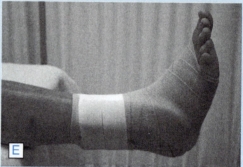

Figure 4-19   *continued*

ACHILLES TENDON STRIPS   Figure 4–20

▶ **Purpose:** The Achilles tendon strip technique reduces shearing forces that may occur when using taping and bracing techniques (Fig. 4–20).

DETAILS

Applying taping and bracing techniques daily to prevent and treat ankle sprains often causes irritation of the skin. Taping technique closure strips and/or brace straps can cause irritation, especially over the Achilles tendon. Abnormal body contours, such as malalignment of the Achilles tendon, may also lead to irritation.

▶ **Materials:**
- ¼ inch or ½ inch foam, taping scissors

▶ **Position of the individual:** Sitting on a taping table or bench with the leg extended off the edge with the foot in 90° of dorsiflexion.

▶ **Preparation:** Apply the strips directly to the skin.

▶ **Application:**
STEP 1: Cut two strips approximately 1–1½ inches in width and 4–6 inches in length, from ¼ inch or ½ inch foam.

STEP 2: Position the strips on each side of the Achilles tendon with the distal end just superior to the tendon's insertion on the calcaneus (Fig. 4–20A).

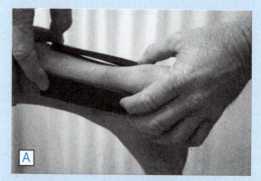

Figure 4-20

STEP 3: When applying a taping technique, cover the strips with pre-tape material or self-adherent wrap and continue with the technique ◄— (Fig. 4–20B).

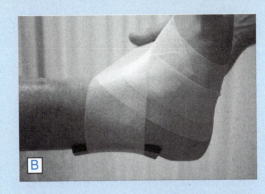

STEP 4: With braces, position the strips and anchor them with a circular pattern of 2 inch self-adherent wrap or pre-tape material and 2 inch elastic tape with mild roll tension ◄— (Fig. 4–20C). Continue by applying a sock, then the brace.

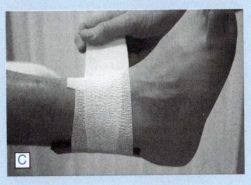

Figure 4-20 *continued*

DONUT PADS

▶ **Purpose:** Donut pads can also be used to reduce shearing forces on the ankle (see Fig. 3–27).
 • Cut pads from ⅛ inch or ¼ inch foam or felt and place them over the medial and/or lateral malleoli.
 • The pad may be used under taping, wrapping, and bracing techniques.
 • With taping techniques, attach the pad directly to the skin with adhesive gauze material (see Fig. 3–13) prior to tape application or with pre-tape material (see Fig. 4–1A) during the taping technique.
 • When applying wrapping techniques, anchor the pad within the technique.
 • With bracing techniques, attach the pad with adhesive gauze material (see Fig. 3–13) or pre-tape material and 2 inch elastic tape, with the heel lock technique (see Fig. 4–2).

Critical Thinking Question 6

After several weeks of treatment and rehabilitation for an ankle sprain/fracture, a salesperson for an automobile dealership returns to work. The physician recommends that all work activities be performed with a semirigid brace on the ankle. Soon, the brace begins to cause skin irritation over the lateral malleolus.

▶ **Question: How can you manage this situation?**

...IF/THEN...

IF using viscoelastic polymer, foam, or felt materials for padding, in combination with an ankle taping, wrapping, or bracing technique, **THEN** choose the appropriate thickness of the material; the material should reduce shear forces, but not affect the fit and support provided by the technique, which can occur with an excessively thick pad.

CASE STUDY

Meghan Stewart is a two-sport athlete at Brown College, participating on the volleyball team in the fall and the softball team in the spring. During the first competitive volleyball match of the season, Meghan jumped to block a spike at the net. When she landed, her right foot struck a teammate's shoe, causing a moderate inversion and plantar flexion force. Meghan has no history of ankle injury and was not wearing a prophylactic tape, brace, or wrap technique. Meghan was taken to the Athletic Training Room for evaluation by Lauren Bargar, ATC, and by the team physician. Following an evaluation and subsequent radiographs, Meghan was diagnosed by the physician with a moderate right ankle inversion sprain. The team physician ordered Meghan to be immobilized at 90° of ankle dorsiflexion, non–weight-bearing, for 5 to 10 days. During this time, Meghan could receive treatment to her ankle. What taping, wrapping, bracing, and/or padding techniques would help to immobilize, support, and control swelling and effusion in Meghan's right ankle?

Meghan is progressing well within the therapeutic exercise program Lauren and the team physician have designed. Meghan is now ready to begin sport-specific drills during volleyball practice. The team physician requests that Meghan's ankle be supported during these drills and for the remainder of the season. What are the appropriate taping, wrapping, and/or bracing techniques that you could use to provide support to the ankle upon a return to activity?

Meghan finishes the volleyball season without further injury and is ready to begin practice with the softball team. Meghan asks Lauren if she can continue with some type of ankle support during softball practices. Lauren agrees and continues applying the technique used for volleyball practices and competitions. During softball practice, a base running drill requires Meghan to sprint from home plate to second base. As she steps on first base, her right ankle is forced into dorsiflexion, and she experiences pain. Meghan finishes practice and returns to the Athletic Training Room to talk to Lauren about a different technique for support. Which techniques can you use to provide support and limit dorsiflexion to allow Meghan to participate pain-free?

WRAP UP

- Ankle sprains are caused by excessive range of motion and are common in athletic activities. Fractures can occur in combination with sprains.
- Blisters can result from repetitive shearing forces caused by footwear and the application of taping, wrapping, and bracing techniques.
- The closed basketweave, heel lock, elastic, open basketweave, Spartan Slipper, subtalar sling, and spatting techniques provide support and reduce range of motion of the subtalar and talocrural joints.
- Cast tape and off-the-shelf fiberglass splints provide immobilization in treating sprains and fractures.
- Elastic wraps, tapes, and sleeves, as well as soft cast compression techniques, control swelling and effusion following injury.

- Cloth wraps provide mild support when preventing ankle sprains.
- Lace-up, semirigid, air/gel bladder, and wrap braces provide support and compression, and limit range of motion when preventing and treating ankle sprains and fractures.
- Walking boots and posterior splints can be used to provide support and immobilization.
- Viscoelastic polymers, donut, and Achilles tendon strip pad techniques reduce shearing forces.
- The horseshoe pad technique provides compression to reduce swelling and effusion.

■ WEB REFERENCES

American Academy of Orthopaedic Surgeons
http://www.aaos.org
· This Web site allows you to search for information about the mechanism, treatment, and rehabilitation of ankle injuries.
The American College of Foot & Ankle Orthopedics & Medicine
http://www.acfaom.org
· This site provides general information on common injuries and conditions.

■ REFERENCES

1. Alt, W, Lohrer, H, and Gollhofer, A: Functional properties of adhesive ankle taping: Neuromuscular and mechanical effects before and after exercise. Foot Ankle Int 20:238–245, 1999.
2. Bahr, R, Karlsen, R, Lian, O, and Ovrebo, RV: Incidence and mechanisms of acute ankle inversion injuries in volleyball: A retrospective cohort study. Am J Sports Med 22:595–600, 1994.
3. Barker, HB, Beynnon, BD, and Renström, AFH: Ankle injury risk factors in sports. Sports Med 23:69–74, 1997.

4. Bocchinfuso, C, Sitler, MR, and Kimura, IF: Effects of two semirigid prophylactic ankle stabilizers on speed, agility, and vertical jump. J Sport Rehabil 3:125–134, 1994.

5. Burks, RT, Bean, BG, Marcus, R, and Barker, HB: Analysis of athletic performance with prophylactic ankle devices. Am J Sports Med 19:104–106, 1991.

6. Cordova, ML, Cardona, CV, Ingersoll, CD, and Sandrey, MA: Long-term ankle brace use does not affect peroneus longus muscle latency during sudden inversion in normal subjects. J Athl Train 35:407–411, 2000.

7. Cordova, ML, and Ingersoll, CD: The effect of chronic ankle brace use on peroneus longus stretch reflex amplitude [abstract]. Med Sci Sports Exerc 32(suppl):274, 2000.

8. Cordova, ML, Ingersoll, CD, and LeBlanc, MJ: Influence of ankle support on joint range of motion before and after exercise: A meta-analysis. J Orthop Sports Phys Ther 30:170–182, 2000.

9. Cordova, ML, Ingersoll, CD, and Palmieri, RM: Efficacy of prophylactic ankle support: An experimental perspective. J Athl Train 37:446–457, 2002.

10. Feuerbach, JW, and Grabiner, MD: Effect of the Aircast on unilateral postural control: Amplitude and frequency variables. J Orthop Sports Phys Ther 7:149–154, 1993.

11. Feuerbach, JW, Grabiner, MD, Koh, TJ, and Weiker, GG: Effect of an ankle orthosis and ankle ligament anesthesia on ankle joint proprioception. Am J Sports Med 22:223–229, 1994.

12. Freeman, MA, Dean, MR, and Hanham, IW: The etiology and prevention of functional instability of the foot. J Bone Joint Surg Br 47:678–685, 1965.

13. Garrick, JG: The frequency of injury, mechanism of injury, and epidemiology of ankle sprains. Am J Sports Med 5:241–242, 1977.

14. Garrick, JG, and Requa, RK: Role of external support in the prevention of ankle sprains. Med Sci Sports 5:200–203, 1973.

15. Gibney, VP: Sprained ankle: A treatment that involves no loss of time, requires no crutches, and is not attended with an ultimate impairment of function. NY Med J 61:193–197, 1985.

16. Goldie, PA, Evans, OM, and Bach, TM: Postural control following inversion injuries of the ankle. Arch Phys Med Rehabil 75:969–975, 1994.

17. Greene, TA, and Hillman, SK: Comparison of support provided by a semirigid orthosis and adhesive ankle taping before, during, and after exercise. Am J Sports Med 18:498–506, 1990.

18. Greene, TA, and Wight, CR: A comparative support evaluation of three ankle orthoses before, during, and after exercise. J Orthop Sports Phys Ther 11:453–466, 1990.

19. Gross, MT, Ballard, CL, Mears, HG, and Watkins, EJ: Comparison of Donjoy Ankle Ligament Protector and Aircast Sport-Stirrup orthoses in restricting foot and ankle motion before and after exercise. J Orthop Sports Phys Ther 16:60–67, 1992.

20. Gross, MT, Batten, AM, Lamm, AL, Lorren, JL, Stevens, JJ, Davis, JM, and Wilkerson, GB: Comparison of DonJoy ankle ligament protector and subtalar sling ankle taping in restricting foot and ankle motion before and after exercise. J Orthop Sports Phys Ther 19:33–41, 1994.

21. Gross, MT, Bradshaw, MK, Ventry, LC, and Weller, KH: Comparison of support provided by ankle taping and semirigid orthosis. J Orthop Sports Phys Ther 9:33–39, 1987.

22. Gross, MT, Clemence, LM, Cox, BD, McMillan, HP, Meadows. AF, Piland, CS, and Powers, WS: Effect of ankle orthoses on functional performance for individuals with recurrent lateral ankle sprains. J Orthop Sports Phys Ther 25:245–252, 1997.

23. Gross, MT, Everts, JR, Roberson, SE, Roskin, DS, and Young, KD: Effect of DonJoy Ankle Ligament Protector and Aircast Sport-Stirrup orthoses on functional performance. J Orthop Sports Phys Ther 19:150–156, 1994.

24. Gross, MT, Lapp, AK, and Davis, JM: Comparison of Swede-O Universal Ankle Support and Aircast Sport-Stirrup orthoses and ankle tape in restricting eversion-inversion before and after exercise. J Orthop Sports Phys Ther 13:11–19, 1991.

25. Heit, EJ, Lephart, SM, and Rozzi, SL: The effect of ankle bracing and taping on joint position sense in the stable ankle. J Sport Rehabil 5:206–213, 1996.

26. Irvin, R, Iverson, D, and Roy, S: Sports Medicine Prevention, Evaluation, Management, and Rehabilitation, ed 2. Allyn & Bacon, Boston, 1998, pp 59–61.

27. Isakov, E, Mizrahi, J, and Solzi, P: Response of the peroneal muscles to sudden inversion of the ankle during standing. Int J Sport Biomech 2:100–109, 1986.

28. Jerosch, J, Hoffstetter, I, Bork, H, and Bischof, M: The influence of orthoses on the proprioception of the ankle joint. Knee Surg Sports Traumatol Arthrosc 3:39–46, 1995.

29. Jerosch, J, Thorwesten, L, Bork, H, and Bischof, M: Is prophylactic bracing of the ankle cost effective. Orthopedics 19:405–414, 1996.

30. Jerosch, J, Thorwesten, L, Frebel, T, and Linnenbecker, S: Influence of external stabilizing devices of the ankle on sport-specific capabilities. Knee Surg Sports Traumatol Arthrosc 5:50–57, 1997.

31. Juvenal, JP: The effects of ankle taping on vertical jumping ability. Athl Train J Natl Athl Train Assoc 7:146–149, 1972.

32. Karlsson, J, and Andreasson, GO: The effect of ankle support in chronic lateral ankle joint instability: An electromyographic study. Am J Sports Med 20:257–261, 1992.

33. Konradsen, L, Voigt, M, and Hojsgaard, C: Ankle inversion injuries: The role of the dynamic defense mechanism. Am J Sports Med 25:54–58, 1997.

34. Laughman, RK, Carr, TA, Chao, EY, Youdas, JW, and Sim, FH: Three-dimensional kinematics of the taped ankle before and after exercise. Am J Sports Med 8:425–431, 1980.

35. Locke, A, Sitler, MR, Aland, C, and Kimura, I: Long-term use of a softshell prophylactic ankle stabilizer on speed, agility, and vertical jump performance. J Sport Rehabil 6:235–245, 1997.

36. Löfvenburg, R, and Kärrholm, J: The influence of an ankle orthosis on the talar and calcaneal motions in chronic lateral instability of the ankle: A stereophotogrammetric analysis. Am J Sports Med 21:224–230, 1993.

37. Lohrer, H, Alt, W, and Golhofer, A: Neuromuscular properties and functional aspects of taped ankles. Am J Sports Med 27:69–75, 1999.

38. MacKean, LC, Bell, G, and Burnham, RS: Prophylactic ankle bracing vs. taping: Effects on functional performance in female basketball players. J Orthop Sports Phys Ther 22:77–81, 1995.

39. Macpherson, K, Sitle, MR, Kimura, I, and Horodyski, M: Effects of a semi-rigid and softshell prophylactic ankle stabilizer on selected performance tests among high school football players. J Orthop Sports Phys Ther 21:147–152, 1995.

40. Malina, RM, Plagenz, LB, and Rarick, GL: Effect of exercise upon the measurable supporting strength of cloth and tape wraps. Res Q 34:158–165, 1963.

41. Manfroy, PP, Ashton-Miller, JA, and Wojtys, EM: The effect of exercise, prewrap, and athletic tape on the maximal active and passive ankle resistance to ankle-inversion. Am J Sports Med 25:156–163, 1997.

42. Martin, N, and Harter, RA: Comparison of inversion restraint provided by ankle prophylactic devices before and after exercise. J Athl Train 28:324–329, 1993.

43. Mayhew, JL: Effects of ankle taping on motor performance. Athl Train J Natl Athl Train Assoc 7:10–11, 1972.

44. McCaw, ST, and Cerullo, JF: Prophylactic ankle stabilizers affect ankle joint kinematics during drop landings. Med Sci Sports Exerc 31:702–707, 1999.

45. McIntyre, DR, Smith, MA, and Denniston, NL: The effectiveness of strapping techniques during prolonged dynamic exercises. J Athl Train 18:52–55, 1983.

46. Metcalfe, RC, Schlabach, GA, Looney, MA, and Renehan, EJ: A comparison of moleskin tape, linen tape, and lace-up brace on joint restriction and movement performance. J Athl Train 32:136–140, 1997.

47. Myburgh, KH, Vaughan, CL, and Isaacs, SK: The effects of ankle guards and taping on joint motion before, during, and after a squash match. Am J Sports Med 12:441–446, 1984.

48. Nishikawa, T, and Grabiner, MD: Peroneal motoneuron excitability increases immediately following application of a semirigid ankle brace. J Orthop Sports Phys Ther 29:168–176, 1999.

49. Palmieri, RP, Ingersoll, CD, Cordova, ML, and Kinzey, SJ: Prolonged ankle brace application does not affect the spectral properties of postural sway [abstract]. Med Sci Sports Exerc 33(suppl):153, 2001.

50. Paris, DL: The effects of the Swede-O, New Cross, and McDavid ankle braces and adhesive taping on speed, balance, agility, and vertical jump. J Athl Train 27:253–256, 1992.

51. Pederson, TS, Ricard, MD, Merrill, G, Schulthies, SS, and Allsen, PE: The effects of spatting and ankle taping on inversion before and after exercise. J Athl Train 32:29–33, 1997.

52. Pienkowski, D, McMorrow, M, Shapiro, R, Caborn, DN, and Stayton, J: The effect of ankle stabilizers on athletic performance: A randomized prospective study. Am J Sports Med 23:757–762, 1995.

53. Rarick, GL, Bigley, G, Karst, R, and Malina, RM: The measurable support of the ankle joint by conventional methods of taping. J Bone Joint Surg Am 44:1183–1190, 1962.

54. Reeves, DA, and Emel TJ, http://www.emedicine.com/sports/topic143.htm, Ankle taping and bracing, 2001.

55. Rovere, GD, Clarke, TJ, Yates, CS, and Burley, K: Retrospective comparison of taping and ankle stabilizers in preventing ankle injuries. Am J Sports Med 16:228–233, 1988.

56. Simoneau, GG, Degner, RM, Kramper, CA, and Kittelson, KH: Changes in ankle joint proprioception resulting from strips of athletic tape applied over the skin. J Athl Train 32:141–147, 1997.

57. Sitler, MR, and Horodyski, M: Effectiveness of prophylactic ankle stabilizers for prevention of ankle injuries. Sports Med 20:53–57, 1995.

58. Surve, I, Schwellnus, MP, Noakes, T, and Lombard, C: A fivefold reduction in the incidence of recurrent ankle sprains in soccer players using the Sport-Stirrup orthosis. Am J Sports Med 22:601–606, 1994.

59. Tropp, H, Askling, C, and Gillquist, J: Prevention of ankle sprains. Am J Sports Med 13:259–262, 1985.

60. Vaes, P, De Boeck, H, Handlberg, F, and Opdecam, P: Comparative radiological study of the influence of ankle joint strapping and taping on ankle stability. J Orthop Sports Phys Ther 7:110–114, 1985.

61. Vaes, PH, Duquet, W, Handelberg, F, Casteleyn, PP, Tiggelen, RV, and Opdecam, P: Influence of ankle strapping, taping, and nine braces: A stress roentgenologic comparison. J Sport Rehabil 7:157–171, 1998.

62. Verbrugge, JD: The effects of semirigid Air-Stirrup bracing vs. adhesive ankle taping on motor performance. J Orthop Sports Phys Ther 23:320–325, 1996.

63. Wilkerson, GB: Biomechanical and neuromuscular effects of ankle taping and bracing. J Athletic Training 37:436–445, 2002.

64. Wilkerson, GB: Comparative biomechanical effects of the standard method of ankle taping and a taping method designed to enhance subtalar stability. Am J Sports Med 19:588–595, 1991.

Lower Leg

1. Explain common injuries that occur to the lower leg.
2. Demonstrate the ability to apply tapes, wraps, braces, and pads to the lower leg when preventing, treating, and rehabilitating injuries.
3. Explain and demonstrate appropriate taping, wrapping, bracing, and padding techniques for the lower leg within a therapeutic exercise program.

INJURIES AND CONDITIONS

Acute and chronic injuries and conditions of the lower leg can result from direct force, excessive range of motion, rapid acceleration and/or deceleration, and repetitive stress. Sudden acceleration, such as that experienced by a sprinter pushing off from the blocks or a softball outfielder chasing a fly ball, can cause excessive plantar flexion and/or dorsiflexion of the ankle and can result in a strain or rupture of the lower leg musculature. Moreover, repetitive running and jumping can cause inflammation of and injury to the soft tissues. Common injuries to the lower leg include:

• Contusions
• Strains
• Ruptures
• Overuse injuries and conditions

Contusions

Contusions to the lower leg are caused by direct forces and typically involve the tibia and/or posterior musculature. The tibia is susceptible to injury because overlying soft tissue does not provide a lot of protection. Direct forces to the tibia often affect the **periosteum** and cause irritation. Contusions to the posterior musculature frequently involve the gastrocnemius (see Illustration 5–1). These injuries are common in many athletic activities as a result of being kicked or struck with equipment.

Strains

Strains to the lower leg musculature are caused by a variety of mechanisms during athletic and work activities. Achilles tendon strains are caused by excessive dorsiflexion of the ankle (Illustration 5–1).[4] For example, a strain can occur as a soccer player suddenly decelerates, changes direction, and accelerates in the opposite direction off the right foot, causing excessive dorsiflexion of the right ankle. An inversion force to the ankle, excessive dorsiflexion, or a direct force to the posterior lateral malleolus can cause a peroneal tendon strain (see Illustration 5–2). With a violent eversion and dorsiflexion or inversion and plantar flexion force, the **peroneal retinaculum** can tear, causing a peroneal tendon **subluxation** and/or **dislocation**

(Illustration 5–2). A subluxation and/or dislocation can result, for example, when a wrestler's left foot is caught on the mat while the trunk is forced forward by an opponent during a takedown, causing eversion and dorsiflexion of the left ankle. Injury to the gastrocnemius, commonly the medial head, can result from activities involving rapid acceleration, deceleration, and jumping. Two common causes of gastrocnemius injury include dorsiflexion of the foot with forced knee extension and extension of the knee with forced foot dorsiflexion.

Ruptures

Complete rupture of the Achilles tendon is caused by the sudden acceleration that is common with many athletic activities. During the toe-off phase of the running gait, the foot is placed in plantar flexion while the knee moves toward full extension. While more common in individuals 30–50 years of age, because of chronic inflammation and degeneration,[1] ruptures have been seen in individuals of all ages.[3]

Overuse

Overload and repetitive stress from weight-bearing activities and structural abnormalities can cause lower leg overuse injuries and conditions. Repetitive tensile stress caused by excessive weight-bearing can result in **Achilles tendinitis.** Repetitive running on a downhill grade may lead to **anterior tibialis tendinitis** (see Illustration 5–3). **Posterior tibialis tendinitis** can be associated with foot pronation. Supination and pronation of the foot can result in **peroneal tendinitis.** Repetitive stress, supination or pronation of the foot, inflexibility and/or weakness of the musculature, and training errors can cause **medial tibial stress syndrome (MTSS).** Excessive running on hard surfaces such as asphalt or concrete in shoes without appropriate support or shock absorption can lead to the development of MTSS. Furthermore, **stress fractures** of the tibia or fibula may result from overload, foot pronation, pes cavus, training errors, **amenorrhea, oligomenorrhea,** and disordered eating and associated nutritional deficiencies. Overload and repetitive stress may also lead to **exertional compartment syndrome.**

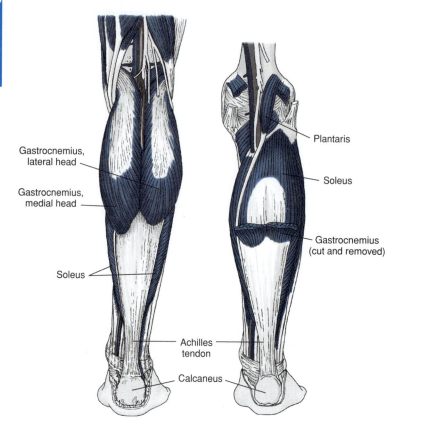

Gastrocnemius, lateral head

Gastrocnemius, medial head

Soleus

Achilles tendon

Calcaneus

Plantaris

Soleus

Gastrocnemius (cut and removed)

Illustration 5-1 Superficial muscles of the posterior lower leg.

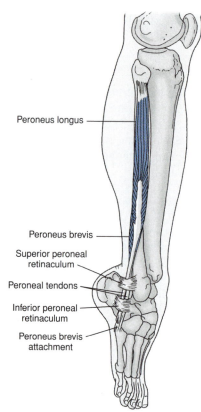

Peroneus longus

Peroneus brevis

Superior peroneal retinaculum

Peroneal tendons

Inferior peroneal retinaculum

Peroneus brevis attachment

Illustration 5-2 Peroneal muscles of the lateral lower leg.

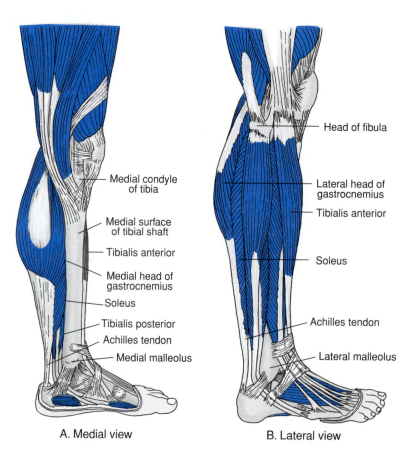

Medial condyle of tibia

Medial surface of tibial shaft

Tibialis anterior

Medial head of gastrocnemius

Soleus

Tibialis posterior

Achilles tendon

Medial malleolus

Head of fibula

Lateral head of gastrocnemius

Tibialis anterior

Soleus

Achilles tendon

Lateral malleolus

A. Medial view

B. Lateral view

Illustration 5-3 Superficial muscles of the lower leg.

Taping Techniques

Use several taping techniques to treat lower leg injuries and conditions, to limit excessive range of motion, support the musculature and soft tissue, and immobilize the foot, ankle, and lower leg.

ACHILLES TENDON Figures 5–1, 5–2

▶ **Purpose:** Use the Achilles tendon technique to treat strains and tendinitis, to limit excessive dorsiflexion and stretch on the tendon. Two interchangeable methods are illustrated in the application of the technique. Choose according to individual preferences (Fig. 5–1).

Achilles Tendon Technique One

▶ **Materials:**
  • 1½ inch non-elastic tape or 2 inch self-adherent wrap, 2 inch and 3 inch elastic tape, 3 inch heavyweight elastic tape, adherent tape spray, thin foam pads, taping scissors

  Option:
  • Pre-tape material

▶ **Position of the individual:** Prone, sitting, or kneeling on a taping table or bench, with the lower leg extended off the edge. Determine the range of dorsiflexion that produces pain by stabilizing the mid-to-distal lower leg. Place a hand on the plantar surface of the distal foot and slowly move the foot into dorsiflexion until pain occurs. Once painful range of motion is determined, place the involved foot in a pain-free range and maintain this position during application.

▶ **Preparation:** Apply adherent tape spray to the distal lower leg and distal plantar surface of the foot. Place a thin foam pad over the heel area to prevent irritation. Apply Technique One directly to the skin.

  Option: *Apply pre-tape material over the area to lessen irritation.*

▶ **Application:**
  STEP 1: Apply two anchors around the distal lower leg, with 1½ inch non-elastic tape or 2 inch self-adherent wrap, and one anchor around the ball of the foot, with 2 inch elastic tape or self-adherent wrap with moderate roll tension ◀▶ (Fig. 5–1A). The lower leg anchor may be placed inferior to the knee, around the upper portion of the gastrocnemius belly. Using this anchor will allow for additional tensile strength of the heavyweight elastic tape in limiting range of motion. Use 2 inch or 3 inch elastic tape for the anchor to prevent constriction.

  STEP 2: Using 3 inch heavyweight elastic tape, anchor a strip on the middle plantar foot and pull up toward the calcaneus (Fig. 5–1B).

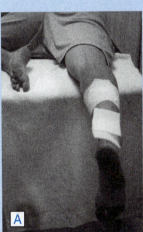

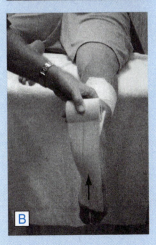

Figure 5-1

Lower Leg

STEP 3: Continue across the middle calcaneus, over the posterior lower leg, and finish on the posterior distal lower leg anchor (Fig. 5–1C). Apply moderate roll tension with the tape and monitor the pain-free position of the foot.

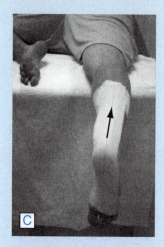

STEP 4: Anchor an additional 3 inch heavyweight elastic tape strip on the plantar foot over the first strip and pull the additional strip toward the distal lower leg anchor (Fig. 5–1D). Cut or tear this strip approximately 3–4 inches beyond the distal lower leg anchor.

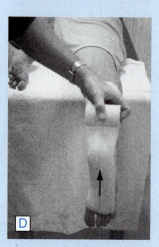

STEP 5: Tear or cut the proximal end of this strip lengthwise down the middle to an area just superior to the insertion of the Achilles tendon on the calcaneus (Fig. 5–1E).

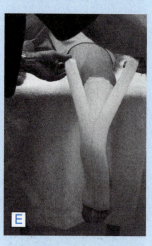

Figure 5-1 *continued*

STEP 6: Apply moderate tension on the tape ends and wrap each, in opposite directions, around the lower leg in a spiral pattern. Finish the pattern on the distal lower leg anchor (Fig. 5–1F).

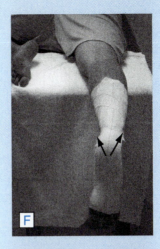

STEP 7: Apply two to four circular strips of 2 inch elastic tape around the midfoot and distal foot and four to six circular strips of 2 inch elastic tape around the lower leg with mild to moderate roll tension ◀▶ (Fig. 5–1G). Additional strips of non-elastic tape are not required.

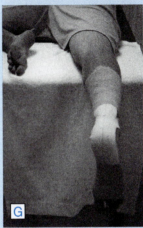

Figure 5-1 *continued*

Achilles Tendon Technique Two

▶ **Materials:**
   • 1½ inch non-elastic tape or 2 inch self-adherent wrap, 2 inch and 3 inch elastic tape, 2 inch heavyweight elastic tape, adherent tape spray, thin foam pads, taping scissors

   Option:
   • Pre-tape material

▶ **Position of the individual:** Prone, sitting, or kneeling on a taping table or bench, with the lower leg extended off the edge. Determine the range of dorsiflexion that produces pain, as explained above. After the painful range of motion has been determined, place the involved foot in a pain-free range and maintain this position during application.

▶ **Preparation:** Apply adherent tape spray to the distal lower leg and distal plantar surface of the foot. Place a thin foam pad over the heel area to prevent irritation. Apply Technique Two directly to the skin.

   Option: *Apply pre-tape material over the area to lessen irritation.*

▶ **Application:**
   STEP 1: Apply anchors as illustrated in Figure 5–1A.
   STEP 2: Anchor a strip of 2 inch heavyweight elastic tape on the middle plantar foot. Proceed over the middle calcaneus, and finish on the distal lower leg anchor (Fig. 5–2A). Apply moderate roll tension during strip application and monitor the pain-free position of the foot.

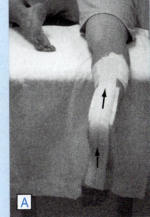

Figure 5-2

STEP 3: Anchor the next 2 inch heavyweight elastic tape strip at an angle over the head of the fifth metatarsal. Continue over the medial calcaneus, and anchor on the medial lower leg (Fig. 5–2B).

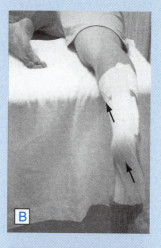

STEP 4: Place the last 2 inch heavyweight elastic tape strip at an angle over the head of the first metatarsal, proceed over the lateral calcaneus, and anchor on the lateral lower leg (Fig. 5–2C).

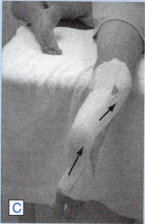

STEP 5: Apply circular strips around the foot and lower leg with 2 inch elastic tape (Fig. 5–2D).

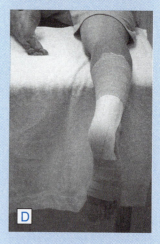

Figure 5-2 *continued*

DORSAL BRIDGE Figure 5–3

▸ **Purpose:** The dorsal bridge technique limits excessive plantar flexion and stretch on the tendon when treating anterior tibialis tendinitis (Fig. 5–3). This technique also can be used with ankle sprains to limit plantar flexion, which is often temporarily lost following injury. When treating sprains, the dorsal bridge may be used in combination with the closed basketweave (see Fig. 4–1), elastic (see Fig. 4–4), Spartan Slipper (see Fig. 4–6), or subtalar sling (see Fig. 4–7) taping techniques to limit excessive plantar flexion further and lessen additional stress on bony and ligamentous structures.

▸ **Materials:**
  • 1½ inch non-elastic tape or 2 inch self-adherent wrap, 2 inch elastic tape, 3 inch heavyweight elastic tape, adherent tape spray, thin foam pads, taping scissors

Option:
• Pre-tape material

▶ **Position of the individual:** Sitting on a taping table or bench with the lower leg extended off the edge. Determine the range of plantar flexion that produces pain by stabilizing the mid-to-distal lower leg. Place a hand on the dorsal surface of the distal foot. Slowly move the foot into plantar flexion until pain occurs. After painful range of motion has been determined, place the involved foot in a pain-free range and maintain this position during application.

▶ **Preparation:** Apply adherent tape spray to the distal lower leg and foot. Place a thin foam pad over the lace area to prevent irritation. Apply the dorsal bridge directly to the skin.

Option: *Apply pre-tape material over the area to lessen irritation.*

▶ **Application:**

STEP 1: Place two anchor strips around the distal lower leg, with 1½ inch non-elastic tape or 2 inch self-adherent wrap, and place one anchor around the ball of the foot, with 2 inch elastic tape or self-adherent wrap.

STEP 2: Anchor a strip of 3 inch heavyweight elastic tape on the middle dorsal foot and pull with moderate tension toward the lower leg. Anchor the strip on the middle anterior lower leg (Fig. 5–3A). Apply an additional bridge over the first strip.

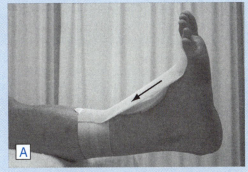

STEP 3: To prevent migration or slippage of the strip(s) during activity, tear or cut the ends lengthwise down the middle and anchor on the distal foot and lower leg in a spiral pattern ✂ (Fig. 5–3B).

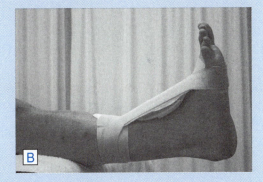

Helpful Hint: If migration of the heavyweight elastic tape strips used with the Achilles tendon or dorsal bridge taping techniques continues, just cut longer strips and anchor in a spiral pattern as before. The longer strips will allow for additional anchoring on the foot and lower leg, and should lessen migration.

STEP 4: Apply two to four circular strips of 2 inch elastic tape around the lower leg and two to three strips of 2 inch elastic tape around the distal foot with mild to moderate roll tension ◀▶ (Fig. 5–3C). Additional strips of non-elastic tape are not required.

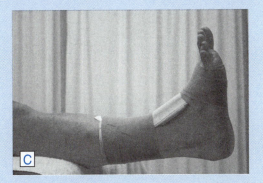

Figure 5-3

STEP 5: Following application of the ankle taping technique, place pre-tape material or self-adherent wrap from the midfoot closure strips to the ball of the foot ◄—► .

STEP 6: Place an anchor around the ball of the foot ◄—► and proceed with the application of the dorsal bridge.

STEP 7: Finish with the application of circular strips with 1½ inch non-elastic or 2 inch elastic tape on the lower leg and foot ◄—► (Fig. 5–3D). A strip of 1½ inch non-elastic tape may be placed over the bridge from the lateral malleolus to the medial malleolus. Do not encircle the ankle with this strip.

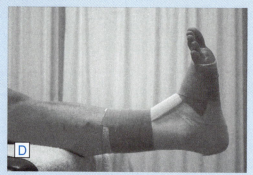

Figure 5-3 *continued*

PERONEAL TENDON Figure 5–4

▶ **Purpose:** The peroneal tendon technique can be used to treat strains when an individual is returning to activity (Fig. 5–4). This technique is effective because it limits excessive inversion and eversion at the subtalar joint and provides moderate support and stability to the tendon as it passes posterior to the lateral malleolus.

▶ **Materials:**
   • 1½ inch non-elastic tape, 2 inch self-adherent wrap, 2 inch elastic tape, 2 inch or 3 inch moleskin, adherent tape spray, thin foam pads, ¼ inch or ½ inch felt, taping scissors

   Option:
   • Pre-tape material

▶ **Position of the individual:** Sitting on a taping table or bench with the leg extended off the edge with the foot in 90° of dorsiflexion.

▶ **Preparation:** Apply adherent tape spray to the distal lower leg and foot. Place a thin foam pad over the heel and lace areas. Apply the peroneal tendon technique directly to the skin.

   Option: *Apply pre-tape material over the area to lessen irritation.*

▶ **Application:**
   STEP 1: With 2 inch elastic tape, apply two anchor strips with mild roll tension around the lower leg over the distal gastrocnemius belly ◄—► ✂ (Fig. 5–4A). An additional midfoot anchor of 1½ inch non-elastic tape or 2 inch self-adherent wrap may be applied, but this is not required ◄—► .

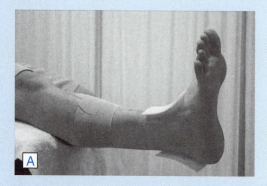

Figure 5-4

Helpful Hint: These anchors are placed in a more proximal position on the lower leg than the anchors used with the ankle taping techniques, to allow for additional tensile strength of the moleskin and non-elastic tape. Monitor roll tension to prevent constriction of the gastrocnemius muscle. Constriction can cause pain, muscle spasm, tingling, and/or numbness in the gastrocnemius and distal lower leg and foot.

STEP 2: Apply a 2 inch or 3 inch moleskin stirrup (see Fig. 4–3C-F). Proceed with the application of the closed basketweave (see Fig. 4–1) or Spartan Slipper (see Fig. 4–6) taping technique to limit excessive inversion and eversion further, omitting heel locks (Fig. 5–4B).

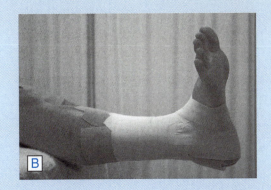

STEP 3: Using ¼ inch or ½ inch felt, cut a pad in the shape of an uppercase "L." The pad provides additional compression and stabilization of the tendon in the fibular groove. The pad extends from 3–4 inches superior to the posterior lateral malleolus, continues distal, and turns in an anterior direction inferior to the malleolus. The pad is approximately 1–1½ inches wide (Fig. 5–4C).

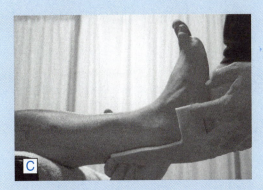

STEP 4: Place the pad around the posterior superior/inferior lateral malleolus and apply a continuous heel lock (see Fig. 4–2) using 2 inch elastic tape with moderate roll tension. Apply an additional heel lock with 1½ inch non-elastic tape (Fig. 5–4D).

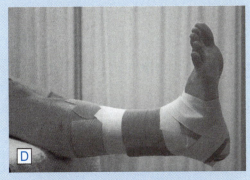

Figure 5-4 *continued*

SPIRAL LOWER LEG Figure 5–5

▶ **Purpose:** Use the spiral lower leg technique to provide mild to moderate compression over the lower leg when treating MTSS (Fig. 5–5). Anecdotally, compression over inflamed areas, such as the lower leg, may lessen pain levels. However, with some individuals, this technique may increase pain. Following application, monitor for an increase in pain levels during activity.

▶ **Materials:**
  • 1½ inch non-elastic tape, adherent tape spray

▶ **Position of the individual:** Standing on a taping table or bench with the majority of the weight on the noninvolved leg and the involved leg in slight knee flexion. Maintain this position by placing a 1½ inch lift under the heel.

▶ **Preparation:** Apply adherent tape spray to the anterior, medial, and lateral lower leg. Apply the spiral technique directly to the skin.

▶ **Application:**

$\boxed{\text{STEP 1:}}$ Apply two anchors to the anterior proximal and distal lower leg with 1½ inch non-elastic tape ◀▶ . Next, apply longitudinal anchors to the medial and lateral lower leg, extending from the proximal to distal anchors ◀▶ (Fig. 5–5A).

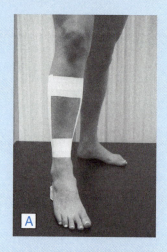

$\boxed{\text{STEP 2:}}$ With 1½ inch non-elastic tape, anchor at an upward angle on the distal lateral lower leg. Continue across the anterior lower leg, pulling in a medial direction with moderate roll tension, and finish on the medial anchor (Fig. 5–5B).

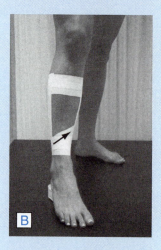

$\boxed{\text{STEP 3:}}$ Apply the next strip on the distal lateral lower leg at a downward angle and proceed across the lower leg to the medial anchor with moderate roll tension, pulling in a medial direction (Fig. 5–5C).

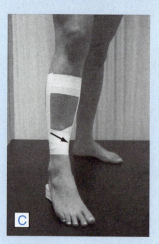

Figure 5-5

STEP 4: Continue to apply strips in this criss-cross pattern to the proximal lower leg anchors, overlapping by ½ of the tape width (Fig. 5–5D).

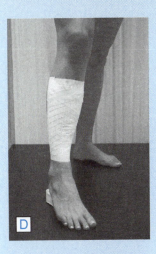

STEP 5: Place a medial and lateral longitudinal anchor over the tape ends ◄━► (Fig. 5–5E).

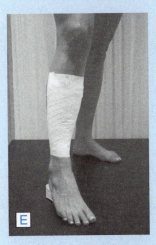

Figure 5-5 *continued*

POSTERIOR SPLINT

▶ **Purpose:** Use the posterior splint technique to immobilize the foot and ankle when treating an Achilles tendon rupture and peroneal tendon subluxation and/or dislocation (see Fig. 4–9). The techniques are commonly used in the acute treatment stages as temporary immobilization, but can also be used for extended periods of immobilization.

• Rigid, padded splints are available off-the-shelf in pre-cut widths and lengths, and can be molded quickly to the individual.
• Use rigid cast tape over stockinet to immobilize the area.
• Off-the-shelf and cast tape splints require an elastic wrap to attach the splint to the lower leg, ankle, and foot.
• The individual will require crutches for non–weight-bearing ambulation.

CAST TAPE

▶ **Purpose:** Orthopedic technicians or physicians commonly apply rigid cast tape to immobilize the foot, ankle, and lower leg completely when treating peroneal tendon subluxations and/or dislocations, Achilles tendon ruptures, gastrocnemius strains, posterior tibialis tendinitis, MTSS, and stress fractures.

• Periods of immobilization are typically determined by a physician.
• The majority of the rigid casts applied for these injuries are referred to as short-leg, extending from the inferior knee to the toes.
• Cast tape is applied over stockinet and soft cast or Gore-Tex padding.

CIRCULAR, "X," LOOP, AND WEAVE ARCH

▸ **Purpose:** When treating MTSS, several arch taping techniques provide support to the foot and correct structural abnormalities.
- Use the circular arch (see Fig. 3–1) technique to provide mild support to the longitudinal arch.
- Use the "X" (see Fig. 3–2), loop (see Fig. 3–3), and weave (see Fig. 3–4) arch techniques to provide mild to moderate support to both the longitudinal arch and forefoot.

LOW-DYE

▸ **Purpose:** Use the Low-Dye technique to provide moderate support of the foot/forefoot and limit excessive pronation when treating peroneal and posterior tibialis tendinitis and MTSS. The two methods are illustrated in Chapter 3 (see Figs. 3–5 and 3–6), in the context of arch strains and plantar fasciitis treatment.

Critical Thinking Question 1

The personnel manager at the local textile manufacturing plant suffers a mild left Achilles tendon strain when playing basketball at the high school gym. You apply the Achilles tendon technique to limit excessive dorsiflexion prior to his athletic activities. Shortly after he begins to play, the taping technique migrates distally, allowing full dorsiflexion.

▸ **Question: How can you manage this problem?**

...IF/THEN...

IF using the circular, "X," loop, or weave arch taping techniques to support the longitudinal arch and/or forefoot when treating MTSS and pain is not lessened, **THEN** consider applying the Low-Dye taping technique or using a soft, semirigid, or rigid orthotic design; these techniques provide support to the longitudinal arch and/or forefoot and correct structural abnormalities, such as excessive pronation in the treatment of MTSS. These techniques also may lessen pain.

Wrapping Techniques

Use compression wrap techniques to control swelling in the acute treatment of Achilles tendon strains and ruptures, peroneal tendon and gastrocnemius strains, and muscle and/or bone contusions. There are three wrapping methods, using elastic wraps and sleeves, that provide mechanical pressure over the lower leg or lower leg and foot following injury, to control and lessen distal migration of swelling.

COMPRESSION WRAP TECHNIQUE ONE Figure 5–6

▸ **Purpose:** The wrap technique for many lower leg strains, ruptures, and distal contusions should include the foot, ankle, and lower leg to assist in controlling swelling and lessening distal migration. This technique controls mild, moderate, or severe swelling (Fig. 5–6).

▸ **Materials:**
- 3 inch, 4 inch, or 6 inch width by 5 or 10 yard length elastic wrap, or 3 inch, 4 inch, and 6 inch width self-adherent wrap, metal clips, 1½ inch non-elastic or 2 inch elastic tape, taping scissors

Options:
- ¼ inch or ½ inch foam or felt

▶ **Position of the individual:** Sitting on a taping table or bench with the leg extended off the edge and the foot in pain-free dorsiflexion.

▶ **Preparation:** Apply the compression wrap directly to the skin.

▶ **Application:**

STEP 1: Anchor the end of the wrap on the distal plantar foot and apply the foot and ankle compression wrap (see Fig. 3–15). Apply the greatest amount of roll tension distally and over the injured area. Lessen the roll tension as the wrap continues proximally from the injured area.

STEP 2: At the distal lower leg, continue the spiral wrap proximally to the inferior knee ◀▶ (Fig. 5–6A). The technique may require using multiple elastic wraps or rolls of self-adherent wrap. Anchor the wrap with Velcro, metal clips, or loosely applied 1½ inch non-elastic or 2 inch elastic tape ◀▶ ✂.

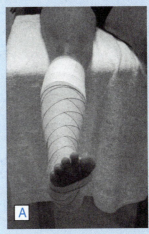

 Helpful Hint: With ambulation, monitor the proximal gastrocnemius and popliteal space for irritation from the wrap, which may occur with repetitive knee flexion.

Option: *The horseshoe pad technique (see Fig. 4–19), along with the compression wrap, may be used when treating peroneal tendon subluxations and/or dislocations to provide additional compression over the area and assist in venous return. Place the pad directly on the skin over the lateral malleolus and cover it with the compression wrap (Fig. 5–6B).*

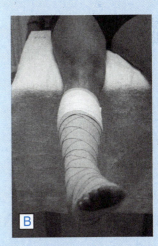

Figure 5-6

COMPRESSION WRAP TECHNIQUE TWO Figure 5–7

▶ **Purpose:** Use this compression wrap technique to assist in reducing mild or moderate swelling in the acute treatment of muscle and/or bone contusions to the mid and proximal lower leg (Fig. 5–7).

▶ **Materials:**
- 3 inch or 4 inch width by 5 yard length elastic wrap or self-adherent wrap, metal clips, 1½ inch non-elastic or 2 inch elastic tape, taping scissors

Options:
• ⅛ inch or ¼ inch foam or felt

▶ **Position of the individual:** Sitting on a taping table or bench with the leg extended off the edge.

▶ **Preparation:** Apply the compression wrap directly to the skin.

Option: Cut a ⅛ inch or ¼ inch foam or felt pad and place it over the inflamed area directly to the skin to provide additional compression and assist in venous return.

▶ **Application:**

STEP 1: Anchor the wrap around the distal lower leg and continue in a distal-to-proximal spiral pattern toward the inferior knee ◀▶ (Fig. 5–7A). Apply the greatest amount of roll tension distally and lessen as the wrap continues proximally.

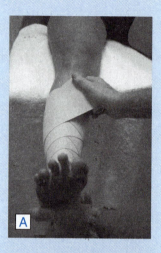

STEP 2: Anchor with Velcro, metal clips, or loosely applied 1½ inch non-elastic or 2 inch elastic tape ◀▶ (Fig. 5–7B).

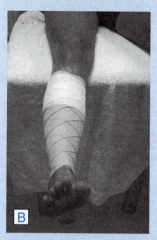

Figure 5-7

COMPRESSION WRAP TECHNIQUE THREE Figure 5–8

▶ **Purpose:** Using an elastic sleeve over the lower leg will also control mild, moderate, or severe swelling (Fig. 5–8). After receiving instructions on application, the individual can apply and remove this compression wrap without assistance.

▶ **Materials:**
• 3 inch elastic sleeve, taping scissors

Options:
• ⅛ inch or ¼ inch foam or felt

▶ **Position of the individual:** Sitting on a taping table or bench with the leg extended off the edge.

▶ **Preparation:** Apply the elastic sleeve directly to the skin.

Option: Cut a ⅛ inch or ¼ inch foam or felt pad and place it over the inflamed area directly to the skin to assist in the control of swelling.

Application:

STEP 1: Cut a sleeve from a roll to extend from the inferior knee to the distal lower leg. A double length sleeve may also be cut and used to provide additional compression.

STEP 2: Pull the sleeve onto the lower leg in a distal-to-proximal direction (Fig. 5–8). If using a double length sleeve, pull the distal end over the first layer to provide an additional layer. No anchors are required. Clean and reuse the sleeve.

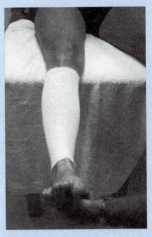

Figure 5-8

Critical Thinking Question 2

Two days ago, a warehouse worker was struck in the proximal right lower leg with a metal cart. He was sent to a physician for evaluation and was diagnosed with a moderate proximal tibial contusion. An elastic wrap was applied over the proximal lower leg to control swelling. Today, he returns with ecchymosis and swelling in the distal lower leg and foot.

▶ **Question: What wrapping techniques can be used in this situation?**

...IF/THEN...

IF an athlete is recovering from a mid tibial contusion and the physician allows a return to practice even though mild swelling remains in the area, **THEN** consider using an elastic sleeve under the protective pad to control the swelling; the sleeve may be more comfortable than an elastic wrap during practice.

Bracing Techniques

Many of these bracing techniques have been discussed previously and can be used to treat a variety of lower leg injuries and conditions. Walking boots and orthotics, discussed in greater detail in Chapter 3, are used to prevent and treat lower leg strains, ruptures, and overuse injuries and conditions. Ankle braces, illustrated in Chapter 4, can be used to treat strains and overuse injuries and conditions.

WALKING BOOT

▶ **Purpose:** Use walking boots (see Fig. 3–23) to provide complete support and immobilization when treating peroneal tendon subluxations and/or dislocations, gastrocnemius strains, Achilles tendon ruptures, posterior tibialis tendinitis, MTSS, and stress fractures.
  • Use the boots to provide lower leg, ankle, and foot support during non–weight-bearing and full weight-bearing rehabilitation periods ♩.

Helpful Hint: When using walking boots in warm, humid environments, place a sock over the involved foot before applying the boot to absorb perspiration and reduce soiling of the inner lining.

• The boots are commonly used in place of rigid casts. The boot allows for removal and treatment, range of motion adjustments, and gait training.

ORTHOTICS

▶ **Purpose:** Soft, semirigid, and rigid orthotic designs provide support, absorb shock, and correct structural abnormalities, while preventing and treating lower leg injuries and conditions.
• Use soft orthotic designs (see Fig. 3–16), such as heel cups and full-length neoprene, silicone, and viscoelastic polymer insoles, to provide shock absorption when treating MTSS and stress fractures. These designs assist in lessening repetitive stress to the lower leg.
• Use semirigid (see Fig. 3–17) and rigid (see Fig. 3–18) orthotics to provide support and correct structural abnormalities, such as excessive foot pronation or supination, when treating Achilles, posterior tibialis, and peroneal tendinitis, stress fractures, MTSS, and exertional compartment syndrome.

NEOPRENE SLEEVE Figure 5–9

▶ **Purpose:** Neoprene sleeves provide compression and mild support when treating gastrocnemius strains, muscle and bone contusions, and MTSS (Fig 5–9). Compression over the injured area may reduce pain levels in some individuals.

▶ **Design:**
• Neoprene sleeves come in off-the-shelf designs in predetermined sizes that correspond to lower leg circumference measurements.
• Extended wear and cleaning of neoprene sleeves may cause them to shrink, resulting in difficulties during daily application .

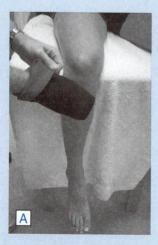

Helpful Hint: Lessen problems with application of neoprene sleeves by first turning the sleeve inside-out (Fig. 5–9A). Next, place the smaller end over the foot (Fig. 5–9B). Pull the sleeve proximally onto the lower leg and stop when the smaller end approaches its normal distal location on the lower leg (Fig. 5–9C). Lastly, pull the larger end proximally and over the sleeve to its normal location (Fig. 5–9D). Talcum powder may also be applied on the inside of the sleeve to lessen problems.

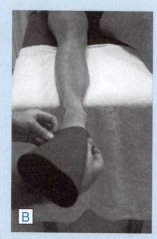
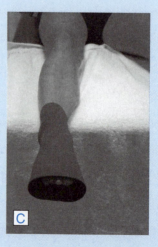
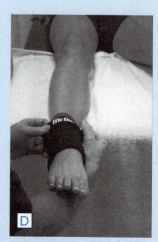

Figure 5-9

▸ **Position of the individual:** Sitting on a taping table or bench with the leg extended off the edge, or in a chair.

▸ **Preparation:** Apply neoprene sleeves directly to the skin; no anchors are required.

▸ **Application:**

STEP 1: To apply, hold each side of the sleeve and place the larger end over the foot (Fig. 5–9E).

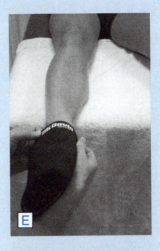

STEP 2: Continue to pull proximally until the sleeve is positioned on the lower leg (Fig. 5–9F).

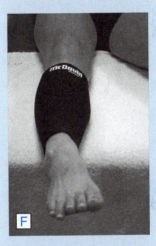

Figure 5-9 *continued*

Critical Thinking Question 3

A cross-country runner begins to develop signs and symptoms of MTSS. The treatment plan includes therapeutic modalities and stretching and strengthening exercises. Along with off-the-shelf soft orthotics, you would like to use a neoprene sleeve to provide compression and support. However, the runner is allergic to several materials used in the manufacturing of neoprene.

▸ **Question: What are the alternative techniques you can use?**

ANKLE BRACES

▸ **Purpose:** Several ankle brace designs can be used to treat peroneal tendon and stress fracture injuries. The braces provide compression and/or moderate support when treating these injuries and can be applied by the individual, following proper instruction.

• Use air/gel bladder braces (see Fig. 4–16) to provide additional compression to control swelling in the acute treatment of subluxations and/or dislocations. These braces may be used in combination with the compression wrap techniques (see Fig. 3–15) to assist in venous return.

Lower Leg

- Air/gel bladder braces are also used when treating stress fractures of the tibia and/or fibula. Lower leg designs are constructed with longer medial and lateral stirrups or shells to provide support to the proximal, mid, and distal lower leg.

RESEARCH BRIEF

Several investigators have demonstrated a reduction in the time required for recreational and competitive athletes who used air/gel bladder braces to return to activity following tibial stress fractures.[2,7,8]

Researchers have suggested that air/gel bladder braces stabilize the tibia and shift some of the weight-bearing forces away from the fracture site to the soft tissues, allowing an earlier return to activity.[7]

- Use lace-up (see Fig. 4–14) and semirigid (see Fig. 4–15) designs during a return to athletic or work activities to limit inversion, eversion, plantar flexion, dorsiflexion, and rotation with peroneal tendon strains.
- Air/gel, lace-up, and semirigid braces are available off-the-shelf in predetermined sizes.

Critical Thinking Question 4

During the second half of the women's basketball game, an official sprints down the court in advance of a fast break. The team misses the layup, and the opponents start a fast break toward their goal. The official quickly stops, turns, and sprints toward the other end of the court. He feels a pop in his left lower leg and immediately stops, suffering a ruptured Achilles tendon. The team physician refers the official to a local orthopedic surgeon for further evaluation.

▶ **Question: What immobilization options are available in this situation and under what circumstances would you choose one option over another?**

...IF/THEN...

IF applying the peroneal tendon taping technique and adequate compression and support is not provided to the tendon in the fibular groove, **THEN** consider using a lace-up or semirigid ankle brace in combination with the taping technique to provide additional compression over the tendon and further limit excessive inversion and eversion at the subtalar joint.

Padding Techniques

Use foam, felt, and thermoplastic materials to offer support, absorb shock, and provide protection when preventing and treating lower leg injuries and conditions. Foam and felt materials can be used to provide support and absorb shock when treating strains, ruptures, and overuse injuries and conditions. Foam and thermoplastic materials are used to prevent and treat contusions. Several high school and intercollegiate sports require mandatory padding of the lower leg. These padding techniques will be discussed in Chapter 13.

OFF-THE-SHELF Figure 5–10

▶ **Purpose:** Padding materials may be molded and attached to off-the-shelf pad designs to provide additional protection following a contusion (Fig. 5–10). Off-the-shelf designs can be found in Chapter 13.

▶ **Materials:**
- ⅛ inch, ¼ inch, or ½ inch open-cell foam, rubber cement, 2 inch elastic tape, thermoplastic material, taping scissors

▶ **Position of the individual:** Sitting on a taping table or bench with the lower leg extended off the edge in a functional position.

▶ **Preparation:** Cut the appropriate size of foam to overlap the shin guard.

▶ **Application:**

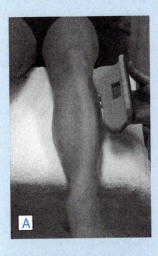

STEP 1: Cut open-cell foam of ⅛ inch, ¼ inch, or ½ inch thickness to the dimensions of a shin guard and attach the foam to the inside surface with rubber cement or 2 inch elastic tape (Fig. 5–10A). Cut a hole or donut in the foam over the contusion to disperse the impact force.

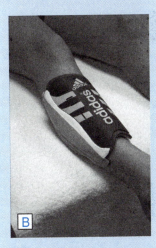

STEP 2: Consider molding and attaching a piece of thermoplastic material with rubber cement or 2 inch elastic tape to a shin guard to protect a medial or lateral contusion (Fig. 5–10B).

Figure 5-10

Helpful Hint: Check to make sure normal range of motion is allowed at the knee, talocrural, and/or subtalar joints when using off-the-shelf or thermoplastic pads over the proximal or distal lower leg.

CUSTOM-MADE Figure 5–11

▶ **Purpose:** Use thermoplastic material to construct custom-made pads to provide protection when preventing and treating lower leg muscle and bone contusions (Fig. 5–11). Many construct these pads when off-the-shelf designs are not available or a comfortable fit cannot be achieved.

▶ **Materials:**
  • Paper, felt tip pen, thermoplastic material, ⅛ inch or ¼ inch foam or felt, taping scissors, a heating source, 2 inch or 3 inch elastic tape or self-adherent wrap, pre-tape material, an elastic wrap, soft, low-density foam, rubber cement

  Options:
  • 1 inch or 1½ inch non-elastic or 2 inch elastic tape

▶ **Position of the individual:** Sitting on a taping table or bench with the lower leg extended off the edge in a functional position.

▶ **Preparation:** Design the pad with a paper pattern (see Fig. 1–14). Cut, mold, and shape the thermoplastic material on the lower leg over the injured area. Attach soft, low-density foam to the inside surface of the material (see Fig. 1–15).

▶ **Application:**

(**STEP 1:**) Attach the pad to the lower leg with 2 inch or 3 inch elastic tape, or self-adherent wrap over pre-tape material, or directly to the skin. Use strips or a circular pattern with moderate roll tension (Fig. 5–11A). One to two circular strips of 1½ inch non-elastic tape may be applied loosely around the pad for additional anchors. Monitor roll tension over the gastrocnemius to prevent constriction.

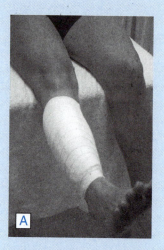

A

Helpful Hint: Anchor the elastic tape directly on the thermoplastic material and continue with application. The tape adhesive bond on the thermoplastic material will lessen migration of the pad during activity.

Option: *Attach the pad to the lower leg by placing the pad underneath a knee-high sock. Apply strips of 1 inch or 1½ inch non-elastic or 2 inch elastic tape over the sock to provide additional anchors* (Fig. 5–11B).

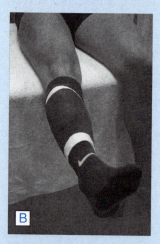

B

Figure 5-11

HEEL LIFT Figure 5–12

▶ **Purpose:** Use this heel lift pad technique to absorb shock, elevate the hindfoot, and lessen the stress and stretch on the tendon and muscle during activity, when treating strains, tendinitis, ruptures of the Achilles tendon, and strains of the gastrocnemius (Fig. 5–12). The heel pad technique, constructed of foam, illustrated in Chapter 3 (see Fig. 3–28), also provides shock absorption when treating MTSS. When soft heel cups are not available, foam heel pads may be used to lessen repetitive stress to the lower leg.

▶ **Materials:**
  • ⅛ inch, ¼ inch, or ½ inch felt, taping scissors

▶ **Position of the individual:** Sitting on a taping table or bench with the leg extended off the edge and the foot in a dorsiflexed position.

▶ **Preparation:** Construct the pads from ⅛ inch, ¼ inch, or ½ inch felt or purchase in pre-cut designs with adhesive backing. The pads should cover the entire heel or shoe liner heel area. To prevent adaptive changes with the use of one pad, such as changes in walking and/or running gaits, place a heel lift on each heel or in each shoe.

Application:

STEP 1: Taper the distal end of the pad and attach it to the heel with adhesive gauze material, 2 inch elastic tape or self-adherent wrap, or cement the pad to the shoe liner (Fig. 5–12).

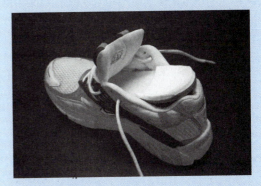

Figure 5-12

○ **DETAILS**

Using certain types of footwear can also elevate the hindfoot and lessen the stress and stretch on the Achilles tendon and gastrocnemius. Shoes with medium heels of 1–2 inches can elevate the hindfoot and lessen stress and stretch on these structures. Cowboy boots are a common shoe design that can be used.

MEDIAL WEDGE Figure 5–13

Purpose: Use the medial wedge pad when treating posterior tibialis tendinitis to prevent excessive foot pronation (Fig. 5–13). The pad elevates the medial aspect of the calcaneus, limiting excessive pronation.

Materials:
- ⅛ inch, ¼ inch, or ½ inch felt, cement, taping scissors

Position of the individual: Sitting on a taping table or bench or chair.

Preparation: Either purchase off-the-shelf designs or construct a medial wedge from ⅛ inch, ¼ inch, or ½ inch felt and attach it to the shoe insole. Outline the dimensions of the insole heel area on the felt.

Application:

STEP 1: When constructing a medial wedge, the dimensions of the wedge should cover the calcaneus and extend distally to the proximal longitudinal arch (Fig. 5–13A).

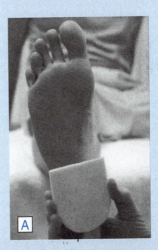

STEP 2: Draw a longitudinal line bisecting the middle of the wedge and cut out the medial portion (Fig. 5–13B). Using taping scissors, taper the medial side of the pad.

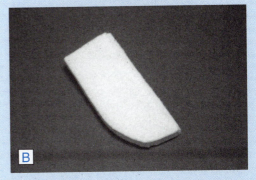

Figure 5-13

STEP 3: Position the wedge pad on the medial aspect of the insole and attach the pad with cement (Fig. 5–13C).

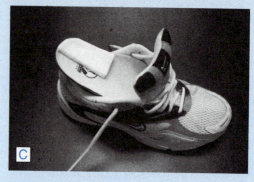

Figure 5-13 *continued*

LONGITUDINAL ARCH

▶ **Purpose:** Use the longitudinal arch pad technique to provide mild to moderate support of the arch when treating MTSS and stress fractures (see Fig. 3–26). The pads are available off-the-shelf or cut from foam or felt. These pads may be used when orthotics are not available. Attach the pad with the circular arch technique (see Fig. 3–1).

MANDATORY PADDING

The NCAA[5] and the NFHS[6] require the use of mandatory protective equipment for the lower leg in several sports. Baseball, field hockey, ice hockey, soccer, and softball athletes are required to wear protective padding on the lower leg during all practices and competitions. The majority of these pads come in off-the-shelf designs. An in-depth discussion of these pads can be found in Chapter 13.

Critical Thinking Question 5

While batting in the fourth inning, the right fielder on the baseball team fouls a ball off his right lateral lower leg. After several days of treatment, the physician allows him to return to activity if protected with padding.

▶ **Question: What padding techniques are appropriate in this situation?**

...IF/THEN...

IF felt heel lifts are effective in lessening the stress and stretch of the Achilles tendon when treating tendinitis, *THEN* consider using custom-made orthotics with heel lifts, which will eliminate the need for daily construction and application of the felt pad.

CASE STUDY

Melissa Hoover is an investment banker at Kozack Financial Services in town. She is currently in week 6 of a 20-week training schedule for the local marathon. Melissa has been running for the past three years, averaging approximately 12–15 miles per week. During the past three years, she has experienced occasional lower leg pain, which she always relieved by purchasing new shoes. Melissa's training schedule was designed by a local running club, specifically for first-time marathoners. Week one began with a total of 16 miles and progressed to 21 miles at week 6. The scheduled mileage peaks at week 18 with a total of 36 miles, then decreases as the marathon approaches. Monday and Friday are rest days, and a long run is scheduled for each Sunday.

During week three, Melissa began to experience a periodic dull ache in her distal right lower leg. She continued training as scheduled. Melissa noticed that the dull ache progressed to constant pain in the area during week 4, especially at night following her morning run. Again, she continued the scheduled training. As week 5 progressed, she began to experience the pain prior to, during, and after each run. The pain was centered in her distal right posteromedial tibia. She also noticed that the medium/high-heeled shoes she wore to work increased the intensity of the pain. Melissa believed that some amount of pain was normal for this type of training and attempted to continue with the training. She decided to take an extra rest day in week 6 and resume training the following day. But Melissa was unable to run the scheduled mileage because of the intense pain in her right lower leg. After obtaining a physician's referral, she contacts a friend, Jennifer Coughlin, who is a PT/ATC at Tolsma Orthopedic Clinic, and schedules an appointment.

Following a static and dynamic evaluation, Jennifer discovers excessive right foot pronation during walking and running gaits. The wear pattern on Melissa's running and work shoes demonstrates the pronation. Jennifer finds point tenderness with palpation, along the distal posteromedial border of the tibia. Bilateral range of motion and strength are normal, but pain is produced with resisted plantar flexion in the right foot. Active weight-bearing movements on the distal right toes also produce pain. Jennifer notes inflexibility of the right heelcord. Jennifer refers Melissa to a physician for further evaluation of suspected medial tibial stress syndrome. The physician finds point tenderness in the distal right tibia with no crepitus, deformity, or neurological symptoms. Radiographs and bone scan reveal no bony pathology. The physician's recommendation is to begin treatment of medial tibial stress syndrome.

Jennifer designs a therapeutic exercise program for Melissa that includes rest, flexibility and strengthening exercises, and modalities for symptomatic treatment. What taping and/or bracing techniques would provide compression, support, shock absorption, and correction of structural abnormalities for Melissa's condition? What padding designs would provide shock absorption, support, and correction of structural abnormalities in the management of this case?

WRAP UP

- Lower leg contusions, strains, ruptures, and overuse injuries and conditions can be caused by excessive range of motion and acute and chronic stresses.
- The Achilles tendon, dorsal bridge, and peroneal tendon taping techniques limit excessive dorsiflexion, plantar flexion, and inversion/eversion of the foot, respectively.
- The Low-Dye and arch taping techniques provide support to the foot and correct structural abnormalities.
- The spiral lower leg technique can be used to provide compression when treating MTSS.
- The posterior splint and cast tape techniques provide immobilization of the foot, ankle, and lower leg.
- Elastic wraps and sleeves and self-adherent wraps provide mechanical pressure to the lower leg in the acute treatment of swelling.
- Walking boots and ankle braces provide support and limit range of motion.
- Orthotics can be used when treating acute and chronic lower leg injuries.
- A neoprene sleeve provides support and compression to the lower leg.
- The heel lift, medial wedge, and longitudinal arch padding techniques provide shock absorption, support, and correction of structural abnormalities.
- Thermoplastic materials provide protection when preventing and treating lower leg contusions.
- The NCAA and NFHS require the use of mandatory protective equipment for the lower leg in several sports.

■ WEB REFERENCES

About
http://sportsmedicine.about.com/
- This site provides access to lower leg information on injuries and conditions as well as prevention and treatment methods.

SportsInjuryClinic.net
http://www.sportsinjuryclinic.net/
- This site allows you to search an injury index for the treatment and rehabilitation of a variety of lower leg injuries and conditions.

■ REFERENCES

1. Brown, DE: Ankle and leg injuries. In Mellion, MB, Walsh, WM, and Shelton, GL (eds): The Team Physician's Handbook. Hanley & Belfus, Philadelphia, 1997.
2. Dickson, TB, Jr, and Kichline, PD: Functional management of stress fractures in female athletes using a pneumatic leg brace. Am J Sports Med 15:86–89, 1987.
3. Leppilahti, I, and Orava, S: Total Achilles tendon rupture: A review. Sports Med 25:79, 1998.
4. Prentice, WE: Arnheim's Principles of Athletic Training, ed 11. McGraw-Hill, Boston, 2003.
5. National Collegiate Athletic Association, http://www.ncaa.org/library/sports_sciences/sports_med_handbook/2003-04/2003-04_sports_med_handbook.pdf, Sports medicine handbook, 2003–2004.
6. National Federation of State High School Associations. 2004–2005 Soccer Rules Book. Indianapolis, IN: National Federation of State High School Associations; 2004.
7. Swenson, EJ, Jr, DeHaven, KE, Sebastianelli, WJ, Hanks, G, Kalenak, A, and Lynch, JM: The effect of a pneumatic leg brace on return to play in athletes with tibial stress fractures. Am J Sports Med 25:322–328, 1997.
8. Whitelaw, GP, Wetzler, MJ, Levy, AS, Segal, D, and Bissonnette, K: A pneumatic leg brace for the treatment of tibial stress fractures. Clin Orthop 270:301–305, 1991.

Knee

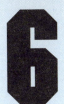

CHAPTER

6

LEARNING OBJECTIVES

1. Discuss common injuries that occur to the knee.
2. Demonstrate the application of taping, wrapping, bracing, and padding techniques when preventing, treating, and rehabilitating knee injuries.
3. Explain and demonstrate appropriate taping, wrapping, bracing, and padding techniques for the knee within a therapeutic exercise program.

INJURIES AND CONDITIONS

Injury to the knee can occur from acute and chronic forces during contact and/or noncontact athletic and work activities. During athletic and work activities, extreme forces are placed on the knee. Because soft tissue structures act as the main stabilizers of the knee joint, injuries occur more frequently to ligaments, menisci, bursae, and tendons as a result of compression, friction, repetitive movements, and rotary and shearing forces. Common injuries to the knee include the following:

- Contusions
- Sprains
- Meniscal tears
- Plica syndrome
- Anterior knee pain
- Nerve contusion
- Fractures
- Dislocations/subluxations
- Bursitis
- Overuse injuries and conditions

Contusions

Contusions to the soft tissue and bone of the knee can be caused by compressive forces. Falling on the knee and being struck by a direct force may result in pain, swelling, and loss of range of motion. A direct blow, chronic compression from kneeling, and being pinched between the tibia, patella, and femur can cause an **infrapatellar fat pad** contusion (see Illustration 6–1).

Sprains

Knee sprains are caused by **unidirectional, multidirectional,** and/or **rotary forces** during contact or noncontact activities. Depending on the force, a sprain of the knee can result in damage to single or multiple ligamentous structures. A valgus force on the lateral aspect of the knee can result in a **medial collateral ligament (MCL)** sprain (see Illustration 6–2). Adduction and internal rotation of the knee is a common mechanism of MCL injury.[85] For example, a sprain can occur as a football offensive linemen pass blocks and another player is pushed or falls against the lateral aspect of the linemen's

right knee, causing a valgus force. The **lateral collateral ligament (LCL)** is injured by a varus force on the medial aspect of the knee, commonly with internal rotation of the tibia. Medial or lateral lower leg rotation on a planted foot, direct force causing hyperextension, and external tibia rotation with the knee in a valgus position can cause injury to the **anterior cruciate ligament (ACL)** (see Illustration 6–3). ACL injuries typically occur with quick deceleration, cutting, twisting, and landing movements. An ACL sprain can result as a lacrosse midfielder sprints down the field and suddenly stops, then pivots on the left foot and quickly turns to the right, causing external rotation of the left tibia and valgus stress at the knee. The **posterior cruciate ligament (PCL)** can be injured by a fall on the anterior knee while in a flexed position with foot plantar flexion, a direct force to the proximal lower leg, hyperextension, or a rotational force (Illustration 6–3). With multidirectional and rotary forces, injury commonly occurs to more than one structure.

Meniscal Tears

Tears to the **medial** and **lateral menisci** are caused by compression and shearing forces (Illustration 6–3). Injury to the medial meniscus is more common because of its connection to the joint capsule surrounding the knee and the deep fibers of the MCL. Tears can occur from twisting or cutting movements on a planted foot during flexion or extension of the knee.[12] Medial meniscal tears are also associated with multiple sprains of the MCL, caused by the loss of medial stability and their structural connection.

Medial Plica Syndrome

The most commonly injured **plica** is the mediopatellar, which originates on the medial knee and crosses the medial femoral condyle (see Illustration 6–1). A direct blow to the medial knee as a result of being kicked, or repetitive friction of the plica over the medial femoral condyle during knee flexion and extension, can cause inflammation and additional thickening.

Anterior Knee Pain

Anterior knee pain is commonly associated with injury or structural abnormalities involving the extensor mechanism,

Knee

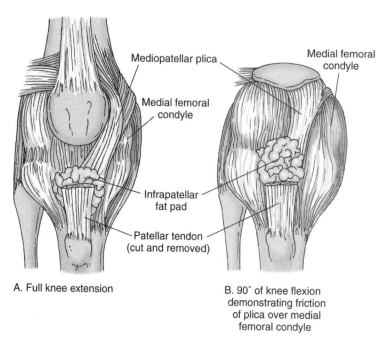

Mediopatellar plica

Medial femoral
condyle

Medial femoral
condyle

Infrapatellar
fat pad

Patellar tendon
(cut and removed)

A. Full knee extension

B. 90° of knee flexion
demonstrating friction
of plica over medial
femoral condyle

Illustration 6-1   Anterior view of the knee.

consisting of the distal quadriceps, quadriceps tendon, patella, and patellar tendon (see Illustration 6–2). **Patellofemoral stress syndrome (PFSS)** is caused by inflexibility of the posterior leg musculature and lateral retinaculum, pronation of the foot, and weakness of the medial quadriceps and hip adductors resulting in lateral tracking and compression of the patella within the femoral groove. Compressive and shear forces and abnormal tracking of the patella caused by pronation of

the foot, external torsion of the tibia, **patella alta,** and degeneration can result in **chondromalacia patella.** **Patellar tendinitis (jumper's knee),** is caused by repetitive jumping, running, or kicking. These movements can also result in tendinitis of the quadriceps tendon. Repetitive tension on the patellar tendon in the adolescent can lead to **Osgood-Schlatter disease (OSD)** or **Sinding-Larsen Johansson disease (SLJ).** Ruptures of the patellar or quadriceps tendon can occur with violent eccentric quadriceps contractions and often follow injuries and conditions that have caused degenerative changes in these structures.

Rectus femoris muscle

Vastus
lateralis
muscle

Vastus
medialis
muscle

Quadriceps
tendon

Patella

Lateral
collateral
ligament

Medial
collateral
ligament

Patellar
tendon

Fibula

Tibia

Illustration 6-2   Anterior view of the ligaments and muscles of the knee.

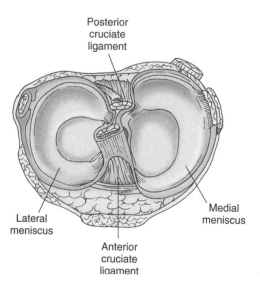

Posterior
cruciate
ligament

Lateral
meniscus

Medial
meniscus

Anterior
cruciate
ligament

Illustration 6-3   Superior view of the cruciate ligaments and menisci.

Nerve Contusion

A direct blow or excessive compression to the inferior aspect of the fibular head can cause a peroneal nerve contusion. The force is commonly a result of being kicked or excessive compression from a wrap or brace.

Fractures

Fractures of the patella can be caused by a direct blow occurring with a fall or a blow to the anterior knee or an eccentric contraction of the quadriceps occurring with jumping or running movements.[6] **Osteochondral** and **chondral fractures** can occur from a direct blow or violent twisting, cutting, or rotational movement. Overuse, direct trauma, or a violent muscular contraction can result in an avulsion fracture. A fracture of the tibial tubercle can be caused by active contraction of the quadriceps with forced flexion of the knee and may follow the development of OSD.[6]

Dislocations/Subluxations

Dislocations of the knee are caused by multidirectional and/or rotary forces and are associated with injury to other structures in and around the knee. Acute patellar subluxations or dislocations can be caused by sudden deceleration with an associated cutting movement, experienced by football wide receivers while running pass routes. Individuals with flat lateral femoral condyles, pronated feet, **genu valgum,** externally rotated patellas, and/or medial knee laxity and lateral knee tightness are predisposed to lateral subluxations or dislocations.[85]

Bursitis

Bursitis of the knee can be caused by direct force or overuse. Compressive force from a direct blow or excessive kneeling can cause inflammation of the **prepatellar bursa** (see Illustration 6–4). Repetitive friction of the patellar tendon can result in inflammation of the **deep infrapatellar bursa** (Illustration 6–4). Compressive force from a direct blow, genu valgum, quadriceps weakness, or inflexibility of the hamstrings can result in inflammation of

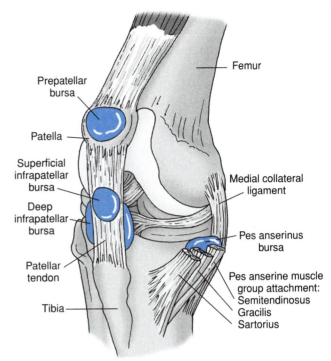

Illustration 6-4   Bursae of the anterior and medial knee.

the **pes anserinus bursa** (Illustration 6–4). Ligamentous or meniscal injuries of the knee can cause inflammation of the **semimembranosus bursa (Baker's cyst).**

Overuse

Overuse injuries and conditions of the knee are caused by repetitive stress and structural abnormalities. **Iliotibial band syndrome** is caused by repetitive stress and friction as the iliotibial band passes over the lateral femoral condyle (see Illustration 7–3). The syndrome is often associated with excessive foot pronation, leg-length discrepancy, **genu varus,** and training errors. Genu valgum, quadriceps weakness, and overuse can cause **pes anserinus tendinitis** (see Illustration 6–4). Stress fractures of the tibial tubercle, tibial plateau, and femoral condyles can be the result of repetitive jumping or running movements and training errors.

Taping Techniques

Provide support and reduce stress to the soft tissue, limit excessive range of motion, and prevent and treat knee injuries and conditions by using several taping techniques. Techniques used following sprains protect against valgus and varus forces and knee hyperextension. For overuse injuries and conditions, several techniques correct structural abnormalities and lessen tension of the patellar tendon on the tibial tubercle. A technique may be effective for one individual but ineffective for another. Prior to application, consider the purpose of the technique, the injury, the individual, and the activity.

McCONNELL TAPING   Figure 6–1

- **Purpose:** The McConnell taping technique[67,69] is used to treat PFSS and to provide relief of pain and correct patellofemoral malalignment (Fig. 6–1). Use the technique within a therapeutic exercise program that consists of stretching tight lateral structures, retraining and strengthening the vastus medialis oblique muscle, mobilizing the patella, and correcting structural foot abnormalities.[33,68,69]
    - Rigid non-elastic tape in 1½ inch width is placed over adhesive gauze material and is used to correct patellar malalignment. Many manufacturers offer the tape; it is also available in kits containing the adhesive gauze material.
    - Design the application of the technique specifically for the individual with regard to the sequence of tape strips and roll tension, or how tightly the tape is applied.
    - Begin the sequence of strips with correction of the most excessive malalignment component. Use additional strips to correct other components if necessary.
    - After applying each strip, re-evaluate the painful activity. There should be an immediate decrease in pain. If the pain does not lessen or if it worsens, reapply the strips or re-evaluate patellar orientation.

- **Materials:**
    - 1½ inch rigid non-elastic tape, 2 inch adhesive gauze material, taping scissors

- **Position of the individual:** Sitting on a taping table or bench with the knee in extension and the quadriceps relaxed.

- **Preparation:** Perform a static and dynamic evaluation of the individual to determine patellar glide, rotation, tilt, and anteroposterior orientation components. Shaving may be necessary for effective application.

- **Application:**

    STEP 1: Apply two strips of 2 inch adhesive gauze material directly to the skin over the patella, extending from the lateral femoral condyle to the posterior aspect of the medial femoral condyle to serve as a base ◀▬▶ (Fig. 6–1A).

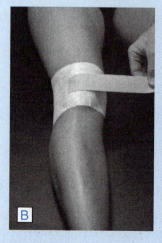

    STEP 2: To correct the glide component (typically a positive lateral glide), anchor a strip of rigid non-elastic tape on the lateral border of the patella (Fig. 6–1B). Pull the strip in a medial direction and push the soft tissue on the medial aspect of the knee toward the patella, and anchor on the adhesive gauze material over the medial femoral condyle (Fig. 6–1C).

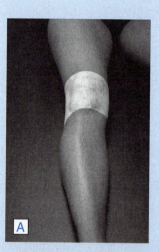

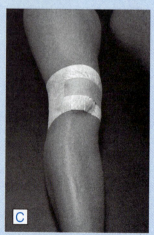

Figure 6-1

STEP 3: To correct the rotation component (commonly positive external rotation of the inferior pole), place a strip of rigid tape on the middle of the inferior pole of the patella at an angle (Fig. 6–1D). Pull the strip upward and medially, and anchor on the medial aspect of the knee (Fig. 6–1E). The superior pole of the patella should rotate laterally.

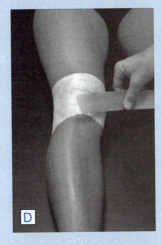
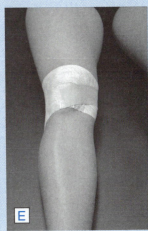

STEP 4: To correct the tilt component (often a positive lateral tilt), anchor a strip of rigid tape on the middle of the patella (Fig. 6–1F). Pull the strip medially, push the medial knee soft tissue toward the patella, and anchor on the medial femoral condyle (Fig. 6–1G).

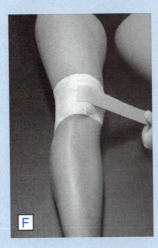
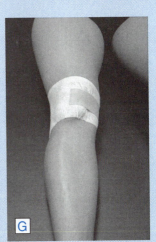

STEP 5: To correct the anteroposterior component (commonly a positive inferior tilt), place a strip of rigid tape across the upper half of the patella and anchor the strip on the lateral and medial femoral condyles (Fig. 6–1H) .

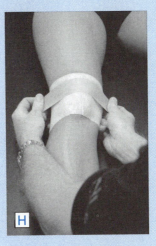

Figure 6-1 *continued*

Helpful Hint: A positive anteroposterior inferior tilt may require correction first in the taping sequence to lift the inferior pole of the patella away from the infrapatellar fat pad to prevent irritation and pain.[33]

RESEARCH BRIEF

The McConnell taping technique is used by many health-care professionals when treating PFSS. While positive outcomes have been demonstrated when the technique has been used in the clinical setting, many questions remain unanswered. Investigators examining the effectiveness of the technique when treating PFSS have demonstrated inconclusive findings.

The influence of patellar taping on pain levels has been well documented in the literature. Researchers [18,26,27,29,31,32,34,46,50,51,83,109] have found an immediate decrease in pain levels during a stimulating task following tape application. However, explanations for the reduction in pain remain unclear. Some researchers have questioned whether the reduction is a result of the actual technique, a placebo effect, a structural correction in patellar alignment, or a neuroinhibitory mechanism.[18,31,45,46,53,55,60]

Research focusing on the effect of taping on patellar alignment with radiographic studies has produced conflicting findings. Examining subjects with PFSS, positional patellar changes were demonstrated following medial taping.[90,98] In healthy subjects, medial taping also resulted in positional changes, but lessened following 15 minutes of intense exercise.[60] Other researchers have found no changes in patellar positioning among subjects with PFSS following tape application.[18,45,108,109]

Studies examining the influence of patellar taping on quadriceps muscle function have demonstrated inconsistent findings. Among subjects with PFSS, patellar taping was found to increase isokinetic concentric[29,49] and eccentric[29] torque of the quadriceps compared with placebo tape and brace. With vertical jump and lateral step-up movements, tape was shown to increase knee extensor moment and power compared with placebo tape, brace, and no tape among subjects with PFSS.[38] Activation of the vastus medialis oblique was shown to increase during a maximal quadriceps contraction following application of patellar tape.[69] Other studies have revealed no change following taping in vastus medialis oblique and vastus lateralis activity during isotonic and isometric quadriceps contractions.[26,51] The timing of vastus medialis oblique activity during ascent and descent of stairs has been shown to occur earlier with patellar taping.[46] During a 4-week therapeutic exercise program, patellar taping was found to have little benefit over a standard rehabilitation program in regard to isokinetic strength and vastus medialis oblique and vastus lateralis activation.[58]

The effect and role of patellar taping in the treatment of PFSS appear to be unclear.[17,33,58] The research suggests that using taping achieves immediate reductions in levels of pain during activity.[17,33,45] However, the effect of taping on other possible causes of PFSS has yet to be answered and warrants further investigation.[17,18,33,46,53,60]

COLLATERAL "X"   Figure 6–2

▶ **Purpose:** The collateral "X" technique is used in the treatment of medial and lateral collateral ligament sprains to provide mild to moderate support and protection against valgus and varus forces at the knee (Fig. 6–2).

▶ **Materials:**
- Pre-tape material, 3 inch heavyweight elastic tape, adherent tape spray, taping scissors

Option:
- 6 inch width by 5 yard length elastic wrap

▶ **Position of the individual:** Standing on a taping table or bench with the majority of the weight on the noninvolved leg and the involved knee placed in slight flexion. Maintain this position by placing a 1½ inch lift under the heel .

 Helpful Hint: You can construct a quick and inexpensive heel lift from paper or plastic tape cores of 1½ inch or 2 inch width tape. Place five to seven of these cores together and apply non-elastic or elastic tape around them, completely covering all sides. You can store the lift in a taping table or bench between uses.

▶ **Preparation:** The leg should be shaved from the mid thigh to the mid lower leg to provide effective support and protection. Apply the technique directly to the skin or over one layer of pre-tape material. Apply adherent tape spray from the mid thigh to mid lower leg area.

▶ **Application:**

STEP 1: Place an anchor of 3 inch heavy-weight elastic tape around the mid thigh and lower leg with mild roll tension ◀▶ (Fig. 6–2A).

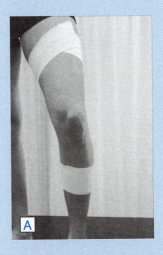

STEP 2: Anchor the first strip of 3 inch heavy-weight elastic tape on the posterior lateral lower leg, proceed up and around the lateral patella with moderate roll tension, and anchor on the medial thigh (Fig. 6–2B).

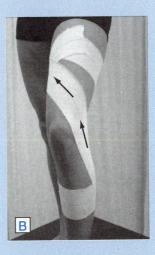

STEP 3: Anchor the second strip on the posterior medial lower leg, continue up and around the medial patella, and finish on the lateral thigh (Fig. 6–2C).

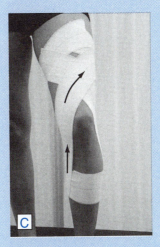

Figure 6-2

STEP 4: Begin the third strip on the anterior medial lower leg, continue up and around the lateral patella, and finish on the lateral thigh (Fig. 6–2D).

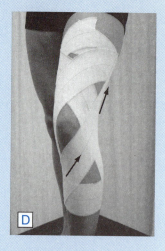

STEP 5: Anchor the fourth strip on the anterior lateral lower leg, proceed up and around the medial patella, and anchor on the medial thigh (Fig. 6–2E).

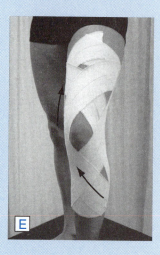

STEP 6: Repeat the strips (see Figs. 6–2B, C, D, and E) with moderate roll tension, overlapping the tape by ⅓ of its width. These strips should resemble an "X" pattern over the medial and lateral joint lines and form a diamond pattern around the patella.

STEP 7: With 3 inch elastic tape, apply a longitudinal strip over the medial and lateral joint line from the lower leg to thigh anchor (Fig. 6–2F).

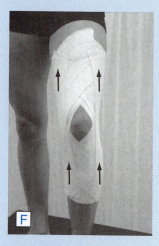

Figure 6-2 *continued*

STEP 8: Starting at the mid thigh anchor, apply three to five circular closure patterns with 3 inch heavyweight elastic tape in a proximal-to-distal direction with mild roll tension, overlapping by ½ of the tape width ◀▶ (Fig. 6–2G).

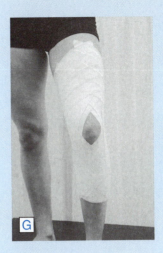

STEP 9: Place three to four circular closure patterns around the lower leg with mild roll tension ◀▶ (Fig. 6–2H). The closure patterns should not enclose or constrict the popliteal space. No additional non-elastic tape anchors are required.

Option: *Consider applying a 6 inch width by 5 yard length elastic wrap in a circular pattern with moderate roll tension in a distal-to-proximal direction over the technique to lessen migration and unraveling of the tape* ◀▶ *. Anchor the wrap with 2 inch or 3 inch elastic tape in a circular pattern* ◀▶ *(Fig. 6–2I).*

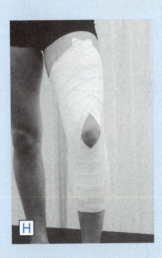

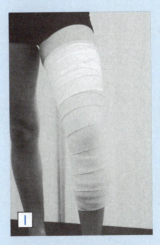

Figure 6-2 *continued*

HYPEREXTENSION Figures 6–3, 6–4

▶ **Purpose:** The hyperextension technique is used to limit hyperextension of the knee and stretch on the soft tissues when treating sprains. Two interchangeable methods are illustrated in the application of the technique; the different methods accommodate individual preferences and available supplies.

Hyperextension Technique One

▶ **Materials:**
  • Pre-tape material, thin foam pads, 3 inch heavyweight elastic tape, adherent tape spray, skin lubricant, taping scissors

  Option:
  • 6 inch width by 5 yard length elastic wrap

▶ **Position of the individual:** Standing on a taping table or bench with the majority of the weight on the noninvolved leg. Determine the range of extension that produces pain by having the individual actively contract the quadriceps and slowly extend the knee until pain occurs. Once painful range of motion is determined, place the involved knee in a pain-free range and, using a heel lift, maintain this position during application.

▶ **Preparation:** Shave the leg from the mid thigh to mid lower leg. The technique is applied directly to the skin or over one layer of pre-tape material. Cover the popliteal space with thin foam pads to prevent irritation. A skin lubricant can also be used. Apply adherent tape spray from the mid thigh to the mid lower leg area.

▶ **Application:**
  STEP 1: Apply two anchors of 3 inch heavyweight elastic tape around the mid thigh and mid lower leg with mild roll tension ◀▬▶ (Fig. 6–3A).

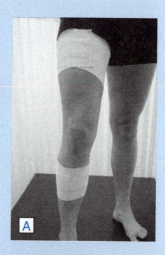

  STEP 2: Using 3 inch heavyweight elastic tape, apply a strip from the middle posterior lower leg to the posterior middle thigh (Fig. 6–3B). Apply moderate roll tension with the tape and monitor the pain-free position of the knee.

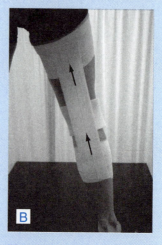

Figure 6-3

STEP 3: Place another strip of 3 inch heavy-weight elastic tape on the anterior lateral lower leg, continue across the popliteal area, and anchor on the anterior medial thigh (Fig. 6–3C).

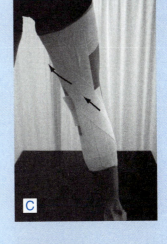

C

STEP 4: Begin the next strip on the anterior medial lower leg, across the popliteal area, and anchor on the anterior lateral thigh (Fig. 6–3D). These strips should form an "X" over the posterior knee. These strips (see Figs. 6–3C and D) can be repeated with moderate tension, overlapping by ⅓ of the tape width.

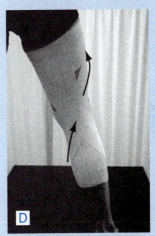

D

STEP 5: Apply three to four circular closure patterns around the thigh and lower leg with mild roll tension, overlapping each ◀▶ (Fig. 6–3E). Non-elastic tape anchors are not necessary.

Option: Consider applying a 6 inch width by 5 yard length elastic wrap in a circular pattern over the technique with moderate roll tension in a distal-to-proximal direction to lessen migration and unraveling of the tape ◀▶. Anchor with elastic tape ◀▶.

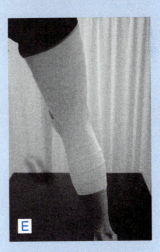

E

Figure 6-3 *continued*

Hyperextension Technique Two

▶ **Materials:**
- Pre-tape material, thin foam pads, 6 inch width heavy resistance exercise band, 3 inch heavyweight elastic tape, adherent tape spray, skin lubricant, taping scissors

Option:
- 6 inch width by 5 yard length elastic wrap

▸ **Position of the individual:** Standing on a taping table or bench with the majority of the weight on the noninvolved leg. Determine the range of extension that produces pain. Once determined, place the involved knee in a pain-free range and maintain this position during application with the use of a heel lift.

▸ **Preparation:** Shave the leg from the mid thigh to mid lower leg. The technique is applied directly to the skin or over one layer of pre-tape material. Cover the popliteal space with thin foam pads to prevent irritation. A skin lubricant can also be used. Apply adherent tape spray from the mid thigh to mid lower leg area ✂.

Helpful Hint: Closely monitor the skin of the thigh and lower leg for irritation from heavyweight elastic tape and/or adherent tape spray with daily application of the collateral "X" and/or hyperextension taping techniques. If irritation occurs, apply the tape over pre-tape material or replace the taping technique with a bracing technique.

▸ **Application:**

STEP 1: Apply anchors as illustrated in Figure 6–3A. Anchor a piece of 6 inch width heavy resistance exercise band around the posterior lower leg with mild roll tension in a circular pattern with 3 inch heavyweight elastic tape. Leave approximately 2–3 inches of the band extending distally beyond the anchor ◀▶ (Fig. 6–4A).

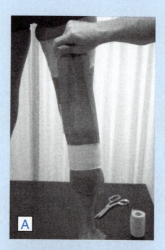

STEP 2: With moderate tension, stretch the band and anchor it on the posterior thigh with 3 inch heavyweight elastic tape, cutting the band approximately 2–3 inches above the anchor ◀▶ (Fig. 6–4B). Monitor the pain-free position of the knee. A second piece of elastic exercise band may be applied directly over the first for additional support.

STEP 3: At the lower leg, fold the excess band up and over the tape anchor and apply three to four closure patterns with 3 inch heavyweight elastic tape with mild roll tension, covering the band ◀▶.

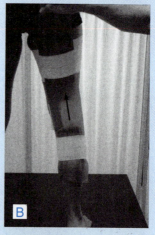

STEP 4: Fold the excess band over onto the thigh anchor and apply three to four closure patterns, also covering the band ◀▶ (Fig. 6–4C). Non-elastic tape anchors are not required.

Option: *Consider applying a 6 inch width by 5 yard length elastic wrap in a circular pattern in a distal-to-proximal direction with moderate roll tension over the technique to prevent migration and unraveling of the tape ◀▶. Anchor with elastic tape ◀▶.*

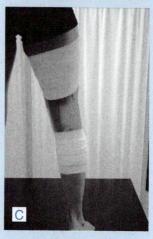

Figure 6-4

PATELLAR TENDON STRAP   Figures 6–5, 6–6, 6–7

▶ **Purpose:** Use the strap technique to treat patellar tendinitis, OSD, PFSS, and chondromalacia and to reduce the tension or pull of the tendon on the inferior pole of the patella and/or tibial tubercle. The straps can be made from taping materials or purchased off-the-shelf. The off-the-shelf designs are illustrated in the Bracing section. Three interchangeable methods are illustrated in the application of the technique. Choose according to individual preferences and available supplies.

Patellar Tendon Strap Technique One

▶ **Materials:**
- 2 inch heavyweight elastic tape, ½ inch non-elastic tape, taping scissors

Option:
- 2 inch self-adherent wrap

▶ **Position of the individual:** Sitting on a taping table or bench, or in a chair, with the knee placed in 90° of flexion.

▶ **Preparation:** Cut a piece of 2 inch heavyweight elastic tape in a 25–30 inch length strip.

Option: *Cut a piece of 2 inch self-adherent wrap in a 25–30 inch length strip.*

▶ **Application:**

STEP 1: Fold the 2 inch heavyweight elastic tape strip over into one piece lengthwise, adhering both sides together. Grasp the ends of this 1 inch strip and rub over a table edge to enhance adhesion (Fig. 6–5A).

Option: *2 inch self-adherent wrap may be used if 2 inch heavyweight elastic tape is not available.*

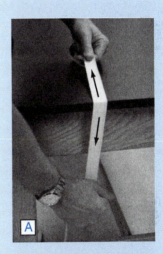

STEP 2: Locate the mid portion of the tendon between the inferior pole of the patella and the tibial tubercle. Anchor the strip directly to the skin on the medial proximal lower leg, continue laterally across the mid portion of the patellar tendon, around the posterior knee, and return to the anchor position (Fig. 6–5B).

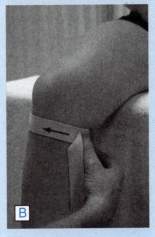

Figure 6-5

STEP 3: Without overlapping, continue to apply the strip around the knee and finish on the medial lower leg, cutting any excess of the strip (Fig. 6–5C). The elastic tape strip should be applied with moderate tension.

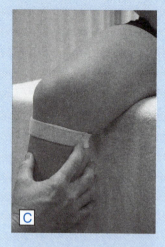

STEP 4: Anchor ½ inch non-elastic tape on the anterior knee and apply two to four continuous strips over the elastic tape in a medial-to-lateral direction (Fig. 6–5D) .

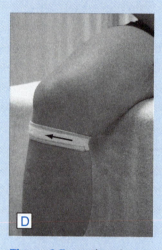

Figure 6-5 *continued*

Helpful Hint: To achieve proper tension and pain relief, the roll tension of the non-elastic tape will vary among individuals. Check the tension of the strips by allowing the individual to perform a previously painful activity. Readjust the tension of the non-elastic strips if necessary. The elastic strip can be reused several times.

Patellar Tendon Strap Technique Two

▶ **Materials:**
  • Pre-tape material, 2 inch lightweight elastic tape, taping scissors

▶ **Position of the individual:** Sitting on a taping table or bench, or in a chair, with the knee placed in 90° of flexion.

▶ **Preparation:** Apply the strap directly to the skin.

Application:

STEP 1: Using pre-tape material, roll the material onto itself and continue until a sausage sized roll is produced (Fig. 6–6A).

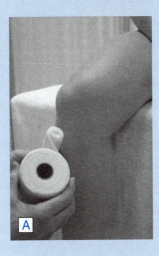

A

STEP 2: Apply 2 inch lightweight elastic tape around the roll (Fig. 6–6B).

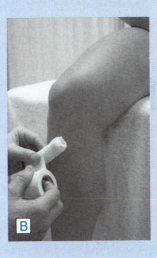

B

STEP 3: Palpate the anterior knee and place the roll over the mid portion of the patellar tendon directly to the skin (Fig. 6–6C).

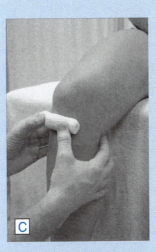

C

Figure 6-6

STEP 4: Attach the roll to the knee by applying pre-tape material in a circular pattern around the proximal lower leg ◄► (Fig. 6–6D).

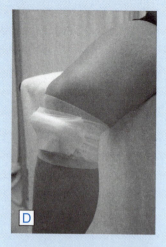

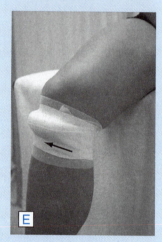

STEP 5: With 2 inch lightweight elastic tape, anchor on the medial lower leg and apply two to four continuous strips over the pre-tape material and roll in a medial-to-lateral direction (Fig. 6–6E). Roll tension will vary among individuals. Additional non-elastic tape strips are not necessary. The pre-tape material roll can be reused.

Figure 6-6 *continued*

Patellar Tendon Strap Technique Three

▶ **Materials:**
  • Pre-tape material

▶ **Position of the individual:** Sitting on a taping table or bench, or in a chair, with the knee placed in 90° of flexion.

▶ **Preparation:** Apply this strap technique directly to the skin.

▶ **Application:**
  STEP 1: Using pre-tape material, encircle the proximal lower leg 10–15 times in a continuous pattern with moderate roll tension ◄► (Fig. 6–7A).

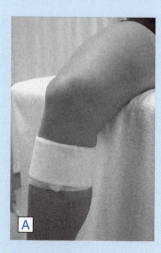

Figure 6-7

STEP 2: Roll the material in a distal-to-proximal fashion and position the roll over the mid portion of the patellar tendon (Fig. 6–7B). No additional tape is required.

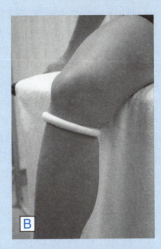

B

Figure 6-7 *continued*

Critical Thinking Question 1

Over the past 6 months, a competitive weightlifter has experienced periodic pain in his left patellar tendon during intense workouts. He has been evaluated by a physician and has undergone treatment for patellar tendinitis that included an off-the-shelf patellar tendon strap. When he initially applies the strap with maximal tension, his pain lessens. However, during workouts the strap loosens when perspiration collects on the neoprene strap and Velcro closure, lessening tension over the patellar tendon.

▶ **Question: What techniques can you use to maintain maximal tension during workouts?**

...IF/THEN...

IF limits in hyperextension are required over several weeks during a return to activity, **THEN** consider the use of a neoprene sleeve with hinged bars brace, which will allow for range of motion control. Most designs will be cost effective.

Wrapping Techniques

Use compression wrap techniques to control swelling and effusion when treating contusions, sprains, meniscal tears, bursitis, iliotibial band friction syndrome, and patellar fractures, dislocations, and subluxations. There are three wrapping methods that provide compression over the knee following injury. Choose a technique based on the amount of swelling and effusion.

COMPRESSION WRAP TECHNIQUE ONE Figure 6–8

▶ **Purpose:** Apply this compression wrap technique for injuries and conditions of the knee that cause mild to moderate swelling and effusion (Fig. 6–8).

▶ **Materials:**
  • 6 inch width by 5 yard length elastic wrap, metal clips, 1½ inch non-elastic or 2 inch elastic tape, taping scissors

Option:
  • ¼ inch or ½ inch open-cell foam

Knee

- **Position of the individual:** Standing on a taping table or bench with the majority of the weight on the noninvolved leg and the involved knee placed in a pain-free, slightly flexed position. Also, sitting on a taping table or bench with the leg extended off the edge.

- **Preparation:** To lessen migration, apply adherent tape spray, tape strips, or anchors directly to the skin (see Fig. 1–7).

- **Application:**

  STEP 1: Anchor the extended end of the wrap directly to the skin around the proximal lower leg and encircle the anchor ◄► (Fig. 6–8A).

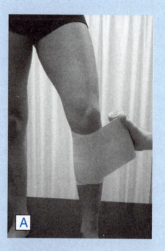

A

  STEP 2: Continue to apply the wrap in a spiral pattern, overlapping by ½ of the wrap width, in a distal-to-proximal direction (Fig. 6–8B). Apply the greatest roll tension distally and lessen tension as the wrap continues proximally.

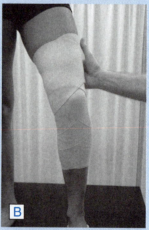

B

  STEP 3: Finish the wrap over the mid thigh area. Anchor the wrap with Velcro, metal clips, or loosely applied 1½ inch non-elastic or 2 inch elastic tape (Fig. 6–8C).

  Option: It is possible to place a ¼ inch or ½ inch open-cell foam pad over the anterior knee, extending from the lateral femoral condyle to the medial femoral condyle, for additional compression around the patella to assist in venous return (see Fig. 6–24A). Place the pad directly on the skin and cover it with the compression wrap.

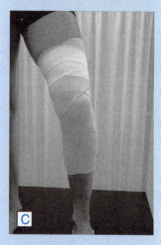

C

Figure 6-8

COMPRESSION WRAP TECHNIQUE TWO Figure 6–9

▶ **Purpose:** With some knee injuries, such as third degree sprains of the ACL, swelling and effusion can be immediate and severe. To lessen the deleterious effects of moderate to severe swelling/effusion and distal migration, use this compression wrap; it incorporates the foot, ankle, lower leg, and knee (Fig. 6–9).

▶ **Materials:**
- 4 inch or 6 inch width by 10 yard length elastic wrap, metal clips, 1½ inch non-elastic or 2 inch elastic tape, taping scissors

Option:
- ¼ inch or ½ inch open-cell foam

▶ **Position of the individual:** Sitting on a taping table or bench with the leg extended off the edge, knee in a pain-free, slightly flexed position, and the ankle placed in 90° of dorsiflexion.

▶ **Preparation:** To lessen migration, apply adherent tape spray, tape strips, or anchors directly to the skin (see Fig. 1–7).

▶ **Application:**

STEP 1: Anchor the end of the wrap on the distal plantar foot and apply the foot, ankle, and lower leg compression wrap directly to the skin (see Fig. 5–6A).

STEP 2: At the inferior knee, continue the spiral wrap proximally to the mid thigh area ◀▶ (Fig. 6–9A). Apply the greatest amount of roll tension distally and lessen as the wrap continues proximally.

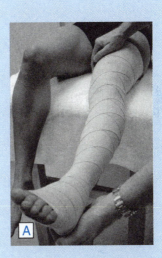

A

STEP 3: Anchor the wrap with Velcro, metal clips, or loosely applied 1½ inch non-elastic or 2 inch elastic tape ◀▶ (Fig. 6–9B).

Option: *Consider using a ¼ inch or ½ inch open-cell foam pad over the anterior knee for additional compression to control swelling and effusion.*

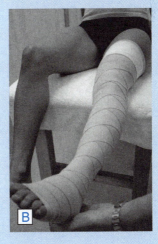

B

Figure 6-9

COMPRESSION WRAP TECHNIQUE THREE   Figure 6–10

- **Purpose:** An elastic sleeve may also be used over the knee to control mild to moderate swelling and effusion (Fig. 6–10). Following proper instruction, this compression wrap can be applied and removed by the individual without assistance.

- **Materials:**
  - 3 inch or 5 inch width elastic sleeve determined by the size of the lower leg and thigh, taping scissors

  Option:
  - ¼ inch or ½ inch open-cell foam

- **Position of the individual:** Sitting on a taping table or bench with the leg extended off the edge.

- **Preparation:** Cut a sleeve from a roll to extend from the proximal lower leg to the mid thigh area or from the distal lower leg to the mid thigh area. Cut and use a double length sleeve to provide additional compression.

- **Application:**

  STEP 1: Pull the sleeve onto the knee in a distal-to-proximal direction. If using a double length sleeve, pull the distal end over the first layer to provide an additional layer (Fig. 6–10). No anchors are required. The elastic sleeve can be cleaned and reused.

  Option: An open-cell foam pad may be cut and placed over the anterior knee to assist in controlling swelling and effusion.

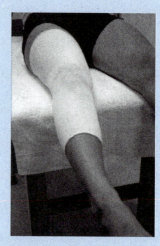

Figure 6-10

Critical Thinking Question 2

Several members of a high school wrestling team practice daily without any type of anterior knee padding. One particular athlete in the 103 lb weight class complains of pain over the prepatellar region with direct compression and passive knee flexion. Swelling has developed over the prepatellar area. Treatment consisting of ice, a compression wrap, and protective pad returns him to pain-free activity. Two weeks later, swelling returns to the prepatellar region and remains despite the use of a compression wrap. He is able to continue practice pain-free.

- **Question: What techniques are available to lessen the swelling?**

...IF/THEN...

IF considering when to use a compression wrap technique safely and effectively, **THEN** remember that an elastic wrap or sleeve can be used immediately following most injuries and/or surgeries to control swelling and effusion.

Bracing Techniques

Bracing techniques for the knee provide immobilization, support, and compression, and they correct structural abnormalities when preventing and treating injuries and conditions. In 1984, the American Academy of Orthopaedic Surgeons (AAOS)[5] classified knee braces into three categories: prophylactic, rehabilitative, and functional. Other bracing techniques—also often used interchangeably within these categories—include neoprene sleeves, neoprene sleeves with hinged bars or buttress pads, and patellar tendon straps. Knee braces are available in off-the-shelf and custom-made designs and can be used for a variety of injuries and conditions.

PROPHYLACTIC Figure 6–11

▶ **Purpose:** Prophylactic braces are designed to prevent or reduce the severity of knee injuries (Fig. 6–11).[5] The braces provide moderate support and are primarily used to protect the knee from valgus forces and injury to the MCL.

⚪ **DETAILS**

Prophylactic knee braces are commonly used when preventing MCL sprains of athletes in collision and contact sports, such as football and hockey. The nonpliable brace materials are covered with padding that meets NCAA[75] and NFHS[76] rules.

▶ **Design:**
- The braces are available off-the-shelf in predetermined sizes, corresponding either to circumference measurements of the thigh and lower leg or the height of the individual.
- The braces are manufactured in a universal fit design and can be used on either knee.
- Most prophylactic designs consist of a stainless steel, polycarbonate, or aircraft aluminum bar with single, dual, or polycentric hinges.
- The braces contain a hyperextension block to prevent excessive range of motion.
- Several designs have additional nylon straps to limit migration.
- To provide additional stability, some designs contain a pressure pad that fits under the hinged bar over the lateral joint line of the knee.

▶ **Materials:**
- 2 inch or 3 inch heavyweight elastic tape, pre-tape material, self-adherent wrap, adherent tape spray, taping scissors

▶ **Position of the individual:** Standing on a taping table or bench with the majority of the weight on the noninvolved leg and the involved knee placed in slight flexion. Maintain this position by placing a 1½ inch lift under the heel.

▶ **Preparation:** Some prophylactic designs are attached directly to the skin over the lateral aspect of the thigh and lower leg with neoprene wraps, cuffs, or sleeves. Other designs are attached directly to the skin with elastic tape, or over one layer of pre-tape material or self-adherent wrap. Apply adherent tape spray underneath neoprene, pre-tape material, or self-adherent wrap to lessen brace migration.

   Application of prophylactic designs should follow manufacturers' instructions, which are included with the braces when purchased. The following application guidelines pertain to most braces.

◗ **Application:**

STEP 1: If using designs with neoprene attachments, begin by loosening the wraps, cuffs, or sleeves. Center the brace hinge over the lateral joint line of the knee with the bars extending proximally over the lateral thigh and distally over the lateral lower leg (Fig. 6–11A) ✂.

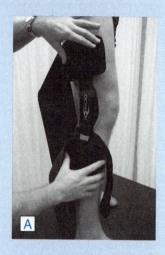

A

✂ **Helpful Hint:** Accommodate for migration during the initial positioning of the brace. After centering the hinge, reposition the hinge slightly superior to the lateral joint line. During activity, the hinge will migrate distally into the correct position over the lateral joint line.

STEP 2: The application of neoprene wraps, cuffs, or sleeves will depend on the specific brace design. Apply most of these designs by wrapping the neoprene around the thigh and lower leg and anchoring with Velcro (Fig. 6–11B). With some designs, anchor additional straps over the neoprene.

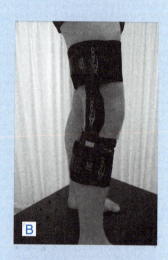

B

STEP 3: With other designs, apply one layer of pre-tape material or self-adherent wrap directly over the distal thigh and proximal leg ◀▶. Anchor 2 inch or 3 inch heavyweight elastic tape directly on the proximal end of the brace bar and proceed around the thigh in a circular pattern with mild to moderate roll tension, overlapping the tape by ½ of its width with each pass ◀▶. Cover the entire end of the bar and anchor on the anterior thigh (Fig. 6–11C). Avoid gaps, wrinkles, or inconsistent roll tension. The tape may also be applied directly to the skin.

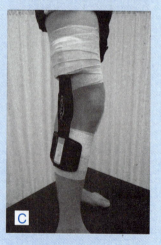

C

Figure 6-11

STEP 4: Anchor 2 inch or 3 inch heavyweight elastic tape on the distal brace bar and proceed around the lower leg in a circular pattern with mild to moderate roll tension ◄—► (Fig. 6–D). Cover the entire end of the bar and anchor on the anterior lower leg. No additional anchors are required.

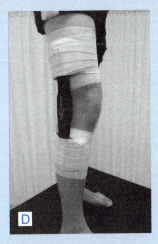

Figure 6-11 *continued*

RESEARCH BRIEF

Prophylactic braces are designed and worn in an attempt to prevent injury to the knee. Health-care professionals have a variety of designs to choose from; decisions regarding their use should be based on empirical data examining their effectiveness. However, past investigations focusing on their use and protection from injurious forces, effects on functional performance, and actual reductions in injuries have produced conflicting findings.

Research examining the amount of protection prophylactic braces can provide against injurious forces to the MCL and ACL has resulted in inconsistent findings. Using mechanical limb models or cadaver specimens, researchers have loaded or applied various forces at multiple angles to determine stress on the ligaments. Examining several designs under various loads and joint angles, prophylactic braces appeared to demonstrate some protection or decrease in injurious loads for the MCL[8,35,42,81] and ACL.[9,81] Under similar conditions, other researchers have shown that the braces did not decrease loads on the MCL[8,9,37,92] and ACL.[37] At low impact levels, the braces did not affect neuromuscular response times, suggesting limited protection during high velocity loads experienced in sports.[42] Some researchers have concluded that prophylactic braces may provide 20% to 30% more protection from a valgus force than no brace,[4] while others believe no conclusions can be drawn at this time.[5,48,74,93]

Efforts to investigate the effects of prophylactic braces on functional performance are numerous in the literature. At best, the findings appear mixed among the multitude of brace designs available off-the-shelf.[93] Among subjects with little or no experience with wearing prophylactic braces, several researchers found a decrease in performance of forward[19,43,48,86] and

backward[43] sprint times and drills consisting of rapid change of direction.[43,48] In contrast, other researchers[48,86] showed that brace wear had no effect on forward and backward sprint times and agility drills. Interestingly, subjects who had previously worn prophylactic braces demonstrated a reduction in forward sprint performance, but the braces had no influence on backward sprint and agility drill performance.[43] Some researchers revealed a decrease in lower extremity muscle activity[77] during treadmill running while others reported no effect on running gait patterns[62] among nonexperienced brace wearers. Examining peak quadriceps torque, several researchers found that brace wear reduced peak torque measurements[19]; others found no influence on performance.[94] The findings appear to suggest that some prophylactic braces have a negative effect on performance and other braces do not. Many researchers have noted that the novelty of wearing the braces may have affected the generalizability of the findings, and further research is needed.[19,43,93]

The majority of research conducted does not support the use of prophylactic braces to prevent knee injuries. The investigations reviewed all involved American football and are varied in regard to methodology and experimental design, which makes control and comparisons difficult. In perhaps one of the best-designed studies, researchers demonstrated a consistent trend of lower injury rates among intercollegiate athletes wearing braces compared to nonbrace-wearers.[2,3] Another well-designed investigation revealed that among West Point cadets participating in intramural tackle football, the use of braces resulted in a reduction in the incidence of knee injury.[96] In contrast, several

(continued)

researchers have shown that brace wear did not lower injury rates. Examining intercollegiate athletes, several[91,101] researchers demonstrated that prophylactic brace wear resulted in injury rates equal to or greater than those of nonbrace-wearers. Among high school athletes, using prophylactic braces resulted in a higher injury rate.[47] Although overall injury rates were decreased with brace wear, some researchers have shown that among at-risk positions such as linemen, tight ends, and linebackers, prophylactic braces had no influence on the reduction of injury.[52] From the data, several researchers have concluded that prophylactic braces are not preventive and may even be harmful, causing an increase in foot and ankle injuries.[47,101]

Preventing knee injuries is a concern for both the individual and health-care professional. For the individual, issues such as lost time from athletic and work activities, quality of life, and cost of medical services must be considered. The health-care professional must examine the personnel required for the application of preventive techniques and subsequent treatment and rehabilitation of injury and the cost effectiveness of prophylactic brace use. The findings from the studies reviewed do not support the use of prophylactic braces to prevent or reduce the severity of injury to the knee. Based on the research and current prophylactic designs, the position statement of the AAOS[5] states "that the routine use of prophylactic knee braces currently available has not been proven effective in reducing the number or severity of knee injuries. In some circumstances, such braces may even have the potential to be a contributing factor to injury." Further research and development of prophylactic designs are needed to determine the exact role and effectiveness of the braces in preventing injury.

REHABILITATIVE Figures 6–12, 6–13

▶ **Purpose:** Rehabilitative braces are designed to support, immobilize, and allow protected range of motion of the knee following injury and surgery.[5] The braces can be used to treat knee sprains, meniscal tears, tendon ruptures, OSD, SLJ, fractures, dislocations, and subluxations. Two rehabilitative designs are illustrated below.

Rehabilitative Technique One

▶ **Purpose:** This rehabilitative brace technique provides mild to moderate support and complete immobilization of the knee (Fig. 6–12).

> ◯ DETAILS
>
> The braces are commonly used (following acute injury or surgery) with crutches for non–weight-bearing ambulation. The braces may be removed for treatment and rehabilitation.
>
> Consider using the braces in combination with the knee compression wrapping techniques to control swelling and effusion (see Figs. 6–8, 6–9, and 6–10).

▶ **Design:**
  • These universal fit designed braces are available in predetermined sizes based on thigh and lower leg circumference measurements.
  • The braces are available in various lengths, measured from the proximal/mid thigh to the mid/distal lower leg, to accommodate the height of the individual.
  • The braces are constructed of foam and nylon/fiber laminate panels with Velcro strap closures.
  • The designs have removable plastic or aluminum stays incorporated into the panels on the medial, lateral, and posterior surfaces.
  • Some designs have popliteal pads to provide additional support and to lessen brace migration.

▶ **Position of the individual:** Sitting on a taping table or bench with the knee in full extension.

▶ **Preparation:** Apply the braces directly to the skin or over tight-fitting pants.

Specific instructions for applying the braces are included with each design. The following general application guidelines apply to most designs.

▶ **Application:**

STEP 1: Begin by loosening the straps and unfolding the brace.

STEP 2: With assistance, position the brace under the involved leg of the individual. Ensure proper alignment of the medial, lateral, and posterior stays as well as the patellar opening (Fig. 6–12A). Reposition the brace if necessary.

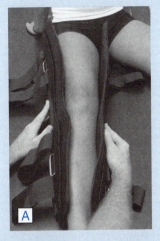

STEP 3: Bring the panels together over the anterior thigh, knee, and lower leg. Beginning at the superior patella, pull the strap tight and secure to the brace with Velcro (Fig. 6–12B). Next, pull the inferior patellar strap and anchor (Fig. 6–12C).

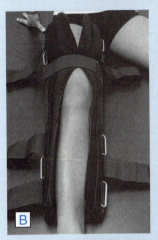
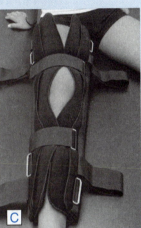

STEP 4: Continue to anchor the straps in this alternating pattern until all straps are anchored (Fig. 6–12D).

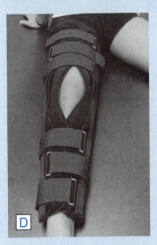

Figure 6-12

Rehabilitative Technique Two

▶ **Purpose:** Use this rehabilitative brace technique to provide mild to moderate support, immobilization, and protected range of motion (Fig. 6–13). These braces can replace a plaster or fiberglass cast or a splint. The advantages of the braces include the following: they are removable, which allows for treatment and rehabilitation; they have adjustable range of motion; they are of lightweight design; and they support and control early weight-bearing.

○ **D E T A I L S**

The braces can be used following acute injury or surgery, with or without the use of crutches.

This design may be used in combination with the compression wrapping techniques to control swelling and effusion (see Figs. 6–8, 6–9, 6–10).

▶ **Design:**
- The braces are manufactured in universal fit designs in predetermined sizes corresponding to thigh and lower leg circumference measurements.
- The designs are available in various lengths depending on the objective of the technique.
- Most designs consist of foam or polyethylene thigh and lower leg wraps or cuffs with medial and lateral hinged aluminum bars, attached with Velcro. The wraps or cuffs may be cut to achieve proper fit.
- The polycentric hinges on most designs allow for control and locking of range of motion. Some designs have easy-to-use dials for quick range of motion settings.
- The designs have straps incorporated into the bars to anchor the brace to the thigh and lower leg.

▶ **Position of the individual:** Sitting on a taping table or bench with the involved knee in a pain-free range of motion.

▶ **Preparation:** Set the brace range of motion at the desired settings of flexion and extension as indicated by a physician and/or therapeutic exercise program. Apply the brace directly to the skin or over tight-fitting pants.

Again, instructions for application are included with each brace. The following guidelines pertain to most designs.

▶ **Application:**

(**STEP 1:**) Begin the application by loosening the straps and unfolding the brace.

(**STEP 2:**) Position the brace under the involved leg. Center the hinges with the joint line and the bars along the medial and lateral thigh and lower leg (Fig. 6–13A). Reposition the bars on the wraps or cuffs with the Velcro attachments if necessary.

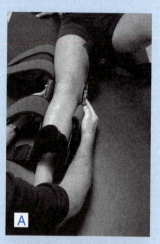

(**STEP 3:**) Anchor the wraps or cuffs around the thigh and lower leg. At the superior patella, pull the strap tight and anchor. Next, anchor the inferior patellar strap. Continue to anchor the remaining straps in this alternating pattern (Fig. 6–13B).

... I F / T H E N ...

IF budget constraints allow for the purchase of only one type of rehabilitative brace technique, **THEN** consider brace technique two, which allows for range of motion adjustments, from complete immobilization (the purpose of technique one) to full protected range of motion.

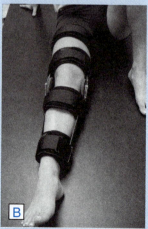

Figure 6-13

RESEARCH BRIEF

Rehabilitative brace designs are used following injury and/or surgery to provide protection for healing structures. Research to determine the effectiveness of the brace is limited in the literature.[41,57,89] It has been suggested that rehabilitative braces are utilized by health-care professionals based on the braces' subjective performance rather than empirical data.[104]

Investigations have shown that rehabilitative braces function best when they fit properly and are constructed of rigid materials.[23,25] The most effective braces were constructed of plastic, conforming shells and lightweight metal hinge bars with multiple straps to attach the shells and bars to the thigh and lower leg. The hinge bars should contact the joint line of the knee and offer an adjustable, rigid stop to range of motion.

Although using rehabilitative braces to treat acute and surgical knee injuries is clinically effective and widely practiced, many health-care professionals utilize functional knee braces to provide support and to allow for range of motion during this period. The AAOS[5] has suggested that rehabilitative braces are more useful in preventing excessive flexion and extension, rather than excessive anterior and posterior translation, and can be effective in many treatment protocols. Decisions regarding which design to use are normally dictated by the physician and/or surgeon. Advancements in surgical procedures and rehabilitation protocols will most likely affect the future design and use of rehabilitative braces in the treatment of knee injuries.

FUNCTIONAL Figures 6–14, 6–15

▶ **Purpose:** Functional braces are designed to provide moderate stability to the unstable knee following injury and surgery (Fig. 6–14).[5] The braces are commonly used when treating ACL, PCL, MCL, and LCL sprains to control anterior tibial translation and rotary stress. Some health-care professionals use functional braces prophylactically with athletes in collision and contact sports to provide optimal protection against unidirectional and multidirectional forces.

○ DETAILS

Functional knee braces are commonly used to provide knee stability for athletes in sports such as baseball, basketball, field hockey, football, gymnastics, ice hockey, lacrosse, soccer, softball, track and field, volleyball, and wrestling, but can also be useful with work and casual activities.

The nonpliable materials of the brace must be padded to meet NCAA and NFHS rules. Off-the-shelf brace covers are available from some manufacturers to meet the standards.

▶ **Design:**
- Functional braces are available in three designs: bilateral hinge-post-shell, bilateral hinge-post-strap, and unilateral hinge-post-shell.[64]
- Bilateral hinge-post-shell designs consist of a rigid frame or shell, medial and lateral hinges, and soft straps. Bilateral hinge-post-strap designs are manufactured with medial and lateral hinges and soft straps. Unilateral hinge-post-shell designs are constructed of a rigid frame or shell, a medial or lateral hinge, and soft straps.
- These braces are available in off-the-shelf and custom-made designs in a right or left style.
- Off-the-shelf designs are manufactured in predetermined sizes corresponding to knee joint and distal thigh circumference measurements. The designs allow for small size adjustments during wear.
- Custom-made designs are manufactured for a specific individual following fitting by a manufacturer representative or orthopedic technician. The size cannot be adjusted after a custom-made brace is constructed.
- Most braces are available in short and standard length designs to accommodate different heights of individuals and activities such as motocross, horseback riding, and skiing.

- Functional brace designs consist of a frame or shell, condyle pads, liners, and straps. With most designs, the liners and straps may be cut to achieve proper fit.
- The frames are constructed of tempered aluminum, carbon composite, metallic plastic composite, carbon fiber titanium, or carbon/graphite laminate materials with monocentric or polycentric hinges.
- The hinges allow control over the range of motion; most designs contain a hyperextension block.
- Most designs have suede and chamois condyle pads and liners, and nylon straps with Velcro closures.
- Some designs have pneumatic condyle pads and liners to enhance fit and comfort.

▶ **Position of the individual:** Sitting in a chair with the knee in approximately 30° to 45° of flexion.

▶ **Preparation:** Apply functional braces directly to the skin or over a Lycra or neoprene sleeve. Set the brace range of motion at the desired settings of flexion and extension. Loosen all straps.

Specific instructions for application of functional braces are included with each design. For proper application and use, follow the step-by-step procedure. The following general application guidelines apply to most functional designs.

▶ **Application:**

(**STEP 1:**) Hold each hinge and guide the individual to place the leg into the brace. Position the condyle pads just superior to the joint line. Push the brace in a posterior direction on the knee (Fig. 6–14A).

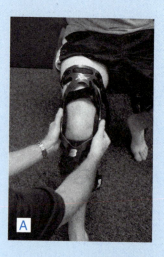

(**STEP 2:**) Applying straps will depend on the specific brace design. Begin application of some designs by anchoring the proximal posterior lower leg strap (Fig. 6–14B). Next, anchor the distal posterior thigh strap, allowing the lower leg cuff to move anteriorly (Fig. 6–14C).

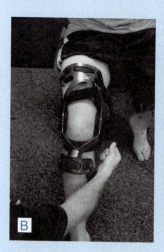 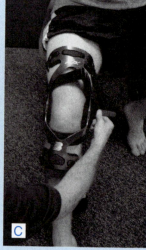

Figure 6-14

STEP 3: Continue and anchor the proximal posterior thigh strap (Fig. 6–14D).

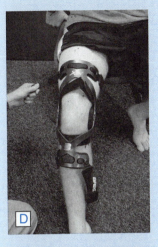

STEP 4: Anchor the distal posterior lower leg strap, pulling the cuff to the lower leg (Fig. 6–14E).

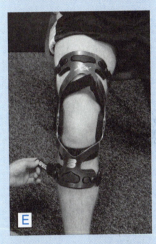

STEP 5: Allow the individual to stand with the quadriceps flexed and anchor the distal anterior thigh strap (Fig. 6–14F). Allow the individual to walk to ensure proper fit. Retighten the straps and/or reposition the brace if necessary.

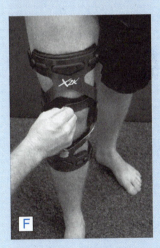

Figure 6-14 *continued*

Custom-Made Functional Knee Brace Fitting

Fitting of custom-made functional knee braces is performed by taking measurements of the individual's leg or by casting the leg in a weight-bearing position (Fig. 6–15).

▸ **Purpose:** Each manufacturer has step-by-step procedures, and many manufacturers use a measurement device that is attached to the leg during fitting. To achieve the best fit, measurements should be taken without the presence of effusion or thigh and lower leg atrophy.

The following guidelines apply to the use of a fitting device to record circumference measurements.

▶ **Procedure:**

STEP 1: Place the individual in a standing position, feet shoulder width apart, and slight knee flexion. Attach the measurement device directly to the skin on the medial and lateral knee (Fig. 6–15A).

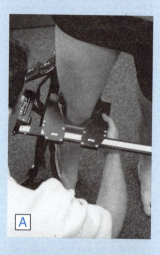

A

STEP 2: Next, pull the condyle pads away from the knee and reposition them over the medial and lateral femoral condyles, just posterior to the midline of the thigh (Fig. 6–15B).

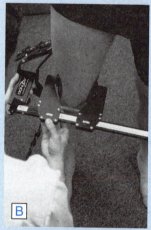

B

STEP 3: Position the measurement tapes against the lateral aspect of the thigh and lower leg. Next, wrap the tapes around the thigh and lower leg with moderate tension. The tapes should be parallel to the floor and not compress the soft tissue (Fig. 6–15C).

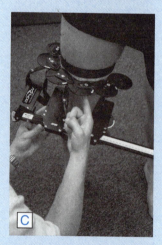

C

Figure 6-15

STEP 4: Depending on the manufacturer, record the various measurements. These may include thigh and lower leg circumference, knee joint angle, knee width, and contour of the anterior thigh and posterior lower leg (Fig. 6–15D).

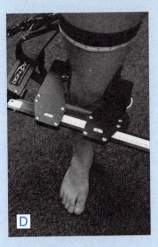

D

Figure 6-15 *continued*

RESEARCH BRIEF

Functional braces are used to protect the unstable knee following injury and/or surgery. These braces have been used for many years by health-care professionals during various phases of the treatment and rehabilitation process, and manufacturers continue to develop new designs. Research conducted to examine the effectiveness of functional bracing techniques has been inconsistent, and many questions remain unanswered. Investigators have focused on the influence of functional brace designs on control of tibial translation, proprioception, muscle response, functional performance, and psychology of the individual.

The control of anterior tibial translation is perhaps one of the most important roles of the functional knee brace. Researchers[7,13,56,72,107] have shown that under low external loads, the braces increased mechanical stability of ACL deficient subjects, reducing anterior translation. These studies were performed on non–weight-bearing knees, excluding body weight forces and muscle contractions.[13] Other studies have demonstrated that with ACL deficient subjects in weight-bearing conditions, the braces also reduced anterior translation under low external loads.[13,107] Some researchers have cautioned that these low loads are below those experienced during daily and, more importantly, athletic activities.[73] With moderate to high loads, several researchers[15,89] have demonstrated that the braces did not significantly reduce anterior translation in ACL deficient subjects, while other researchers found a reduction.[97] Researchers have also examined the influence of functional braces during the transition from non–weight-bearing to weight-bearing positions. Past studies have shown that during this transition, the tibia translates anteriorly.[14,103] The findings demonstrated that functional braces did not reduce anterior translation of the tibia in ACL

deficient subjects to levels of the normal knee.[13,87] The results from the investigations appear to suggest that functional knee braces can reduce anterior tibial translation under low load conditions, such as during the early postoperative period.[20,30] However, the effect on translation during functional load conditions warrants further investigation.

Few studies have examined the effect of functional knee braces on lower extremity proprioception. Several methods have been utilized in the investigations; comparisons of the findings are difficult to make. Investigators[65] have reported improvements in motor control with static and dynamic tests among ACL deficient subjects following 1 month of functional brace wear. Other studies have demonstrated a more erect posture at 3 weeks post-ACL reconstruction[36] and improved static knee joint angle reproduction (active reproduction of a joint position) at 5 months post-ACL reconstruction[110] with brace use. Researchers[16] have also revealed small improvements in threshold to detection of passive motion values (active detection of a change in joint position) with brace wear among ACL deficient subjects. These results were not significant. However, several researchers[21,22] measured dynamic EMG activity among ACL deficient subjects and revealed that functional braces did not improve proprioception. Many researchers have proposed that the improvements could have been due to cutaneous stimulation, increased mechanical stability, and ACL deficiency, but the mechanism is unclear.[16,110]

Previous research has produced conflicting findings with regard to the effects of functional braces on muscular response. Researchers[1,54,89] have demonstrated that the braces decreased isokinetic peak torque of the quadriceps among post-ACL

(continued)

reconstruction subjects with 1–2 years of brace wear and subjects without instability symptoms. Other studies[1] revealed an increase in peak torque among subjects with symptoms of knee instability. In contrast, some researchers[94,110] have found that functional braces did not influence peak torque. Researchers[1] suggested that improvements in peak torque may be a result of anterior tibial translation control during contraction of the quadriceps. Investigators[107] have also shown that bracing hampers normal hamstring function, causing a delay in normal firing patterns. Interestingly, the longest delay was related to the brace designs that provided the most control of anterior tibial translation.

Numerous studies have examined the effects of functional braces on overall functional performance. Researchers[20,54,59,105] have demonstrated that the brace designs result in higher energy expenditures for wearers, which may affect functional performance. However, some researchers[79,99,100] have revealed that the braces had no effect on performance while other researchers[30,88] found an increase in the performance of various functional activities. Although functional braces have been shown to control anterior tibial translation, some investigators[74,95] caution that episodes of recurrent buckling of the knee may occur during activity.

A review of the literature examining the psychological effects of functional braces appears to create a discrepancy between subjective and objective findings.[110] The majority of the research suggests that braces are only effective in providing mechanical stability at low external loads. However, ACL deficient and post-ACL reconstruction subjects have reported that functional braces improved function,[30,88,89] reduced feelings/perceptions of knee instability or buckling episodes,[10,28,89] increased confidence,[24,41,59] and were beneficial[28] during performance of various activities. Health-care professionals should monitor the individual's activities and stress the importance of adherence to a comprehensive therapeutic exercise program to protect the healing structures and restore preinjury function.

Health-care professionals can choose from a variety of off-the-shelf and custom-made functional brace designs when treating and rehabilitating knee injuries. Examining brace effectiveness, researchers[15,64,66,106] have found no differences between off-the-shelf and custom designs. Among functional braces, the bilateral hinge-post-shell design provided the greatest restriction to anterior tibial translation.[40,63,74] Overall, the research appears to support using functional brace techniques in the protection of knee instability. The AAOS[5] states "that functional knee braces can be effective in many treatment programs, and that this efficacy has been demonstrated by long-term scientifically conducted studies." Currently, there is no one or best brace design available. Additional research is needed to answer questions regarding brace effectiveness and to assist health-care professionals in decisions regarding brace use.

...IF/THEN...

IF protection from valgus and varus forces is needed following a sprain, **THEN** use a functional brace design; remember that most prophylactic braces are constructed with a single hinged bar designed to prevent or lessen injury only from valgus forces.

Critical Thinking Question 3

A rookie defensive end on a professional football team sustains a first degree MCL sprain of the left knee during training camp. His history includes two previous first degree MCL sprains of the same knee that occurred during his four-year intercollegiate career. After completing a rehabilitation program, he is allowed to return to practice. The team physician is concerned about laxity of the MCL and the risk of trauma to other structures in the left knee.

▶ **Question: What techniques can be used in this situation?**

NEOPRENE SLEEVE Figure 6–16

▶ **Purpose:** Neoprene sleeves provide compression and mild support when treating contusions, sprains, meniscal tears, PFSS, quadriceps tendinitis, chondromalacia, plica, bursitis, and overuse injuries and conditions (Fig. 6–16).

◯ **DETAILS**

The sleeves may be used during rehabilitative, athletic, work, and casual activities.

▶ **Design:**
- The off-the-shelf sleeves are manufactured in universal fit designs in predetermined sizes corresponding to thigh and knee circumference measurements.
- Some designs cover the patella (closed patella), while others are cut-out (open patella) over the area.
- Several designs also have a cut-out area over the popliteal space (open popliteal).

▶ **Position of the individual:** Sitting on a taping table or bench with the leg extended off the edge, or in a chair, with the knee in approximately 45° of flexion.

▶ **Preparation:** Apply neoprene sleeves directly to the skin; no anchors are required.

▶ **Application:**

(STEP 1:) Hold each side of the sleeve and place the larger end over the foot. Pull in a proximal direction until the sleeve is positioned on the knee (Fig. 6–16).

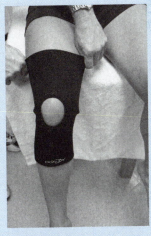

Figure 6-16

RESEARCH BRIEF

Neoprene knee sleeves are typically used to provide warmth, compression, and mild support following injury. There is a limited amount of research in the literature regarding the effectiveness of these sleeves.[11,82,84] The investigations reviewed focused on the effects of sleeve use on proprioception, specifically joint position sense and threshold to detection.

Past investigations examining the effects of neoprene knee sleeves on proprioception have resulted in overall positive findings. Examining joint position sense, researchers have demonstrated improvements in accuracy and awareness among healthy[70] and post-ACL reconstruction[61] subjects. Other researchers have shown that among ACL deficient subjects, the threshold to detection of passive motion was not changed with the use of a sleeve.[16]

These results appear to indicate that neoprene sleeves influence knee proprioception. Some investigators have suggested that the improvements in proprioception from sleeve use may assist in reducing injury to the knee.[93]

NEOPRENE SLEEVE WITH HINGED BARS Figure 6–17

▶ **Purpose:** Neoprene sleeves with hinged bars provide compression and mild to moderate support to the knee following injury (Fig. 6–17). These braces are commonly used when treating mild and moderate MCL and LCL and mild ACL and PCL sprains to control valgus, varus, and rotary stresses.

○ **DETAILS**────────────────

Use the sleeves during rehabilitative, athletic, work, and casual activities. The nonpliable materials, commonly the hinges, must be padded to meet NCAA[75] and NFHS[76] rules.

▶ **Design:**
- The universal fit sleeves are available off-the-shelf in predetermined sizes corresponding to thigh and knee circumference measurements.
- The sleeves are manufactured in standard and short length designs to accommodate individual height differences.
- Most designs consist of a one-piece neoprene sleeve with medial and lateral hinged aluminum bars, and two nylon strap closures.
- Some designs use a contoured sleeve that wraps around the knee to accommodate hard-to-fit leg shapes. These designs are anchored on the anterior thigh and lower leg with Velcro.
- The sleeves are constructed with an open patella front; some sleeves also have an open popliteal space cut-out.
- Most designs have a polycentric hinge that allows for range of motion control. A hyperextension block is also available.
- Some designs have a small adjustable hinge similar to the rehabilitative brace.
- Most designs are constructed with proximal and distal pockets or pouches that anchor the medial and lateral bars to the sleeve. Outer nylon straps provide further support to the bars.
- To provide additional support, some designs have condyle pads located under the hinges at the joint line, attached to the sleeve with Velcro.

▶ **Position of the individual:** Sitting on a taping table or bench with the leg extended off the edge, or in a chair, with the knee in approximately 45° of flexion.

▶ **Preparation:** Apply neoprene sleeves with hinged bars directly to the skin; no anchors are required. Set the brace range of motion at the desired settings of flexion and extension.

Follow the instructions of the manufacturer when applying the sleeves. The following application guidelines pertain to most sleeves.

▶ **Application:**

STEP 1: Begin by loosening the thigh and lower leg straps.

STEP 2: Grasp the loops above the proximal ends of the bars and pull the brace in a proximal direction over the knee. Center the hinges over the joint line with the cut-out positioned over the patella (Fig. 6–17A).

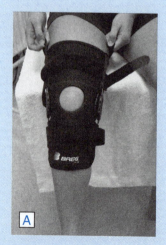

A

Figure 6-17

STEP 3: With the contoured or wrap around design, position the brace on the posterior thigh and lower leg. Wrap the sleeve around and anchor on the anterior thigh and lower leg with Velcro closures (Fig. 6–17B). Center the hinges over the joint line.

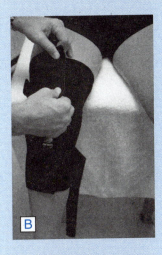

B

STEP 4: The application of straps will depend on the specific sleeve design. Apply most by pulling the straps tight and anchoring with Velcro (Fig. 6–17C).

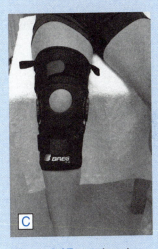

C

Figure 6-17 *continued*

Helpful Hint: Elastic wrap, clothing fibers, and debris from playing surfaces often adhere to the male ends of the Velcro closures and lessen adherence. To increase adherence, clean the male ends of fibers and debris with small, pointed scissors or tweezers.

...IF/THEN...

IF support and protection are needed following a MCL sprain and taping is not an option, **THEN** consider using a prophylactic or neoprene sleeve with hinged bars brace design, which will protect against valgus forces and further injury.

Critical Thinking Question 4

A forward on an intercollegiate ice hockey team suffers a first degree LCL sprain of the right knee. Following a short period of rehabilitation, the athlete is allowed to return to activity. The team physician requests that the knee be supported and protected from further injury for a period of 2 weeks during all practices and competitions. During this 2-week period, 10 practices and 2 competitions will occur.

▶ **Question:** Which taping or bracing technique can you use? Which technique would be cost effective?

NEOPRENE SLEEVE WITH BUTTRESS   Figures 6–18, 6–19

- **Purpose:** Neoprene sleeves with buttresses provide compression, reduce friction and stress, provide mild to moderate support, and correct structural abnormalities when treating PFSS, chondromalacia, patellar dislocations and subluxations, patellar tendinitis, and OSD. A variety of buttress sleeve designs are available to treat these injuries and conditions.

> **○ DETAILS**
>
> Fixed and adjustable sleeves can be used with athletic, work, and casual activities.

- These sleeves may be purchased off-the-shelf in right and left styles, with predetermined sizes corresponding to thigh and knee circumference measurements.
- The designs consist of a neoprene sleeve with a fixed or adjustable buttress with various straps.

Fixed Buttress

- **Design:**
  - Fixed buttresses are incorporated into the brace and do not allow for adjustments during application or activity (Fig. 6–18).
  - Fixed buttress sleeves are constructed with an open patella front, surrounded by a felt, silicone, rubber, foam, or pneumatic buttress in the shape of an uppercase "C," "H," "J," or "U," or circular pattern.
  - The "C"- and "J"-shaped buttresses are designed to limit lateral movement of the patella.
  - The "H"-shaped buttress is designed to limit inferior and superior patellar movement, while the "U"-shaped buttress limits inferior movement.
  - Circular buttresses are designed to stabilize the patella in multidirectional ranges of motion.
  - Many designs are available with an open popliteal space.
  - Some designs have proximal and distal straps with Velcro closures to anchor the brace to the thigh and lower leg.

- **Position of the individual:** Sitting on a taping table or bench with the leg extended off the edge, or in a chair, with the knee in approximately 45° of flexion.

- **Preparation:** Apply fixed buttress sleeves directly to the skin; no anchors are required.

- **Application:**
  STEP 1: Place the larger end of the sleeve over the foot and pull in a proximal direction. Position the cut-out over the patella and the buttress against the patella. Following the manufacturer's instructions, pull the straps tight and secure to the sleeve with Velcro (Fig. 6–18).

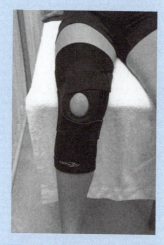

Figure 6-18

Adjustable Buttress

▶ **Design:**
- • These designs allow adjustment of the buttress that is incorporated into the sleeve and/or adjustment of various straps to provide additional support to the patella (Fig. 6–19).
- • The sleeves are manufactured with an open patella front; some sleeves also have an open popliteal space.
- • Many adjustable designs contain a "C," "H," "J," "U," or circular buttress that one can reposition and/or trim to achieve the desired compression and support.
- • Some designs use various straps with Velcro attachments incorporated into the sleeve to limit excessive patellar range of motion.
- • Several other sleeves are manufactured with a fixed buttress and adjustable straps.
- • Most strap designs are attached on the lateral aspect of the sleeve. The straps are normally pulled in a medial direction to limit lateral movement of the patella.
- • Some adjustable designs use both a buttress incorporated into the sleeve and an external buttress to limit excessive patellar range of motion.
- • Another design uses an external buttress plate attached to a tension hinge to adjust support to the patella throughout knee range of motion.

▶ **Position of the individual:** Sitting on a taping table or bench with the leg extended off the edge, or in a chair, with the knee in approximately 45° of flexion.

▶ **Preparation:** Apply adjustable buttress sleeves directly to the skin; no anchors are required.

The manufacturer includes specific instructions for fitting and application. For proper fit and support, follow the step-by-step procedures. The following application guidelines apply to most sleeves.

▶ **Application:**

STEP 1: To apply, pull the sleeve over the foot and onto the knee. Adjust the cut-out and buttress over and around the patella (Fig. 6–19A).

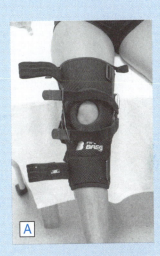

STEP 2: Applying straps will depend on the specific brace design. Generally, pull these straps tightly in a medial direction over the thigh and lower leg and anchor on the medial or lateral sleeve with Velcro (Fig. 6–19B).

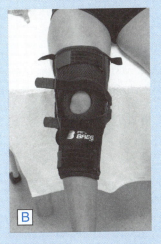

Figure 6-19

STEP 3: Position the external buttresses just next to the lateral patella and pull the straps across the superior and inferior patella; anchor on the medial or lateral sleeve (Fig. 6–19C).

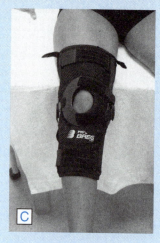

C

Figure 6-19 *continued*

...IF/THEN...

IF an athlete requires support of the patella in the treatment of PFSS or patellar subluxation, **THEN** use a neoprene sleeve with buttress brace; although a neoprene sleeve does provide support, a fixed or adjustable buttress brace provides greater support and stabilization of the patella and surrounding soft tissues, lessening excessive movement.

RESEARCH BRIEF

Neoprene sleeves with buttresses are designed to influence patellar tracking in the trochlear groove and lessen friction and pain in the treatment of many anterior knee injuries and conditions.[17,104] Research to support the use of these braces is lacking in the literature, which perhaps can be attributed to the plethora of causes of anterior knee pain.[74]

Investigations conducted with the brace designs have produced conflicting results. Some researchers demonstrated a reduction in pain and improvement in function[78,102] and a reduction in the occurrence of anterior knee pain[11] with the use of buttress and strap sleeves. Other investigators have shown that these designs did not reduce pain levels.[39,71] Many researchers have suggested that neoprene sleeves with buttresses and straps compress soft tissue and limit patellar movement,[80] reduce loads and increase proprioceptive feedback,[11] apply a sustained force,[44,80] and should be used within a comprehensive therapeutic exercise program.[17] Based on the available findings, further research is warranted to determine the beneficial effects of neoprene sleeves with buttresses and straps.

PATELLAR TENDON STRAP Figure 6–20

▶ **Purpose:** Several patellar tendon strap brace designs exist to lessen tension on the tendon at the inferior pole of the patella and/or at the tibial tubercle, to treat patellar tendinitis, OSD, PFSS, and chondromalacia (Fig. 6–20).

○ **DETAILS**

Use the straps with athletic, work, or casual activities. Patellar tendon straps may be used in combination with neoprene sleeves to provide compression and support.

▶ **Design:**
- The straps are available off-the-shelf in universal styles and predetermined sizes that correspond to inferior knee circumference measurements. Some designs are available in universal sizes.
- The straps are constructed of neoprene or foam composite materials with Velcro closures.
- Most designs contain a semi-tubular or tubular foam, foam/air cell, or padded plastic buttress incorporated into the strap.

- **Position of the individual:** Sitting on a taping table or bench with the leg extended off the edge, or in a chair, with the knee in approximately 45° of flexion.

- **Preparation:** Apply patellar tendon straps directly to the skin; no anchors are required.

- **Application:**

  STEP 1: To apply, place the semi-tubular/tubular buttress over the patellar tendon, between the inferior pole of the patella and tibial tubercle (Fig. 6–20A).

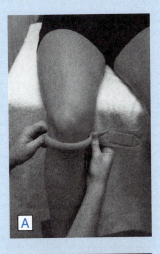

  STEP 2: Pull the ends snugly together and anchor on the posterior knee with the Velcro closures (Fig. 6–20B). Allow the individual to perform a previously painful activity. Readjust the strap if necessary.

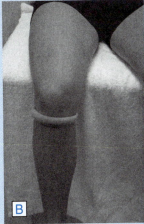

Figure 6-20

ORTHOTICS

- **Purpose:** Orthotics provide support, absorb shock, and correct structural abnormalities when treating knee injuries and conditions.
  - Use soft orthotic designs (see Fig. 3–16) to absorb shock and lessen stress on the patellar tendon to treat OSD and SLJ. The soft designs can also be used to absorb shock when preventing and treating stress fractures of the tibial tubercle, tibial plateau, and femoral condyles. Heel cups and full-length neoprene, silicone, and viscoelastic polymer insoles are available in off-the-shelf designs.
  - Use semirigid (see Fig. 3–17) and rigid (see Fig. 3–18) orthotics to provide support and correct structural abnormalities like excessive foot pronation, leg-length discrepancy, genu varus or valgum, or external tibial torsion when treating iliotibial band friction syndrome, chondromalacia, PFSS, and pes anserinus bursitis and tendinitis. The designs can be purchased off-the-shelf or custom-made.

> **Critical Thinking Question 5**
>
> The first mate on a charter fishing boat sustains a torn ACL of the left knee. After imaging studies and a clinical examination by a surgeon, the surgeon schedules ACL reconstruction. The surgeon schedules the procedure 2 weeks post-injury to allow for a reduction in effusion and an increase in range of motion. The first mate will receive daily therapy at a local outpatient orthopedic clinic and can ambulate as tolerated.
>
> - **Question: What wrapping and bracing techniques can you use during the 2-week period?**

Padding Techniques

A variety of off-the-shelf padding techniques can prevent and treat injuries and conditions of the knee. Another option is using foam, felt, viscoelastic polymers, and thermoplastic materials to construct custom-made padding techniques. The use of padding for the knee is mandatory with several interscholastic and intercollegiate sports. These mandatory techniques will be discussed further in Chapter 13.

OFF-THE-SHELF   Figures 6–21, 6–22

▶ **Purpose:** Off-the-shelf padding techniques are available from manufacturers in a variety of designs. These techniques provide shock absorption and protection when preventing and treating bursitis, OSD, SLJ, and contusions of the soft tissue and bone of the knee. Following is a description of two basic designs.

Soft, Low-Density

> **DETAILS**
>
> Soft, low-density pads are commonly used to provide shock absorption to the knees of athletes in sports such as baseball, basketball, football, ice hockey, lacrosse, softball, volleyball, and wrestling. Use the pads with work and casual activities.

▶ **Design:**
  • The pads are manufactured in a universal fit design in predetermined sizes, corresponding either to circumference measurements of the thigh or the weight of the individual (Fig. 6–21A).
  • Most pads are constructed of varying thicknesses of high-impact open- and closed-cell foams, covered with polyester/spandex or woven fabric materials.
  • Several designs consist of a neoprene sleeve with additional foam incorporated on the anterior aspect.
  • Some designs have an open popliteal space, while others have a closed space.

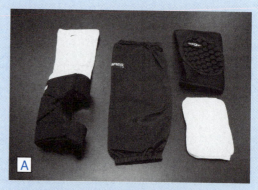

A

Figure 6-21A   Variety of soft, low-density pads. (Bottom left) Pad with open popliteal space. (Middle) Padded cover for a functional ACL knee brace.

▶ **Position of the individual:** Sitting on a taping table or bench with the leg extended off the edge, or in a chair, with the knee in approximately 45° of flexion.

▶ **Preparation:** Apply the soft, low-density designs directly to the skin or over tight-fitting clothing.

▶ **Application:**

STEP 1: To apply the pad, place the larger end over the foot and pull in a proximal direction onto the knee (Fig. 6–21B) ✂.

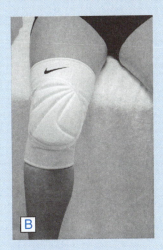

B

Figure 6-21 *continued*

 Helpful Hint: Off-the-shelf soft, low-density pads can cause irritation in the popliteal space. To lessen the chance of irritation, apply a skin lubricant and/or thin foam pads over the area or purchase pad designs with an open popliteal space.

Hard, High-Density

○ DETAILS

Hard, high-density pads are commonly used to provide shock absorption to the knees of athletes in sports such as baseball, ice hockey, and softball. Use the pads in work and casual activities, such as kneeling, which may result in chronic or prolonged compression.

▶ **Design:**

• The universal fit designs are available in predetermined sizes based on lower leg circumference measurements or age of the individual (Fig. 6–22A).
• Most designs are constructed of a polycarbonate or plastic material outer shell pre-molded to the contours of the knee.
• The outer shell is lined with open- and closed-cell foams and is incorporated into a vinyl pad that extends in all directions to provide shock absorption.
• Another design uses a polycarbonate cup lined with foam that attaches to the hinges of functional knee braces to protect the patella.
• The pads are available in various lengths depending on the technique objective.
• Hard, high-density pads are attached to the knee with various adjustable nylon straps with Velcro or buckle closures.

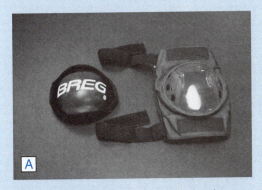

A

Figure 6-22A Variety of hard, high-density pads. (Left) Pad that can be attached to a functional ACL knee brace to protect the anterior knee.

▶ **Position of the individual:** Sitting on a taping table or bench with the leg extended off the edge, or in a chair, with the knee in approximately 45° of flexion.

▶ **Preparation:** Apply the hard, high-density designs directly to the skin or over tight-fitting clothing.

▶ **Application:**

STEP 1: Place the pad over the anterior knee. Applying straps will depend on the specific design. Normally, pull the straps across the posterior knee and anchor on the pad with Velcro or buckle closures (Fig. 6–22B). Readjust the straps if necessary for proper fit. Pad all nonpliable materials to meet NCAA and NFHS rules.

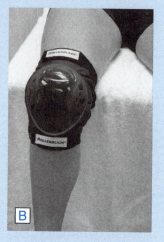

B

Figure 6-22 *continued*

CUSTOM-MADE Figure 6–23

▶ **Purpose:** Use thermoplastic material to mold custom-made pads to absorb shock and provide protection when preventing and treating knee contusions (Fig. 6–23). Consider using these designs when off-the-shelf pads are not available or when a custom fit is needed.

▶ **Materials:**
• Paper, felt tip pen, thermoplastic material, ⅛ inch or ¼ inch foam or felt, a heating source, 2 inch or 3 inch elastic tape, an elastic wrap, soft, low-density foam, rubber cement, taping scissors

▶ **Position of the individual:** Sitting on a taping table or bench with the leg and knee in a functional position.

▶ **Preparation:** Construction begins by designing the pad with a paper pattern (see Fig. 1–14). Next, cut, mold, and shape the thermoplastic material on the knee over the injured area. Attach soft, low-density foam to the inside surface of the pad (see Fig. 1–15). Pre-cut, pre-padded designs off-the-shelf are also available. Following immersion in water, mold the material to the knee.

▶ **Application:**

STEP 1: Attach the pad to the knee with loosely applied 2 inch or 3 inch elastic tape or self-adherent wrap over pre-tape material, or directly to the skin ◀▬▶. Use strips or a circular pattern (Fig. 6–23A).

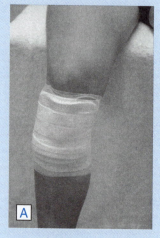

A

Figure 6-23

STEP 2: Another option is to attach the pad to the knee with a compression wrapping technique (see Figs. 6–8 and 6–23B).

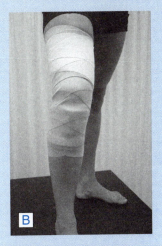

B

Figure 6-23 *continued*

COMPRESSION WRAP PAD   Figure 6–24

▸ **Purpose:** The compression wrap pad technique helps to reduce mild, moderate, or severe swelling and effusion in the acute treatment of knee contusions, sprains, meniscal tears, fractures, dislocations/subluxations, bursitis, and overuse conditions (Fig. 6–24).

▸ **Materials:**
  • ¼ inch or ½ inch open-cell foam, taping scissors

▸ **Position of the individual:** Sitting on a taping table or bench with the leg extended off the edge.

▸ **Preparation:** To lessen migration, apply adherent tape spray, tape strips, or anchors directly to the skin.

▸ **Application:**
  STEP 1: Extend the pad across the anterior knee, from the medial to lateral joint line, and from the suprapatellar pouch to the tibial tubercle (Fig. 6–24A).

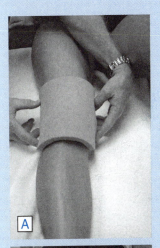

A

  STEP 2: Position the pad over the anterior knee and apply the compression wrap technique to anchor (see Figs. 6–8, 6–9, 6–10, and 6–24B).

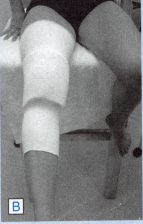

B

Figure 6-24

HEEL LIFT

▶ **Purpose:** The heel lift pad technique (see Fig. 5–12) reduces stress in the treatment of an infrapatellar fat pad contusion. The heel lift elevates the hindfoot and lessens stress on the fat pad that may occur during knee extension.

- Construct the heel lift pads from ½ inch or 1 inch felt, or purchase heel lift pads with an adhesive backing.
- Cut the pad to cover the heel or shoe liner area.
- Use a pad on each heel or in each shoe to prevent adaptive changes.
- Apply the pad to the heel or shoe liner (see Fig. 5–12A).

DONUT PADS

▶ **Purpose:** Use the donut pad technique (see Fig. 3–27) to lessen the amount of stress over an inflamed area when treating contusions and bursitis.

- Make the pads from ⅛ inch or ¼ inch foam or felt or purchase them pre-cut with adhesive backing.
- Another option is to purchase pre-cut viscoelastic donuts in a variety of sizes.
- Attach the pad directly to the skin over the prepatellar, infrapatellar, pes anserinus, or semimembranosus bursa, the infrapatellar fat pad, or the peroneal nerve with adhesive gauze material (see Fig. 3–13), or in a circular pattern with loosely applied 2 inch elastic tape.
- Consider anchoring the pad with the compression wrapping techniques (see Figs. 6–8, 6–9, and 6–10).

MANDATORY PADDING

Mandatory protective equipment for the knee is required by the NCAA[75] and the NFHS[76] in several sports. Athletes participating in baseball, field hockey, football, ice hockey, and softball must wear protective padding during all practices and competitions. These padding techniques are available in a variety of off-the-shelf designs. Chapter 13 provides a full discussion of these padding techniques.

Critical Thinking Question 6

Over the past week, a tile layer has noticed tingling and numbness along the lateral aspect of his lower leg that radiates in a distal direction toward his foot. The pain is worse at the end of the work day. Recently, his company issued new hard, high-density knee pads to all employees that fit snugly around the proximal lower knee.

▶ **Question: How can you manage this situation?**

CASE STUDY

Over the past several weeks, Ron Daubenmire has experienced a progressively worsening dull aching pain in the right anterior knee. Ron is a science teacher at Helmick High School and rides with a local cycling club on Saturdays. He first noticed the pain at school when descending stairs and rising from a prolonged sitting position. The pain has progressed and is now present during walking, running, and squatting movements. During most weeks, he runs 5 to 6 miles and cycles 20–35 miles in preparation for a 30–50 mile Saturday club ride. However, his schedule has not allowed him to visit a fitness center or gym for strengthening and flexibility exercises. Ron enjoys cycling with the club and does not want to take any time off to treat his right anterior knee pain. Last Saturday during a club ride, he noticed that he was unable to perform to the level of the other members because of muscular fatigue and pain in the right knee.

Ron decided to walk down to the football stadium after school the next week to seek assistance from the sports medicine staff. He enters the athletic training room and speaks with Angela Waybright, the ATC at the high school. After gathering a history from Ron, Angela tells him to return later that afternoon for an evaluation. During the evaluation, Angela finds point tenderness along the lateral facet of the right patella, tightness of the lateral retinaculum, and lateral tracking of the patella. Compression of the patella into the patellofemoral groove also produces pain. Angela discovers inflexibility of the right posterior leg musculature with bilateral range of motion testing. Manual muscle testing reveals weaknesses in the right medial quadriceps and hip adductors. Ron is placed on a treadmill for a dynamic evaluation and Angela finds excessive pronation of the right foot during walking and running gaits. Angela begins to discuss her findings with Ron as the team physician arrives in the athletic training room for the afternoon injury clinic. Angela continues talking with Ron; when she is finished, the team physician examines Ron. The evaluation produces the same positive findings, and the team physician and Angela agree that Ron is suffering from PFSS. The team physician recommends that Ron be placed into a comprehensive treatment program for the condition.

Angela and the team physician decide to place Ron into a therapeutic exercise protocol that utilizes rest, avoidance of painful activities, flexibility exercises for tight structures, retraining and strengthening of weak musculature, correction of structural abnormalities, and modalities for symptomatic treatment. What taping techniques would support and correct the structural abnormalities and lessen stress and pain associated with PFSS in this case? What bracing techniques would provide compression, reduce stress, and support and correct the structural abnormalities to allow Ron to continue to ride with the cycling club?

WRAP UP

- Unidirectional, multidirectional, rotary, and compression forces; structural abnormalities; inflexibility and weakness of soft tissue; and repetitive stress can cause injury to the knee.
- The McConnell taping technique provides support when correcting patellofemoral malalignment.
- The collateral "X" and hyperextension taping techniques can be used to provide support and reduce range of motion when treating sprains.
- The patellar tendon strap taping and bracing techniques lessen the tension of the tendon on the inferior pole of the patella and/or the tibial tubercle.
- Elastic wraps and sleeves control swelling and effusion following injury.
- Prophylactic knee braces provide protection and reduce severity of injury, rehabilitative braces provide support and protected range of motion following injury/surgery, and functional braces provide stability following injury/surgery.
- The neoprene sleeve and sleeve with hinged bars bracing techniques provide compression and support to the knee.
- Neoprene sleeves with buttress braces provide compression, reduce stress, and correct structural abnormalities when treating acute and chronic injuries.
- Orthotics and the heel lift padding technique can be used to provide support, absorb shock, and correct structural abnormalities.
- Soft, low-density; hard, high-density; donut; and thermoplastic padding techniques provide shock absorption, protection, and compression, and reduce stress.
- Mandatory protective equipment is required for the knee in several sports by the NCAA and NFHS.

■ WEB REFERENCES

American Academy of Orthopaedic Surgeons
http://www.aaos.org/
- This Web site allows you to search for information on the mechanism, treatment, and rehabilitation of knee injuries.

International Society of Arthroscopy, Knee Surgery and Orthopaedic Sports Medicine
http://www.isakos.com/
- This site provides access to ISAKOS Meeting abstracts and summaries.

United States National Library of Medicine
http://www.nlm.nih.gov/
- This Web site provides access to knee injury prevention, treatment, and rehabilitation information among a variety of populations.

WorldOrtho
http://www.worldortho.com/
- This site provides you with access to full online textbooks, pictures, and other educational materials.

■ REFERENCES

1. Acierno, SP, D'Ambrosia, C, Solomonow, M, Baratta, RV, and D'Ambrosia, RD: Electromyography and biomechanics of a dynamic knee brace for anterior cruciate ligament deficiency. Orthopedics 18:1101–1107, 1995.
2. Albright, JP, Powell, JW, Smith, W, Martindale, A, Crowley, E, Monroe, J, Miller, R, Connolly, J, Hill, BA, Miller, D, Helwig, D, and Marshall, J: Medial collateral ligament knee sprains in college football: Brace wear preferences and injury risk. Am J Sports Med 22:2–11, 1994.
3. Albright, JP, Powell, JW, Smith, W, Martindale, A, Crowley, E, Monroe, J, Miller, R, Connolly, J, Hill, BA, Miller, D, Helwig, D, and Marshall, J: Medial collateral ligament knee sprains in college football: Effectiveness of preventive braces. Am J Sports Med 22:12–18, 1994.
4. Albright, JP, Saterbak, A, and Stokes, J: Use of knee braces in sport: Current recommendations. Sports Med 20:281–301, 1995.
5. American Academy of Orthopaedic Surgeons. http://www.aaos.org/wordhtml/papers/position/1124.htm, Position statement, 2004.
6. Anderson, MK, Hall, SJ, and Martin, M: Sports Injury Management, ed 2. Lippincott Williams & Wilkins, Philadelphia, 2000.

7. Anderson, K, Wojtys, EM, Loubert, PV, and Miller, RE: A bio-mechanical evaluation of taping and bracing in reducing knee joint translation and rotation. Am J Sports Med 20:416–421, 1992.

8. Baker, BE, VanHanswyk, E, Bogosian, S, IV, Werner, FW, and Murphy, D: The effect of knee braces on lateral impact loading of the knee. Am J Sports Med 17:182–186, 1989.

9. Baker, BE, VanHanswyk, E, Bogosian, S, IV, Werner, FW, and Murphy, D: A biomechanical study of the static stabilizing effect of knee braces on medial stability. Am J Sports Med 15:566–570, 1987.

10. Beard, DJ, Kybeed, PJ, Ferguson, CM, and Dodd, CA: Proprioception after rupture of the ACL: An objective indication of the need for surgery. J Bone Joint Surg 75:311–315, 1993.

11. BenGal, S, Lowe J, Mann, G, Finsterbush, A, and Matan, Y: The role of the knee brace in the prevention of anterior knee pain syndrome. Am J Sports Med 25:118–122, 1997.

12. Bernstein, J: Meniscal tears of the knee: Diagnosis and individualized treatment. Phys Sportsmed 28:83, 2000.

13. Beynnon, BD, Fleming, BC, Churchill, DL, and Brown, D: The effect of anterior cruciate ligament deficiency and functional bracing on translation of the tibia relative to the femur during nonweightbearing and weightbearing. Am J Sports Med 31:99–105, 2003.

14. Beynnon, BD, Fleming, BC, Labovitch, R, and Parsons, B: Chronic anterior cruciate ligament deficiency is associated with increased anterior translation of the tibia during the transition from non-weightbearing to weightbearing. J Orthop Res 20:332–337, 2002.

15. Beynnon, BD, Pope, MH, Wertheimer, CM, Johnson, R, Fleming, B, Nichols, C, and Howe, J: The effect of functional knee-braces on strain on the anterior cruciate ligament in vivo. J Bone Joint Surg 74A:1298–1312, 1992.

16. Beynnon, BD, Ryder, SH, Konradsen, L, Johnson, RJ, Johnson, K, and Renström, PA: The effect of anterior cruciate ligament trauma and bracing on knee proprioception. Am J Sports Med 27:150–155, 1999.

17. Bizzini, M, Childs, JD, Piva, SR, and Delitto, A: Systematic review of the quality of randomized controlled trials for patellofemoral pain syndrome. J Orthop Sports Phys Ther 33:4–20, 2003.

18. Bockrath, K, Wooden, C, Worrell, T, Ingerson, CD, and Farr, J: Effects of patella taping on patella position and perceived pain. Med Sci Sports 25:989–992, 1993.

19. Borsa, PA, Lephart, SM, and Fu, FH: Muscular and functional performance characteristics of individuals wearing prophylactic knee braces. JNATA 28:336–340, 1993.

20. Branch, TP, and Hunter, RE: Functional analysis of anterior cruciate ligament braces. Clin Sports Med 9:771–797, 1990.

21. Branch, TP, Hunter, R, and Donath, M: Dynamic EMG analysis of anterior cruciate deficient knees with and without bracing during cutting. Am J Sports Med 17:35, 1989.

22. Branch, TP, Indelicato, PA, Riley, S, and Miller, G: Kinematic analysis of anterior cruciate deficient subjects during side-step cutting with and without a functional knee brace. Clin J Sports Med 3:86, 1993.

23. Cawley, PW: Post-operative knee bracing. Clin Sports Med 9:763–770, 1990.

24. Cawley, PW, France, EP, and Paulos, LE: The current state of functional knee bracing research: A review of the literature. Am J Sports Med 19:226–233, 1991.

25. Cawley, PW, France, EP, and Paulos, LE: Comparison of rehabilitative knee braces: A biomechanical investigation. Am J Sports Med 17:141–146, 1989.

26. Cerny, K: Vastus medialis oblique/vastus lateralis muscle activity ratios for selected exercises in persons with and without patellofemoral pain syndrome. Phys Ther 75:672–682, 1995.

27. Clark, DI, Downing, N, Mitchell, J, Coulson, L, Syzpryt, EP, and Doherty, M: Physiotherapy for anterior knee pain: A randomised controlled trial. Ann Rheum Dis 59:700–704, 2000.

28. Colville, MR, Lee, CL, and Ciullo, JV: The Lenox Hill brace: An evaluation of effectiveness in treating knee instability. Am J Sports Med 14:257–261, 1986.

29. Conway, A, Malone, T, and Conway, P: Patella alignment/tracking alteration: Effect on force output and perceived pain. Isokinet Exerc Sci 2:9–17, 1992.

30. Cook, FF, Tibone, JE, and Redfern, FC: A dynamic analysis of a functional brace for anterior cruciate ligament insufficiency. Am J Sports Med 17:519–524, 1989.

31. Crossley, K, Bennell, K, Green, S, Cowan, S, and McConnell, J: Physical therapy for patellofemoral pain: A randomized, double-blinded, placebo-controlled trial. Am J Sports Med 30:857–865, 2002.

32. Crossley, K, Bennell, K, Green, S, and McConnell, J: A systematic review of physical interventions for patellofemoral pain syndrome. Clin J Sport Med 11:103–110, 2001.

33. Crossley, K, Cowan, SM, Bennell, KL, and McConnell, J: Patellar taping: Is clinical success supported by scientific evidence? Man Ther 5:142–150, 2000.

34. Cushnaghan, J, McCarthy, R, and Dieppe, P: The effect of taping the patella on pain in the osteoarthritic patient. BMJ 308:753–755, 1994.

35. Daley, BJ, Ralston, JL, Brown, TD, and Brand, RA: A parametric design evaluation of lateral prophylactic knee braces. J Biomech Eng 115:131–136, 1993.

36. DeVita, P, Lassiter, T, Jr, Hortobagyi, T, and Torry, M: Functional knee brace effects during walking in patients with anterior cruciate ligament reconstruction. Am J Sports Med 26:778–784, 1998.

37. Erickson, AR, Yasuda, K, Beynnon, B, Johnson, R, and Pope, M: An in vitro dynamic evaluation of prophylactic knee braces during lateral impact loading. Am J Sports Med 21:26–35, 1993.

38. Ernst, GP, Kawaguchi, J, and Saliba, E: Effect of patellar taping on knee kinetics of patients with patellofemoral pain syndrome. J Orthop Sports Phys Ther 29:661–667, 1999.

39. Finestone, A, Radin, EL, Lev, B, Shlamkovitch, N, Wiener, M, and Milgrom, C: Treatment of overuse patellofemoral pain: Prospective randomized controlled clinical trial in a military setting. Clin Orthop 293:208–210, 1993.

40. France, EP, Cawley, PW, and Paulos, LE: Choosing functional knee braces. Clin Sports Med 9:743–759, 1990.

41. France, EP, and Paulos, LE: Knee bracing. J Am Acad Orthop Surg 2:281–287, 1994.

42. France, EP, Paulos, LE, Jayaraman, G, and Rosenberg, TD: The biomechanics of lateral knee bracing: Part II: Impact response of the braced knee. Am J Sports Med 15:430–438, 1987.

43. Fujiwara, LM, Perrin, DH, and Buxton, BP: Effects of three lateral knee braces on speed and agility in experienced and non-experienced wearers. Athl Train JNATA 25:160–161, 1990.

44. Fulkerson, JP: Diagnosis and treatment of patients with patellofemoral pain. Am J Sports Med 30:447–456, 2002.

45. Gigante, A, Pasquinelli, FM, Paladini, P, Ulisse, S, and Greco, F: The effects of patellar taping on patellofemoral incongruence: A computed tomography study. Am J Sports Med 29:88–92, 2001.

46. Gilleard, W, McConnell, J, and Parsons, D: The effect of patellar taping on the onset of vastus medialis obliquus and vastus lateralis muscle activity in persons with patellofemoral pain. Phys Ther 78:25–32, 1998.

47. Grace, TG, Skipper, BJ, Newberry, JC, Nelson, MA, Sweetser, ER, and Rothman, ML: Prophylactic knee braces and injury to the lower extremity. J Bone Joint Surg 70-A:422–427, 1988.

48. Greene, DL, Hamson, KR, Bay, RC, and Bryce, CD: Effects of protective knee bracing on speed and agility. Am J Sports Med 28:453–459, 2000.

49. Handfield, T, and Kramer, J: Effect of McConnell taping on perceived pain and knee extensor torques during isokinetic exercise performed by patients with patellofemoral pain syndrome. Physiother Can Winter:39–44, 2000.

50. Harrison, EL, Sheppard, MS, and McQuarrie, AM: A randomized controlled trial of physical therapy treatment programs in patellofemoral pain syndrome. Physiother Can 51:93–100, 1999.

51. Herrington, L, Payton, C: Effects of corrective taping of the patella on patients with patellofemoral pain. Physiotherapy 83:566–572, 1997.

52. Hewson, GF, Mendini, RA, and Wang, JB: Prophylactic knee bracing in college football. Am J Sports Med 14:262–266, 1986.

53. Hilyard, A: Recent developments in the management of patellofemoral pain: The McConnell programme. Physiotherapy 76:559–565, 1990.

54. Houston, ME, and Goemans, PH: Leg muscle performance of athletes with and without knee support braces. Arch Phys Med Rehabil 63:431–432, 1982.

55. Jessell, TM, and Kelly, DD: Somatic sensory system IV: Central representation of pain and analgesia. In Kandel, ER, Schwartz, JH, and Jessell, TM (eds): Principles of Neural Science, ed 3. Elsevier Science Publishing, New York, 1991, pp 385–399.

56. Jonsson, H, and Karrholm, J: Brace effects on the unstable knee in 21 cases: A roentgen stereophotogrammetric comparison of three designs. Acta Orthop Scand 61:313–318, 1990.

57. Kartus, J, Stener, S, Kohler, K, Sern, N, Eriksson, BI, and Karlson, J: Is bracing after anterior cruciate ligament reconstruction necessary? A 2-year follow-up of 78 consecutive patients rehabilitated with or without a brace. Knee Surg Sports Traumatol Arthrosc 5:157–161, 1997.

58. Kowall, MG, Kolk, G, Nuber, GW, Cassisi, JE, and Stern, SH: Patellar taping in the treatment of patellofemoral pain. Am J Sports Med 24:61–66, 1996.

59. Kramer, JF, Dubowitz, T, Fowler, P, Schachter, C, and Birmingham, T: Functional knee braces and dynamic performance: A review. Clin J Sport Med 7:32–39, 1997.

60. Larsen, B, Andreasen, E, Urfer, A, Mickelson, MR, and Newhouse, KE: Patellar taping: A radiographic examination of the medial glide technique. Am J Sports Med 23:465–471, 1995.

61. Lephart, SM, Kocher, MS, Fu, FH, Borsa, PA, and Harner, CD: Proprioception following ACL reconstruction. J Sports Rehabil 1:188–196, 1992.

62. Liggett, CL, Tandy, RD, and Young, JC: The effect of prophylactic knee bracing on running gait. J Athl Train 30:159–161, 1995.

63 Liu SH, Lunsford T, Gude S, and Vangsness, CT: Comparison of functional knee braces for control of anterior tibial displacement. Clin Orthop 303:203–210, 1994.

64. Liu, SH, and Mirzayan, R: Current review: Functional knee bracing. Clin Orthop Relat Res 317:273–281, 1995.

65. Losse, GM, Howard, ME, and Cawley, PW: Effect of functional knee bracing on neurosensory function in the lower extremity in a group of anterior cruciate deficient knees. American Academy of Orthopedic Surgeons. 63rd Annual Meeting, Atlanta, GA, February 1996.

66. Marans, HJ, Jackson, RW, Piccinin, J, Silver, RL, and Kennedy, DK: Functional testing of braces for anterior cruciate ligament-deficient knees. Can J Surg 34:167–172, 1991.

67. McConnell, J, http://www.mcconnell-institute.com/kneearticle.html, Management of patellofemoral pain, 1999.

68. McConnell, J: A novel approach to pain relief pre-therapeutic exercise. J Sci Med Sport 3:325, 2000.

69. McConnell, JS: The management of chondromalacia patellae: A long term solution. Austr J Physiother 32:215–233, 1986.

70. McNair, PJ, Stanley, SN, and Strauss, GR: Knee bracing: Effects on proprioception. Arch Phys Med Rehabil 77:287–289, 1996.

71. Miller, MD, Hinkin, DT, and Wisnowski, JW: The efficacy of orthotics for anterior knee pain in military trainees: A preliminary report. Am J Knee Surg 10:10–13, 1997.

72. Mishra, DK, Daniel, DM, and Stone, ML: The use of functional knee braces in the control of pathologic anterior knee laxity. Clin Orthop 241:213–220, 1989.

73. Morrison, JB: The mechanics of the knee joint in relation to normal walking. J Biomech 3:51–61, 1970.

74. Munns, SW: Knee orthoses. Phys Med Rehabil: State of the Art Reviews 14:423–433, 2000.

75. National Collegiate Athletic Association, http://www.ncaa.org/library/sports_sciences/ sports_med_handbook/2003-04/index.html, Sports medicine handbook, 2003-2004.

76. National Federation of State High School Associations: 2004 Football Rules Book. Indianapolis, IN: National Federation of State High School Associations; 2004.

77. Osternig, LR, and Robertson, RN: Effects of prophylactic knee bracing on lower extremity joint position and muscle activation during running. Am J Sports Med 21:733–737, 1993.

78. Palumbo, PM, Jr: Dynamic patellar brace: a new orthosis in the management of patellofemoral disorders: A preliminary report. Am J Sports Med 9:45–49, 1981.

79. Paluska, SA, and McKeag, DB: Prescribing functional braces for knee instability. Phys Sportsmed 27:117–118, 1999.

80. Paluska, SA, McKeag, DB, and Roberts, WO: Using patellofemoral braces for anterior knee pain. Phys Sportsmed 27:81–82, 1999.

81. Paulos, LE, Cawley, PW, and France, EP: Impact biomechanics of lateral knee bracing: The anterior cruciate ligament. Am J Sports Med 19:337–342, 1991.

82. Powers, CM: Rehabilitation of patellofemoral joint disorders: A critical review. J Orthop Sports Phys Ther 5:345–354, 1998.

83. Powers, CM, Landel, R, Sosnick, T, Kirby, J, Mengel, K, Cheney, A, and Perry, J: The effects of patellar taping on stride characteristics and joint motion in subjects with patellofemoral pain. J Orthop Sports Phys Ther 26:286–291, 1997.

84. Powers, CM, Shellock, FG, Beering, TV, Garrido, DE, Goldbach, RM, and Molnar, T: Effect of bracing on patellar kinematics in patients with patellofemoral joint pain. Med Sci Sports Exerc 31:1714–1720, 1999.

85. Prentice, WE: Arnheim's Principles of Athletic Training, ed 11. McGraw-Hill, Boston, 2003.

86. Prentice, WE, and Toriscelli, T: The effects of lateral knee stabilizing braces on running speed and agility. JNATA 21:112–113, 1986.

87. Ramsey, DK, Lamontange, M, Wrentenberg, PF, Valentin, A, Engström, B, and Németh, G: Assessment of functional knee bracing: An in vivo three-dimensional kinematic analysis of the anterior cruciate deficient knee. Clin Biomech 16:61–70, 2001.

88. Rink, PC, Scott, RA, Lupo, RL, and Guest, SJ: A comparative study of functional bracing in the anterior cruciate deficient knee. Orthop Rev 18:719–727, 1989.

89. Risberg, MA, Holm, I, Steen, H, Eriksson, J, and Ekeland, A: The effect of knee bracing after anterior cruciate ligament reconstruction: A prospective, randomized study with two years' follow-up. Am J Sports Med 27:76–83, 1999.

90. Roberts, JM: The effect of taping on patellofemoral alignment-a radiological pilot study. Manipulative Therapists Association of Australia Conference, Adelaide, 1989, pp 146–151.

91. Rovere, GD, Haupt, HA, and Yates, CS: Prophylactic knee bracing in college football. Am J Sports Med 15:111–116, 1987.

92. Salvaterra, G, Wang, M, Mourehouse, C, and Buckley, W: An in vitro biomechanical study of the static stabilizing effect of lateral prophylactic knee bracing on medial stability. J Athl Train 28:113–119, 1993.

93. Sauers, EL, and Harter, RA: Efficacy of prophylactic knee braces: Current research perspectives. Athl Ther Today 3:14–20, 1998.

94. Sforzo, GA, Chen, NM, Gold, CA, and Frye, PA: The effect of prophylactic knee bracing on performance. Med Sci Sports Exerc 21:254–257, 1989.

95. Shelton, WR, Barrett, GR, and Dukes, A: Early season anterior cruciate ligament tears. Am J Sports Med 25:656–658, 1997.

96. Sitler, M, Ryan, J, Hopkinson, W, Wheeler, J, Santomier, J, Kolb, R, and Polley, D: The efficacy of a prophylactic knee brace to reduce knee injuries in football: A prospective, randomized study at West Point. Am J Sports Med 18:310–315, 1990.

97. Soma, CA, Vangsness, CT, Cawley, PW, and Liu, SH: Functional knee braces: The effects of rate of force application on anterior tibial translation in custom fit versus

premanufactured braces. American Academy of Orthopedic Surgeons. 62nd Annual Meeting, Orlando, FL, May 1995.

98. Somes, S, Worrell, TW, Corey, B, and Ingersol, CD: Effects of patellar taping on patellar position in the open and closed kinetic chain: A preliminary study. J Sports Rehabil 6:299–308, 1997.

99. Stephens, DL: The effects of functional knee braces on speed in collegiate basketball players. J Orthop Sports Phys Ther 22:259–262, 1995.

100. Tegner, Y, and Lysholm, J: Derotation braces and knee function in patients with anterior cruciate ligament tears. Arthroscopy 1:264–267, 1985.

101. Teitz, CC, Hermanson, BK, Kronmal, RA, and Diehr, PH: Evaluation of the use of braces to prevent injury to the knee in collegiate football players. J Bone Joint Surg 69-A:2–9, 1987.

102. Timm, KE: Randomized controlled trial of Protonics on patellar pain, position, and function. Med Sci Sports Exerc 30:665–670, 1998.

103. Torzilli, PA, Deng, X, and Warren, RF: The effect of joint-compressive load and quadriceps muscle force on knee motion in the intact and anterior cruciate ligament-sectioned knee. Am J Sports Med 22:105–112, 1994.

104. Washington, RL, Bernhardt, DT, Gomez, J, Johnson, MD, Martin, TJ, Rowland, TW, and Small, E: Technical report: Knee brace use in the young athlete. Pediatrics 108:503–507, 2001.

105. Wilson, LQ, Weltman, JY, Martin, DE, and Weltman, A: Effects of a functional knee brace for ACL insufficiency during treadmill running. Med Sci Sports Exerc 30:655–664, 1998.

106. Wojtys, EM, and Huston, LJ: "Custom-fit" versus "off-the-shelf" ACL functional braces. Am J Knee Surg 14:157–162, 2001.

107. Wojtys, EM, Kothari, SU, and Huston, LJ : Anterior cruciate ligament functional brace use in sports. Am J Sports Med 24:539–546, 1996.

108. Worrell, T, Ingersoll, CD, Bockrath-Pugliese, K, and Minis, P: Effect of patellar taping and bracing on patellar position as determined by MRI in patients with patellofemoral pain. J Athl Train 1998;33:16–20, 1998.

109. Worrell, TW, Ingersoll, CD, and Farr, J: Effect of patellar taping and bracing on patellar position: An MRI case study. J Sport Rehabil 3:146–153, 1994.

110. Wu, GKH, Ng, GYF, and Mak, AFT: Effects of knee bracing on the sensorimotor function of subjects with anterior cruciate ligament reconstruction. Am J Sports Med 29:641–645, 2001.

Thigh, Hip, and Pelvis

LEARNING OBJECTIVES

1. Discuss common injuries that occur to the thigh, hip, and pelvis.
2. Demonstrate the ability to apply tapes, wraps, braces, and pads to the thigh, hip, and pelvis when preventing, treating, and rehabilitating injuries.
3. Explain and demonstrate appropriate taping, wrapping, bracing, and padding techniques for the thigh, hip, and pelvis within a therapeutic exercise program.

INJURIES AND CONDITIONS

Acute and chronic injuries can occur to the thigh, hip, and pelvis in athletic and work activities. Thigh and hip contusions are common in athletic activities, but vary in severity. Many athletes are able to return to activity following a mild contusion with additional padding, while a severe contusion may require hospitalization. Strains of the thigh and hip musculature can occur in athletic and work activities and are typically caused by rapid movements. Repetitive stress to the thigh, hip, and pelvis can result in chronic inflammation and/or stress fractures. Common injuries to the thigh, hip, and pelvis include:

- Contusions
- Strains
- Overuse injuries and conditions

Contusions

Contusions to the thigh, hip, and pelvis are caused by direct forces. These areas are susceptible to injury in many sports that do not require protective padding. Thigh contusions (**charleyhorse**) typically involve the anterior and/or lateral aspect (see Illustration 7–1). A contusion can result, for instance, when a soccer sweeper is struck in the anterior or right thigh by an opponent's knee while attempting to stop a breakaway. **Myositis ossificans** may result from a single, violent direct force or repeated direct forces to the anterior or lateral thigh.[1,6,13] Improper use of thermotherapy modalities, forceful manipulation, or a quick return to activity following a quadriceps contusion can also lead to the development of myositis ossificans.[8,9] A direct force or fall on the hip can cause an iliac crest contusion (**hip pointer**) with associated injury to the abdominal soft tissue (Illustrations 7–2 and 12–12) These contusions are common in collision and contact sport activities.

Strains

Strains to the thigh, hip, and pelvis are caused by a variety of mechanisms during athletic and work activities. A rapid stretch, contraction, or change in direction, eccentric overload, fatigue, and muscular weakness and imbalance can

DETAILS

The name charleyhorse was created by major league baseball players in the early 20th century when horses were used to pull lawn mowers, including a horse known as Charley at Ebbets Field in New York. Charley suffered from a chronic limp; when a player sustained a thigh contusion that caused a limp, others reportedly said the player was limping like Charley the horse.[10]

result in a quadriceps, hamstrings, adductor, gluteal, and iliopsoas strain (see Illustrations 7–1, 7–2, 7–3). Abnormal posture and leg-length discrepancy may contribute to a hamstring strain. Strains occur more frequently to the hamstrings; these injuries often have a chronic history.[3,4] For example, a quadriceps strain can occur as a volleyball player jumps to spike the ball at the net, causing an explosive contraction of the quadriceps. A hamstring strain can result when a sprinter increases the stride length at the finish line, causing a violent stretch of the musculature.

Overuse

Structural abnormalities and repetitive stress can cause overuse injuries to the hip, thigh, and pelvis. Repetitive running on banked surfaces, training errors, leg-length discrepancy, and an increased **Q angle** can result in **greater trochanteric bursitis**.[2] A single direct force to the trochanteric bursa causing chronic inflammation can also lead to bursitis.[14] **Osteitis pubis** is caused by repetitive tension from the adductor or rectus abdominis musculature on the pubic symphysis,[2] which occurs with repeated twisting and change in direction activities. The repetitive kicking and pivoting on one leg experienced by rugby players may lead to the development of osteitis pubis. Stress fractures of the femur, hip, and pelvis may arise from overload, training errors, amenorrhea, oligomenorrhea, and disordered eating. For example, repetitive distance running without appropriate footwear, recovery, and caloric and nutrient intake could cause a stress fracture.

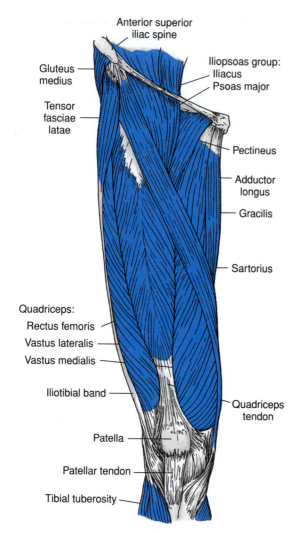

Anterior superior
iliac spine

Gluteus
medius

Tensor
fasciae
latae

Iliopsoas group:
Iliacus
Psoas major

Pectineus

Adductor
longus

Gracilis

Sartorius

Quadriceps:
Rectus femoris
Vastus lateralis
Vastus medialis

Iliotibial band

Quadriceps
tendon

Patella

Patellar tendon

Tibial tuberosity

Illustration 7-1 Superficial muscles of the anterior thigh.

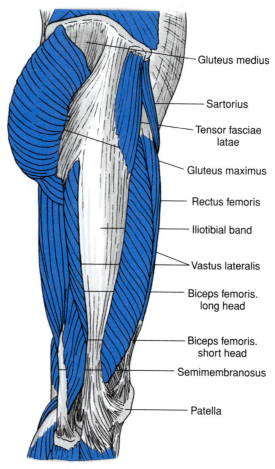

Gluteus medius

Sartorius

Tensor fasciae
latae

Gluteus maximus

Rectus femoris

Iliotibial band

Vastus lateralis

Biceps femoris.
long head

Biceps femoris.
short head

Semimembranosus

Patella

Illustration 7-2 Superficial muscles of the lateral thigh and hip.

Taping Techniques

Taping techniques are used to anchor protective padding to the thigh, hip, and pelvis following a quadriceps contusion or hip pointer. Protective padding techniques are illustrated in the Padding section.

CIRCULAR THIGH Figure 7–1

▶ **Purpose:** The circular thigh technique provides mild support and anchors protective padding to the thigh (Fig. 7–1). Use this technique with off-the-shelf and custom-made pads upon a return to activity, to absorb shock and prevent further injury for a quadriceps contusion or myositis ossificans.

▶ **Materials:**
• Pre-tape material or self-adherent wrap, 3 inch elastic tape, adherent tape spray, taping scissors
Option:
• 1½ inch non-elastic tape

▶ **Position of the individual:** Standing on a taping table or bench with the majority of the weight on the noninvolved leg and the involved leg placed in a neutral position with slight knee flexion. Maintain this position during application, with the use of a heel lift.

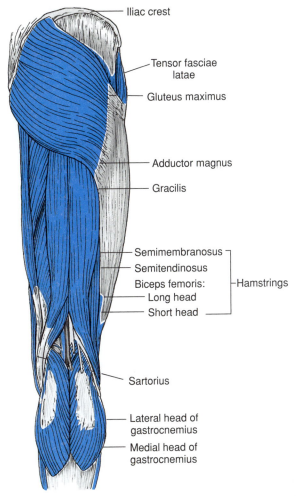

— Iliac crest

— Tensor fasciae
latae

— Gluteus maximus

— Adductor magnus

— Gracilis

— Semimembranosus
— Semitendinosus
Biceps femoris:
— Long head
— Short head

—Hamstrings

— Sartorius

— Lateral head of
gastrocnemius

— Medial head of
gastrocnemius

Illustration 7-3 Superficial muscles of the posterior thigh
and hip.

▶ **Preparation:** Apply adherent tape spray to the thigh, then pre-tape material or self-adherent wrap.

▶ **Application:**

(**STEP 1:**) Place the pad over the injured area.
Anchor 3 inch elastic tape directly on the
distal pad (Fig. 7–1A).

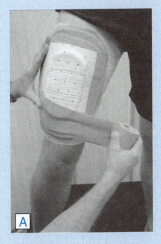

A

Figure 7-1

STEP 2: Continue around the thigh with moderate roll tension in a circular, distal-to-proximal pattern, overlapping the tape by ½ of its width (see Fig. 7–1B). Cover the entire pad and anchor on the top of the pad to prevent irritation. Avoid gaps, wrinkles, or inconsistent roll tension.

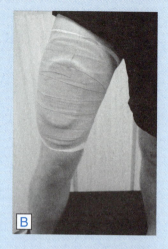

STEP 3: To prevent migration, a distal circular strip of elastic tape may be applied with distal-to-proximal tension or apply the proximal portion of the elastic tape partially on the skin (Fig. 7–1C).

Option: *Apply one to two circular strips of 1½ inch non-elastic tape loosely around the pad for additional anchors* *.*

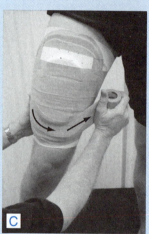

Helpful Hint: Near the completion of the technique, angle a strip distally, across the distal portion of the pad with moderate roll tension. Then continue sharply in a proximal direction, and finish the circular pattern (Fig. 7–1D).

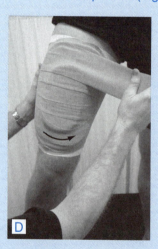

Figure 7-1 *continued*

This strip provides additional tension and support to lessen distal migration of the pad.

HIP POINTER TAPE   Figure 7–2

▶ **Purpose:** Use the hip pointer technique to absorb shock when preventing and treating contusions, and to anchor off-the-shelf and custom-made pads to the iliac crest (Fig. 7–2).

▶ **Materials:**
  • 2 inch or 3 inch heavyweight elastic tape, adherent tape spray, taping scissors

▶ **Position of the individual:** Standing on a taping table, bench, or floor with the majority of the weight on the noninvolved leg and the involved leg placed in a neutral position with slight knee flexion. Maintain this position during application with the use of a heel lift.

▶ **Preparation:** Apply the hip pointer technique directly to the skin.

▶ **Application:**

STEP 1: Apply adherent tape spray over the pad area and 4–6 inches beyond, over the hip and low back (Fig. 7–2A). Allow the spray to dry.

STEP 2: Cut several strips of 2 inch or 3 inch heavyweight elastic tape in lengths that will cover the pad and extend 4–6 inches beyond the pad on the two sides. Place the pad over the injured area.

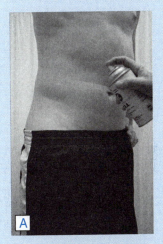

A

STEP 3: Anchor the first tape strip on the abdomen or anterior hip 4–6 inches from the edge of the pad and pat down (Fig. 7–2B). Do not stretch the tape as the anchor is applied.

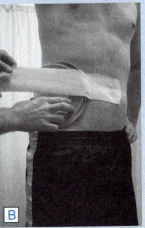

B

STEP 4: Continue to apply the strip to the edge of the pad. At the edge, hold the strip on the abdomen/anterior hip and pad with one hand and pull the strip over the pad with tension on the tape (Fig. 7–2C).

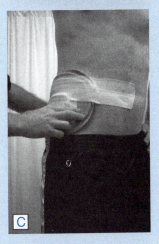

C

Figure 7-2

STEP 5: When the strip completely covers the pad, release the tension in the tape and anchor to the low back and pat down (Fig. 7–2D). This technique is the release-stretch-release sequence illustrated in Figure 1–13A–G.

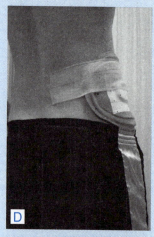

STEP 6: Continue with additional strips in the same manner, overlapping each by ½ the width of the tape (Fig. 7–2E).

STEP 7: Apply enough strips to cover the majority of the pad.

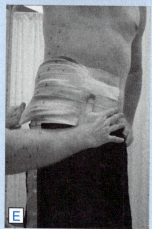

Figure 7-2 *continued*

Wrapping Techniques

Use wrapping techniques to provide compression and support, and to attach protective pads to the thigh, hip, and pelvis to prevent and treat quadriceps contusions and strains; hamstrings, adductor, hip flexor, and gluteal strains; iliac crest contusions; and myositis ossificans.

COMPRESSION WRAP TECHNIQUE ONE Figure 7–3

▶ **Purpose:** Apply this compression wrap technique to control mild to moderate swelling with mild thigh contusions and strains (Fig. 7–3).

▶ **Materials:**
  • 4 inch or 6 inch width by 5 yard length elastic wrap determined by the size of the thigh, metal clips, 1½ inch non-elastic or 2 inch or 3 inch elastic tape, taping scissors

  Options:
  • ¼ inch or ½ inch foam or felt
  • 4 inch or 6 inch width self-adherent wrap

▶ **Position of the individual:** Standing on a taping table or bench with the majority of the weight on the noninvolved leg and the involved leg placed in a pain-free, slightly flexed position. Maintain this position during application with the use of a heel lift.

▶ **Preparation:** To lessen migration, apply adherent tape spray, tape strips, or anchors directly to the skin (see Fig. 1–7).

Option: *Cut a ¼ inch or ½ inch foam or felt pad and place it over the inflamed area directly to the skin to provide additional compression and assist in venous return.*

▸ **Application:**

STEP 1: Anchor the wrap around the distal thigh directly to the skin and encircle the anchor ◀▶ (Fig. 7–3A).

Option: *Four inch or 6 inch self-adherent wrap may be used if an elastic wrap is not available.*

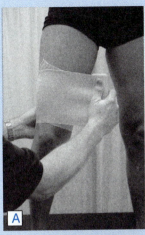

STEP 2: Continue to apply the wrap in a spiral pattern in a distal-to-proximal direction, overlapping the wrap by ½ of its width (Fig. 7–3B). Apply the greatest amount of roll tension distally and over the inflamed area. Lessen the roll tension as the wrap continues proximally from the injured area.

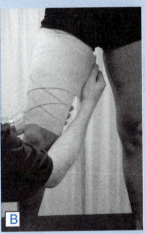

STEP 3: Finish the wrap over the proximal thigh and anchor with Velcro, metal clips, or loosely applied 1½ inch non-elastic or 2 inch or 3 inch elastic tape ◀▶ (Fig. 7–3C).

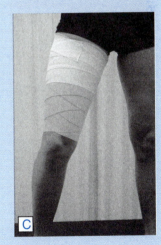

Figure 7-3

COMPRESSION WRAP TECHNIQUE TWO Figure 7–4

▸ **Purpose:** With second and third degree thigh contusions and strains, swelling can be severe. Use this compression wrap technique that includes the foot, ankle, lower leg, knee, and thigh to control moderate to severe swelling and prevent distal migration of postinjury swelling (Fig. 7–4).

▶ **Materials:**
- 4 inch or 6 inch width by 10 yard length elastic wrap, metal clips, 1½ inch non-elastic or 2 inch or 3 inch elastic tape, taping scissors

Option:
- ¼ inch or ½ inch foam or felt

▶ **Position of the individual:** Sitting on a taping table or bench with the leg extended off the edge, knee in a pain-free, slightly flexed position, and the ankle placed in 90° of dorsiflexion.

▶ **Preparation:** To lessen migration, apply adherent tape spray, tape strips, or anchors directly to the skin.

Option: *Cut a ¼ inch or ½ inch foam or felt pad and place it over the inflamed area directly to the skin to assist in controlling swelling.*

▶ **Application:**

STEP 1: Anchor the elastic wrap on the distal plantar foot and apply the foot, ankle, lower leg, and knee compression wrap directly to the skin (see Fig. 6–9).

STEP 2: At the mid thigh, continue the spiral wrap to the proximal thigh ◀▬ (Fig. 7–4A). Apply the greatest amount of roll tension distally and lessen tension as the wrap continues proximally.

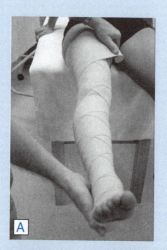

A

STEP 3: Anchor the wrap with Velcro, metal clips, or loosely applied 1½ inch non-elastic or 2 inch or 3 inch elastic tape ◀▬ (Fig. 7–4B) ✂.

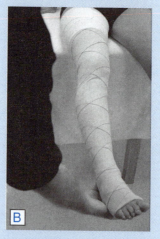

B

Figure 7-4

 Helpful Hint: When treating a quadriceps contusion, place the knee in maximal pain-free flexion to stretch the quadriceps. Use a 4 inch or 6 inch width by 10 yard length elastic wrap to provide compression, anchor an ice bag, and maintain knee flexion by encircling the thigh and proximal lower leg.

COMPRESSION WRAP TECHNIQUE THREE Figure 7–5

▶ **Purpose:** Use an elastic sleeve to provide compression to the thigh in controlling mild to moderate swelling (Fig. 7–5). The benefit of this wrap is that the individual can apply this technique without assistance following application instruction.

▶ **Materials:**
- 5 inch width elastic sleeve, taping scissors

Option:
- ¼ inch or ½ inch foam or felt

▶ **Position of the individual:** Sitting on a taping table or bench with the leg extended off the edge.

▶ **Preparation:** Cut an elastic sleeve from a roll to extend from the superior knee to the proximal thigh area. Cut and use a double length sleeve to provide additional compression.

Option: *Cut a ¼ inch or ½ inch foam or felt pad and place it over the inflamed area directly to the skin to assist in venous return.*

▶ **Application:**
(**STEP 1:**) Pull the sleeve onto the thigh in a distal-to-proximal pattern. If using a double length sleeve, pull the distal end over the first layer (Fig. 7–5). No anchors are required; the sleeve can be cleaned and reused.

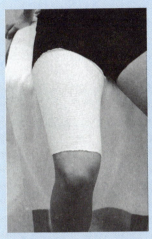

Figure 7-5

QUADRICEPS STRAIN WRAP Figures 7–6, 7–7

▶ **Purpose:** The quadriceps strain technique is used to provide compression and mild to moderate circular support when treating strains. This technique may be used to anchor protective padding for a quadriceps contusion or myositis ossificans. Two methods are illustrated in the application of the technique to accommodate individual preferences and available supplies. Protective padding techniques are illustrated in the Padding section (see Fig. 7–18).

Quadriceps Strain Technique One

▶ **Materials:**
- 4 inch or 6 inch width by 5 yard length elastic wrap, metal clips, 1½ inch non-elastic tape, 2 inch or 3 inch elastic tape, taping scissors

▶ **Position of the individual:** Standing on a taping table or bench with the majority of the weight on the noninvolved leg and the involved leg placed in a neutral position with slight knee flexion. Maintain this position during application with the use of a heel lift.

▶ **Preparation:** To lessen migration, apply adherent tape spray, tape strips, or anchors directly to the skin. To anchor a pad, place the pad over the injured area.

▶ **Application:**

STEP 1: Anchor the extended end of the elastic wrap on the lateral distal thigh directly to the skin and proceed around the thigh in a medial direction to encircle the anchor (Fig. 7–6A).

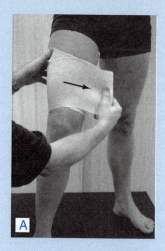

STEP 2: Continue to apply the wrap in a lateral-to-medial circular pattern with moderate roll tension, overlapping by ½ of the wrap width, moving in a distal-to-proximal direction (Fig. 7–6B). Avoid gaps, wrinkles, or inconsistent roll tension.

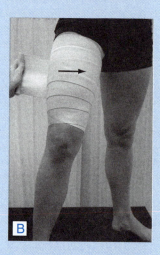

STEP 3: Finish the wrap over the proximal thigh. The wrap should extend above and below the injured area. During nonathletic or nonwork activities, anchor the wrap with Velcro, metal clips, or loosely applied 1½ inch non-elastic tape (Fig. 7–6C).

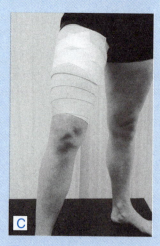

Figure 7-6

STEP 4: With athletic or work activities, anchor 2 inch or 3 inch elastic tape on the lateral distal thigh and apply two to four continuous lateral-to-medial circular patterns with moderate roll tension, finishing on the proximal thigh (Fig. 7–6D). To ensure adherence, anchor the loose end of the elastic tape on the circular tape pattern rather than on the wrap. Additional anchors are not required.

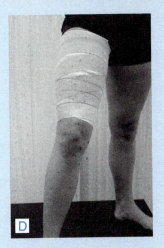

Figure 7-6 *continued*

Quadriceps Strain Technique Two

▶ **Materials:**
- 4 inch or 6 inch width by 10 yard length elastic wrap, metal clips, 1½ inch non-elastic tape, 2 inch or 3 inch elastic tape, taping scissors

▶ **Position of the individual:** Standing on a taping table, bench, or floor with the majority of the weight on the noninvolved leg and the involved leg placed in a neutral position with slight knee flexion. Maintain this position during application.

▶ **Preparation:** To lessen migration, apply adherent tape spray, tape strips, or anchors directly to the skin. If using a pad, place it over the injured area.

▶ **Application:**
STEP 1: Anchor the wrap on the lateral distal thigh directly to the skin and apply technique one.

STEP 2: At the proximal thigh, continue to apply the wrap in a lateral-to-medial direction across the lateral hip and abdomen with mild roll tension (Fig. 7–7A). Continue the wrap to encircle the waist and return to the proximal thigh (Fig. 7–7B). Monitor roll tension to prevent constriction and irritation of the lower abdominal and back soft tissue.

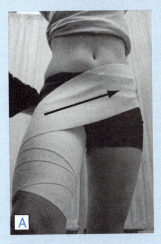 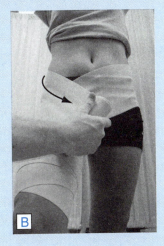

Figure 7-7

STEP 3: Next, apply one to two additional circular patterns around the mid-to-proximal thigh (Fig. 7–7C) and encircle the waist (Fig. 7–7D).

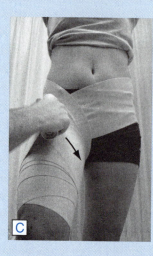
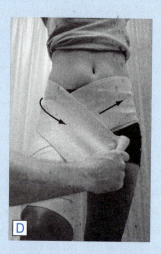

STEP 4: Anchor the wrap over the mid thigh. Use Velcro, metal clips, or 1½ inch non-elastic tape to anchor, for nonathletic or nonwork activities. During athletic or work activities, anchor 2 inch or 3 inch elastic tape on the lateral distal thigh and apply two to four continuous lateral-to-medial circular patterns around the thigh with moderate roll tension.

STEP 5: At the proximal thigh, continue to apply the elastic tape with mild roll tension to encircle the waist and anchor on the circular tape pattern on the mid thigh (Fig. 7–7E). No additional anchors are required.

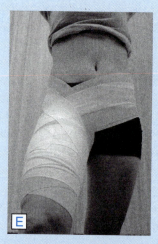

Figure 7-7 *continued*

HAMSTRINGS STRAIN WRAP Figures 7–8, 7–9

▶ **Purpose:** Use the hamstrings strain technique to provide compression and mild to moderate circular support when treating strains. Two methods are illustrated to accommodate individual preferences and available supplies.

Hamstrings Strain Technique One

▶ **Materials:**
- 4 inch or 6 inch width by 5 yard length elastic wrap, metal clips, 1½ inch non-elastic tape, 2 inch or 3 inch elastic tape, taping scissors

▶ **Position of the individual:** Standing on a taping table or bench with the majority of the weight on the noninvolved leg and the involved leg placed in a neutral position with slight knee flexion. Maintain this position during application with the use of a heel lift.

◗ **Preparation:** To lessen migration, apply adherent tape spray, tape strips, or anchors directly to the skin.

◗ **Application:**

STEP 1: When treating a medial hamstrings strain, anchor the extended end of the wrap on the distal, posterior medial thigh directly to the skin and proceed in a lateral direction around the thigh to encircle the anchor (Fig. 7–8A).

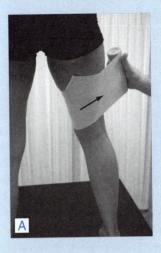

STEP 2: Continue to apply the wrap with moderate roll tension in a medial-to-lateral circular pattern. Overlap the wrap by ½ of the width and apply it in a distal-to-proximal direction (Fig. 7–8B). Avoid gaps, wrinkles, or inconsistent roll tension.

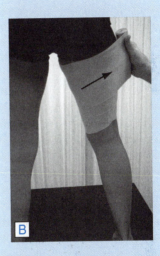

STEP 3: Finish the wrap over the proximal thigh, extending above and below the injured area. Anchor the wrap as illustrated in Figures 7–6C or 7–6D, but apply the 1½ inch non-elastic or 2 inch or 3 inch elastic tape in a medial-to-lateral circular pattern (Fig. 7–8C). Additional anchors are not necessary.

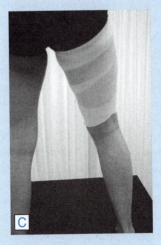

Figure 7-8

Thigh, Hip, and Pelvis

STEP 4: When treating a lateral hamstrings strain, anchor the extended end of the wrap on the distal, posterior lateral thigh directly to the skin and proceed around the thigh in a medial direction to encircle the anchor (Fig. 7–8D).

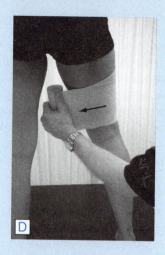

STEP 5: Continue to apply the wrap in a lateral-to-medial circular pattern, overlapping the wrap by ½ of the width, moving in a distal-to-proximal direction with moderate roll tension (Fig. 7–8E).

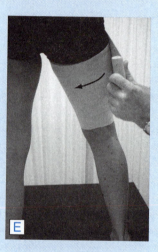

STEP 6: Finish over the proximal thigh and anchor as shown in Figures 7–6C or 7–6D, applying the 1½ inch non-elastic or 2 inch or 3 inch elastic tape in a lateral-to-medial circular pattern (Fig. 7–8F).

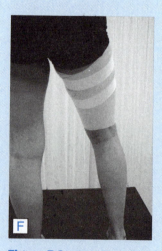

Figure 7-8 *continued*

Hamstrings Strain Technique Two

▶ **Materials:**
  • 4 inch or 6 inch width by 10 yard length elastic wrap, metal clips, 1½ inch non-elastic tape, 2 inch or 3 inch elastic tape, taping scissors

- **Position of the individual:** Standing on a taping table, bench, or floor with the majority of the weight on the noninvolved leg and the involved leg placed in a neutral position with slight knee flexion. Maintain this position during application.

- **Preparation:** To lessen migration, apply adherent tape spray, tape strips, or anchors directly to the skin.

- **Application:**

  STEP 1: When treating a medial hamstrings strain, anchor the extended end of the wrap on the distal, posterior medial thigh and apply technique one.

  STEP 2: At the proximal thigh, continue to apply the wrap in a medial-to-lateral direction across the lateral hip and encircle the waist with mild roll tension (Fig. 7–9A), returning to the proximal thigh (see Fig. 7–9B). Monitor roll tension to prevent constriction and irritation of the soft tissue.

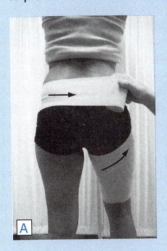 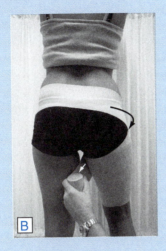

  STEP 3: Next, apply one to two additional circular patterns around the mid-to-proximal thigh and encircle the waist (Fig. 7–9C).

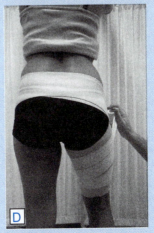

  STEP 4: Anchor the wrap over the mid thigh. Use Velcro, metal clips, or 1½ inch non-elastic tape to anchor with nonathletic or nonwork activities ◀▬. With athletic or work activities, anchor 2 inch or 3 inch elastic tape on the posterior medial thigh and apply two to four continuous medial-to-lateral circular patterns with moderate roll tension around the thigh (Fig. 7–9D).

Figure 7-9

STEP 5: At the proximal thigh, continue to apply the elastic tape with mild roll tension to encircle the waist and anchor on the circular tape pattern on the mid thigh (Fig. 7–9E). No additional anchors are required.

STEP 6: When treating a lateral hamstrings strain, anchor the extended end of the wrap on the distal, posterior lateral thigh directly to the skin and apply technique one.

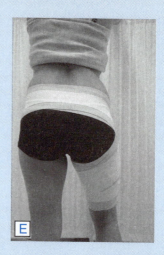

STEP 7: At the proximal thigh, continue to apply the wrap in a lateral-to-medial direction across the lateral hip and encircle the waist with mild roll tension (Fig. 7–9F), returning to the proximal thigh (see Fig. 7–9G).

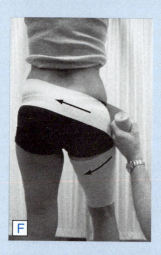
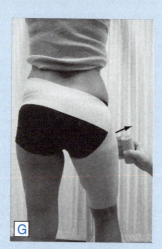

STEP 8: Next, apply one to two additional circular patterns around the mid-to-proximal thigh and encircle the waist (Fig. 7–9H). Anchor the wrap over the mid thigh with Velcro, metal clips, or 1½ inch non-elastic tape ◀▶, or as illustrated in Figure 7–9D and Figure 7–9E. Apply the 1½ inch non-elastic or 2 inch or 3 inch elastic tape in a lateral-to-medial circular pattern (Fig. 7–9I).

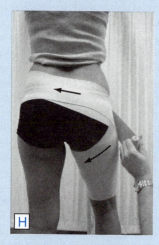
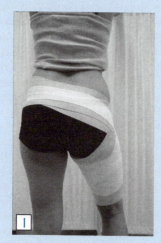

Figure 7-9 *continued*

> **...IF/THEN...**
>
> **IF** the quadriceps and/or hamstrings strain wrapping technique one migrates distally during activity, **THEN** consider applying technique two, incorporating the waist, to lessen migration.

ADDUCTOR STRAIN WRAP   Figure 7–10

▶ **Purpose:** The adductor strain technique is used to provide compression and mild to moderate support of hip adduction when treating strains (Fig. 7–10).

▶ **Materials:**
  • 4 inch or 6 inch width by 10 yard length elastic wrap, metal clips, 1½ inch non-elastic tape, 2 inch or 3 inch elastic tape, taping scissors

▶ **Position of the individual:** Standing on a taping table, bench, or floor with the majority of the weight on the noninvolved leg and the involved leg in an internally rotated position with slight knee flexion. Maintain this position during application.

▶ **Preparation:** To lessen migration, apply adherent tape spray, tape strips, or anchors directly to the skin.

▶ **Application:**
  STEP 1: Anchor the extended end of the elastic wrap on the lateral distal thigh directly to the skin and continue in a medial direction to encircle the anchor (Fig. 7–10A).

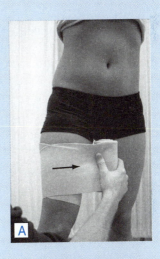

  STEP 2: Continue to apply the wrap in a lateral-to-medial circular pattern with moderate roll tension, supporting internal rotation of the leg (Fig. 7–10B). Move in a distal-to-proximal direction and overlap the wrap by ½ of the width. Avoid gaps, wrinkles, or inconsistent roll tension.

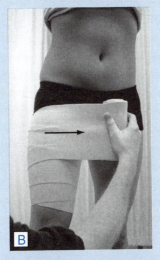

Figure 7-10

STEP 3: At the proximal thigh, continue in a lateral-to-medial direction across the lateral hip, abdomen, and waist with mild roll tension (Fig. 7–10C). Next, continue to apply the wrap distally across the medial proximal thigh with a moderate internal rotation pull, then continue around the proximal thigh (Fig. 7–10D). Monitor roll tension to prevent constriction and irritation of the lower abdominal and back and medial thigh soft tissue.

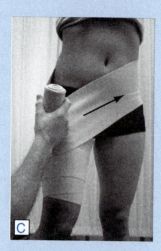
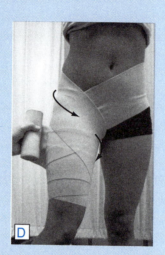

STEP 4: Apply one circular pattern around the mid-to-proximal thigh, encircle the waist, then cross the medial proximal thigh, supporting internal rotation of the leg (Fig. 7–10E). Repeat this pattern one to two times.

STEP 5: Finish the wrap over the mid thigh. Anchor with Velcro, metal clips, or 1½ inch non-elastic tape for nonathletic or nonwork activities ◀━ .

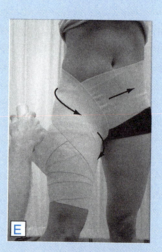

STEP 6: Use 2 inch or 3 inch elastic tape to anchor for athletic or work activities. Start at the lateral distal thigh and apply two to four continuous lateral-to-medial circular patterns around the thigh with moderate roll tension, again supporting internal rotation of the leg. Continue to apply the elastic tape to encircle the hip and waist with mild roll tension, across the medial proximal thigh with a moderate internal rotation pull, encircle the thigh, and anchor on the circular tape pattern on the mid thigh (Fig. 7–10F). No additional anchors are required. When the adductor strain wrapping technique is properly applied, the individual should feel an internal rotation pull from the wrap on the leg.

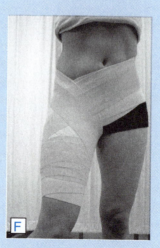

Figure 7-10 *continued*

HIP FLEXOR STRAIN WRAP Figure 7–11

▶ **Purpose:** The hip flexor strain technique provides compression and mild to moderate support of hip flexion when treating iliopsoas strains (Fig. 7–11).

▶ **Materials:**
  • 4 inch or 6 inch width by 10 yard length elastic wrap, metal clips, 1½ inch non-elastic tape, 2 inch or 3 inch elastic tape, taping scissors

▶ **Position of the individual:** Standing on a taping table, bench, or floor with the majority of the weight on the noninvolved leg and the involved leg placed in a neutral position with slight knee flexion. Maintain this position during application.

▶ **Preparation:** To lessen migration, apply adherent tape spray, tape strips, or anchors directly to the skin.

▶ **Application:**

(STEP 1:) Anchor the extended end of the wrap on the mid medial thigh directly to the skin and proceed in a lateral direction around the thigh to encircle the anchor (Fig. 7–11A).

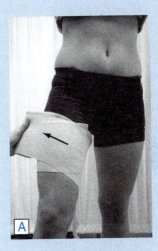

(STEP 2:) Continue to apply the wrap with moderate roll tension in a medial-to-lateral circular pattern. Overlap the wrap by ½ of the width and apply in a distal-to-proximal direction (Fig. 7–11B). Avoid gaps, wrinkles, or inconsistent roll tension.

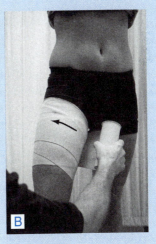

Figure 7-11

STEP 3: At the proximal thigh, apply the wrap in a medial-to-lateral direction across the lateral hip with a moderate upward pull (Fig. 7–11C). Continue to encircle the waist with mild roll tension and return to the proximal thigh. Monitor roll tension to prevent constriction and irritation of the soft tissue.

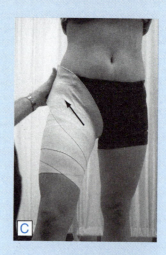

STEP 4: Apply one circular pattern around the mid-to-proximal thigh, across the lateral hip with a moderate upward pull, encircle the waist, and return to the proximal thigh (Fig. 7–11D). Repeat this pattern one to two times.

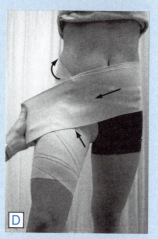

STEP 5: Anchor the wrap over the mid thigh. Use Velcro, metal clips, or 1½ inch non-elastic tape to anchor with nonathletic or nonwork activities 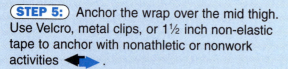.

STEP 6: With athletic or work activities, anchor 2 inch or 3 inch elastic tape on the mid medial thigh and apply two to four continuous medial-to-lateral circular patterns around the thigh with moderate roll tension. At the proximal thigh, continue to apply the elastic tape across the lateral hip with a moderate upward pull, encircle the waist with mild roll tension, and anchor on the circular tape pattern on the mid thigh (Fig. 7–11E). No additional anchors are required.

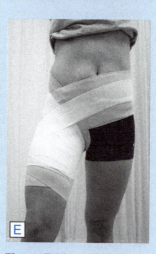

Figure 7-11   *continued*

GLUTEAL STRAIN WRAP Figure 7–12

▶ **Purpose:** Use the gluteal strain technique to provide compression and mild to moderate support and to limit stretch on the gluteal musculature when treating strains (Fig. 7–12).

▶ **Materials:**
- 4 inch or 6 inch width by 10 yard length elastic wrap, metal clips, 1½ inch non-elastic tape, 2 inch or 3 inch elastic tape, taping scissors

- **Position of the individual:** Standing on a taping table, bench, or floor with the majority of the weight on the noninvolved leg and the involved leg placed in a neutral position with slight knee flexion. Maintain this position during application.

- **Preparation:** To lessen migration, apply adherent tape spray, tape strips, or anchors directly to the skin.

- **Application:**

    STEP 1: Anchor the extended end of the wrap on the proximal lateral thigh directly to the skin and proceed in a medial direction around the thigh to encircle the anchor (Fig. 7–12A).

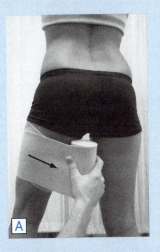

STEP 2: At the anterior thigh, apply the wrap with moderate roll tension in a lateral-to-medial direction across the lateral hip, proximal buttocks, and low back (Fig. 7–12B). Continue around the waist and lateral hip with mild roll tension, then distally across the medial buttocks with a moderate downward pull, around the medial thigh (Fig. 7–12C), and finish on the anterior thigh. Monitor roll tension to prevent constriction and irritation of the soft tissue.

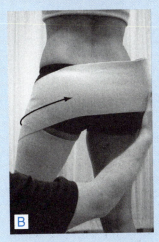
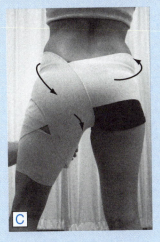

STEP 3: Repeat this pattern two to four times, overlapping the wrap by ½ of the width (Fig. 7–12D). Avoid gaps, wrinkles, or inconsistent roll tension.

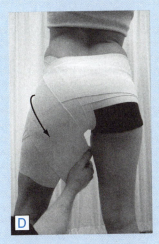

Figure 7-12

STEP 4: Anchor the wrap over the proximal thigh. Use Velcro, metal clips, or 1½ inch non-elastic tape to anchor with nonathletic or nonwork activities ◄══► . With athletic or work activities, anchor 2 inch or 3 inch elastic tape on the proximal lateral thigh and apply two to three continuous lateral-to-medial circular patterns around the thigh with moderate roll tension (Fig. 7–12E).

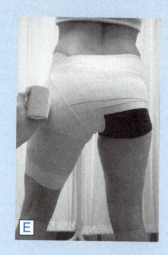

STEP 5: At the anterior thigh, continue to apply the elastic tape with mild roll tension across the lateral hip and proximal buttocks, encircle the waist, then apply distally across the medial buttocks with a moderate downward pull and around the thigh (Fig. 7–12F). Anchor on the circular tape pattern on the proximal thigh. No additional anchors are required.

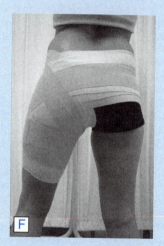

Figure 7-12 *continued*

HIP POINTER WRAP Figures 7–13, 7–14

▸ **Purpose:** The hip pointer technique is commonly used to anchor off-the-shelf and custom-made pads to the iliac crest to absorb shock when preventing and treating contusions. Two interchangeable methods are illustrated in the application of the hip pointer technique to accommodate individual preferences and available supplies.

Hip Pointer Technique One

▸ **Materials:**
  • 4 inch or 6 inch width by 5 yard length elastic wrap, 2 inch or 3 inch elastic tape, taping scissors

▸ **Position of the individual:** Standing on a taping table, bench, or floor with the majority of the weight on the noninvolved leg and the involved leg placed in a neutral position with slight knee flexion. Maintain this position during application.

▸ **Preparation:** To lessen migration, apply adherent tape spray, tape strips, or anchors directly to the skin.

▶ **Application:**

STEP 1: Place the pad over the injured area. Anchor the extended end of the wrap on the anterior hip directly to the skin and proceed over the pad and around the waist to encircle the anchor ◀━ (Fig. 7–13A).

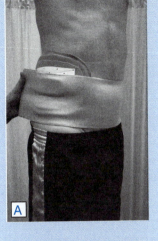

A

STEP 2: Continue to apply the wrap with moderate roll tension over the pad and around the waist (Fig. 7–13B). Overlap the wrap by ½ of the width and avoid gaps, wrinkles, or inconsistent roll tension. Monitor roll tension to prevent constriction and irritation of the soft tissue.

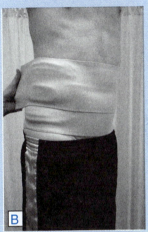

B

STEP 3: Anchor the wrap with 2 inch or 3 inch elastic tape. Apply two to three continuous circular patterns with the tape around the pad and waist with moderate roll tension ◀━ (Fig. 7–13C). Finish the loose end of the tape on the circular tape pattern to ensure adherence. No additional anchors are required.

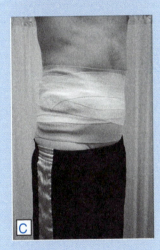

C

Figure 7-13

Hip Pointer Technique Two

▶ **Materials:**
- 4 inch or 6 inch width by 10 yard length elastic wrap, 2 inch or 3 inch elastic tape, taping scissors

▶ **Position of the individual:** Standing on a taping table, bench, or floor with the majority of the weight on the noninvolved leg and the involved leg placed in a neutral position with slight knee flexion. Maintain this position during application.

▶ **Preparation:** To lessen migration, apply adherent tape spray, tape strips, or anchors directly to the skin.

▶ **Application:**

(**STEP 1:**) Place the pad over the injured area. Anchor the extended end of the wrap on the mid medial thigh directly to the skin and apply the hip flexor strain technique over the pad. Note that achieving the moderate upward pull used with the strain technique is not necessary.

(**STEP 2:**) Anchor the wrap with 2 inch or 3 inch elastic tape. Apply one to two continuous medial-to-lateral circular patterns with moderate roll tension around the thigh, hip, and waist. Finish and anchor on the mid thigh circular tape pattern (Fig. 7–14A). No additional anchors are required.

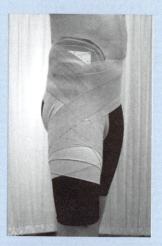

Figure 7-14

> ...**IF/THEN**...
>
> **IF** using the hip pointer wrap technique one or two to anchor an off-the-shelf or custom-made pad and migration occurs during activity, **THEN** consider the hip pointer taping technique; anchoring the pad directly to the skin with heavyweight elastic tape will lessen migration.

Bracing Techniques

Bracing techniques provide compression and support when treating injuries and conditions of the thigh, hip, and pelvis. To provide compression, neoprene sleeves and shorts are used when treating contusions, strains, and overuse injuries and conditions. Combination braces provide compression and support for the thigh and hip when treating strains.

NEOPRENE SLEEVE Figure 7–15

▶ **Purpose:** Neoprene sleeves are designed to provide compression and mild support when treating quadriceps strains and contusions, hamstrings strains, and myositis ossificans (Fig. 7–15).

> ○ **DETAILS**
>
> Use the sleeves during rehabilitative, athletic, work, and casual activities.

▶ **Design:**
- Off-the-shelf sleeves are manufactured in universal fit designs in predetermined sizes corresponding to thigh circumference measurements.
- Several designs have an oval neoprene pad incorporated into the sleeve to provide additional compression over the injured area.

▶ **Position of the individual:** Sitting on a taping table or bench with the leg extended off the edge, or in a chair, with the knee in approximately 45° of flexion.

▶ **Preparation:** Apply neoprene sleeves directly to the skin. No anchors are required.

▶ **Application:**

STEP 1: Hold each side of the sleeve and place the larger end over the foot. Pull in a proximal direction until the sleeve is positioned on the thigh (Fig. 7–15). After use, clean and reuse the sleeves.

STEP 2: If the design has an oval pad, position the pad over the injured area to provide additional compression.

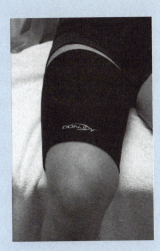

Figure 7-15

Critical Thinking Question 1

An outside hitter on the volleyball team sustained a second degree hamstrings strain during a match 4 weeks ago. Her recovery has progressed without any setbacks. The therapeutic exercise program the athlete is following includes the addition of aquatic therapy. The athlete is anxious about the water and wants to have some type of support around her thigh during the exercises.

▶ **Question: What techniques can you apply to provide support?**

NEOPRENE SHORTS Figure 7–16

▶ **Purpose:** Neoprene shorts provide compression and mild support when treating quadriceps, hamstrings, adductor, gluteal, and iliopsoas strains; quadriceps contusions; myositis ossificans; greater trochanteric bursitis; and osteitis pubis (Fig. 7–16).

○ DETAILS ─────────

The shorts may be used during rehabilitative, athletic, work, and casual activities.

▶ **Design:**
- Off-the-shelf shorts are manufactured in predetermined sizes and universal fit designs according to waist circumference measurements.
- The designs extend from the mid-to-distal thigh to the waist, with a Velcro or elastic waistband.

▶ **Position of the individual:** Sitting in a chair or standing.

▶ **Preparation:** Apply neoprene shorts directly to the skin or over an athletic supporter or girdle. No additional anchors are required.

▶ **Application:**

STEP 1: To apply, place the feet into the shorts and pull in a proximal direction until the shorts are positioned on the thigh and waist (Fig. 7–16). Adjust the shorts and waistband if needed. The shorts may be washed and reused.

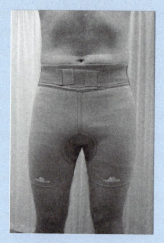

Figure 7-16

THIGH, HIP, AND PELVIS COMBINATION BRACES Figure 7–17

▶ **Purpose:** Thigh, hip, and pelvis combination braces are used when treating quadriceps, hamstrings, adductor, and iliopsoas strains to provide compression and mild to moderate support and to limit excessive range of motion and stretch on the musculature (Fig. 7–17).

▶ **Design:**
- The braces are manufactured in universal fit designs in predetermined sizes corresponding to waist circumference measurements (Fig. 7–17A).
- The designs extend from the mid-to-distal thigh to the waist and are constructed of neoprene or cotton/spandex materials. Some designs have an elastic waistband and others an adjustable buckle at the waist.
- One design uses elastic straps with Velcro attachments to allow for several individual applications based on the injury.
- Another design is manufactured with rubber tubing attached to adjustable straps. The straps allow for adjustments in the tension of the tubing.

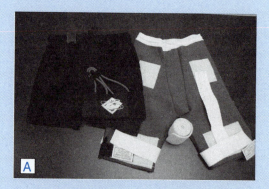

Figure 7-17A Thigh, hip, and pelvis combination braces. (Left) Brace with rubber tubing straps. (Right) Brace with elastic straps.

▶ **Position of the individual:** Sitting in a chair or standing.

▶ **Preparation:** Apply the thigh, hip, and pelvis combination braces directly to the skin or over an athletic supporter or girdle. No additional anchors are required.

Specific instructions for fitting and application of the braces are included with each design. For proper fit and support, carefully follow the manufacturer's step-by-step procedures. The following application guidelines pertain to most braces.

▶ **Application:**

<u>STEP 1:</u> Begin by placing the feet into the shorts and pulling in a proximal direction until the brace is positioned on the thigh, hip, pelvis, and waist (Fig. 7–17B). Adjust the shorts and waistband if needed. The braces may be washed and reused.

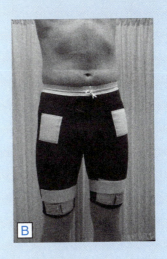

B

<u>STEP 2:</u> Applying and adjusting the straps will depend on the specific brace design. When treating adductor strains, continue application of some designs by wrapping an elastic strap around the thigh, hip, pelvis, and waist in a lateral-to-medial pattern. Anchor the strap with Velcro on the thigh (Fig. 7–17C). Two elastic straps may also be applied in a crisscross pattern around the distal thighs to treat adductor strains (Fig. 7–17D). Apply an elastic strap in a vertical pattern over either the anterior thigh to treat iliopsoas strains (Fig. 7–17E) or the posterior thigh to treat hamstrings strains (Fig. 7–17F). Retighten the straps and/or reposition the shorts if necessary.

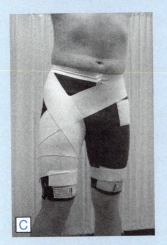

C

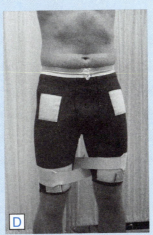

D

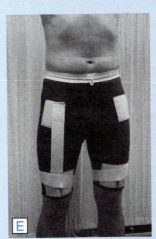

E

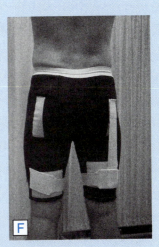

F

<u>STEP 3:</u> With other designs, to treat adductor strains, continue applying by tightening or loosening the straps until the appropriate amount of tension is placed on the rubber tubing (Fig. 7–17G). Adjust the straps or shorts if necessary.

> **...IF/THEN...**
>
> **IF** support is needed when treating an adductor strain for an athlete during a return to sport activities, **THEN** consider using a thigh, hip, and pelvis combination brace; neoprene shorts can be used, but a combination brace provides greater support and limits excessive range of motion because of the adjustable elastic straps and/or rubber tubing.

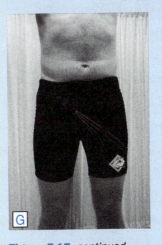

G

Figure 7-17 *continued*

ORTHOTICS

▶ **Purpose:** Orthotics provide support, absorb shock, and correct structural abnormalities when treating thigh, hip, and pelvis injuries and conditions.

- Use soft orthotic designs (see Fig. 3–16) to absorb shock and lessen stress to prevent and treat bursitis and stress fractures. Heel cups and full-length neoprene, silicone, and viscoelastic polymer insoles are available in off-the-shelf designs.
- Use semirigid (see Fig. 3–17) and rigid (see Fig. 3–18) orthotics to provide support and correct structural abnormalities—such as leg-length discrepancy or an increased Q angle—to treat bursitis. The designs are available off-the-shelf or custom-made.

Critical Thinking Question 2

During a baseball game, a concessionaire at the local university slipped on ice in the concession stand and immediately experienced sharp pain in the right quadriceps. Following an evaluation by a physician, the concessionaire has been receiving treatment at an outpatient orthopedic clinic for a mild quadriceps strain. Treatment has progressed normally, and he has returned to work with an elastic wrap applied to his right thigh to provide compression and support. However, the effectiveness of the wrap diminishes 1 to 2 hours after application.

▶ **Question: How can you manage this situation?**

Padding Techniques

Off-the-shelf padding techniques are available in a variety of designs to prevent and treat injuries and conditions of the thigh, hip, and pelvis. Custom-made padding techniques constructed of foam and thermoplastic materials are also used with thigh, hip, and pelvis injuries and conditions. Mandatory padding of the thigh, hip, and pelvis is required in only one interscholastic and intercollegiate sport—football. These padding techniques will be discussed further in Chapter 13.

RESEARCH BRIEF

Most studies recommend using protective padding for 3 to 6 months upon a return to athletic activity following a thigh contusion.[4,6,7,12] Whether the pad is purchased off-the-shelf or custom-made, it should cover and protect the injured area; disperse forces to surrounding, healthy tissues; be comfortable to the individual; and remain in place during activity.[7] The pad lessens the risk of reinjury and the development of myositis ossificans.

OFF-THE-SHELF Figure 7-18

▶ **Purpose:** Off-the-shelf padding techniques absorb shock and provide protection when preventing and treating quadriceps and iliac crest contusions and myositis ossificans (Fig. 7–18). The padding techniques are available from manufacturers in a variety of designs.

DETAILS

Off-the-shelf pads are commonly used following injury to provide shock absorption to the thigh, hip, and pelvis of athletes in sports such as baseball, basketball, field hockey, football, ice hockey, lacrosse, soccer, softball, volleyball, and wrestling. Use the pads with athletic or work activities.

▶ **Design:**
- Individual and universal fit designs are manufactured in predetermined sizes, corresponding either to circumference measurements of the thigh or waist, or age of the individual.
- Several universal fit thigh designs are constructed of plastic inserts covered by varying thicknesses of high-density open- and closed-cell foams. The pads are contoured to the thigh; some are coated with vinyl. Universal fit hip and pelvis designs are constructed of open- and closed-cell foams (Fig. 7–18A).
- Some individual fit designs consist of a plastic material outer shell pre-molded to the contours of the thigh and hip. This outer shell is lined with open- and closed-cell foams extending in all directions to absorb shock (Fig. 7–18B).
- Other thigh and hip designs are manufactured specifically for use following injury. These pads are larger in size with additional padding to cover the thigh, hip, and pelvis (Fig. 7–18C). Some designs have neoprene straps with Velcro closures to attach the pads.
- Another thigh design consists of a high-density shell lined with foam incorporated into a neoprene sleeve.
- Some athletic pant designs, such as those for ice hockey, are available with pads incorporated into the thigh, hip, and pelvis area.

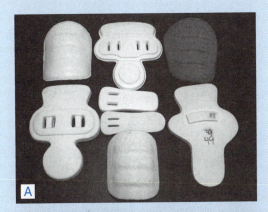

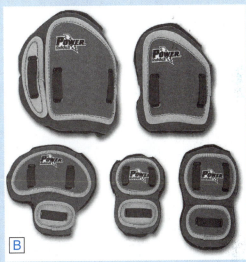

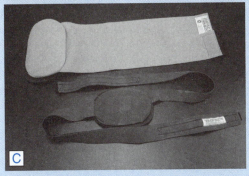

Figure 7-18 **A** Variety of universal fit thigh, hip, and pelvis pads. **B** (Top) Individual fit thigh pads. (Courtesy of Riddell, Elyria, OH). (Bottom) Individual fit hip and pelvis pads. (Courtesy of Riddell, Elyria, OH). **C** Postinjury thigh, hip, and pelvis pads.

▶ **Position of the individual:** Standing on a taping table, bench, or on the ground with the majority of the weight on the noninvolved leg and the involved leg placed in a neutral position with slight knee flexion. Maintain this position during application.

▶ **Preparation:** Apply the off-the-shelf designs over pre-tape material or self-adherent wrap, directly to the skin, under tight-fitting clothing, or within athletic clothing.

▶ **Application:**
STEP 1: With taping techniques, place the pad over the injured area and attach to the thigh over pre-tape material or self-adherent wrap with elastic tape, using the circular thigh technique (see Figs. 7–1A–D). Apply the pad directly to the skin over the iliac crest with elastic tape, using the hip pointer technique (see Figs. 7–2A–E).

STEP 2: The pad may also be applied directly to the skin and attached to the thigh using the quadriceps strain wrapping technique one or technique two (Fig. 7–18D). Attach the pad to the iliac crest with the hip pointer wrapping technique one or technique two.

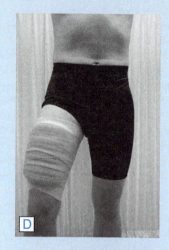

STEP 3: With the strap designs, apply the pad directly to the skin and anchor the neoprene straps around the thigh or hip with Velcro (Fig. 7–18E).

STEP 4: The pad may also be attached to the thigh, hip, and/or pelvis by placing the pad underneath tight-fitting clothing such as spandex or Lycra shorts.

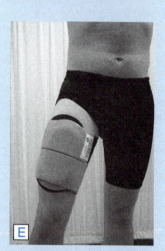

STEP 5: Nylon/polyester girdles with pad pockets are available to attach the pads to the thigh, hip, and/or pelvis (Fig. 7–18F) . These girdles are commonly worn by football athletes.

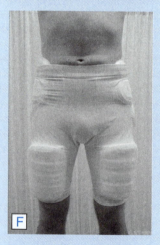

Figure 7-18 *continued*

Helpful Hint: When using off-the-shelf thigh pads in right and left designs, ensure proper placement before activity; typically, the angled side of the pad is positioned over the medial thigh.

CUSTOM-MADE Figure 7–19

▸ **Purpose:** Mold thermoplastic material to absorb shock and provide protection to prevent and treat quadriceps and iliac crest contusions, and myositis ossificans (Fig. 7–19). Use these pads when off-the-shelf designs are not available.

▸ **Materials:**
- Paper, felt tip pen, thermoplastic material, ⅛ inch or ¼ inch foam or felt, a heating source, 2 inch or 3 inch elastic tape, an elastic wrap, soft, low-density foam, rubber cement, taping scissors

▸ **Position of the individual:** Standing on a taping table, bench, or on the ground with the majority of the weight on the noninvolved leg and the involved leg placed in a neutral position with slight knee flexion. Maintain this position during application.

▸ **Preparation:** Design the pad with a paper pattern (see Fig. 1–14). Cut, mold, and shape the thermoplastic material on the thigh, hip, or pelvis over the injured area. Attach soft, low-density foam to the inside surface of the material (see Fig. 1–15).

▸ **Application:**

(STEP 1:) Attach the pad to the thigh with the circular thigh taping technique, quadriceps strain wrapping technique one or technique two, or under tight-fitting clothing or an athletic girdle. Attach the pad to the iliac crest with the hip pointer taping technique, hip pointer wrapping technique one or technique two, or under tight-fitting clothing or an athletic girdle.

(STEP 2:) Consider molding and attaching a piece of thermoplastic material with cement or elastic tape to an off-the-shelf thigh, hip, or pelvis pad to provide additional protection for a contusion (Fig. 7–19).

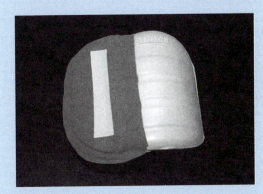

Figure 7-19

MANDATORY PADDING

▸ The NCAA[11] and the NFHS[12] require athletes to use mandatory protective padding for the thigh, hip, and pelvis during all football practices and competitions . The majority of these pads are available in off-the-shelf designs and can be purchased in a set. A more in-depth discussion of these pads can be found in Chapter 13.

Helpful Hint: Among football athletes, closely monitor the proper use and wear of mandatory thigh, hip, and pelvis padding. Many football players cut the pads to smaller sizes for additional comfort, reducing the protection provided.

Critical Thinking Question 3

With 8 minutes remaining in the Conference Championship game, the starting center on your basketball team defends against a layup and is struck in the left anterior thigh by the opponent's knee. An evaluation on the bench reveals general tenderness over the anterior quadriceps. The athlete has full bilateral range of motion, strength, and functional movement, indicating a mild contusion. Your team physician agrees.

▸ **Question: Within the limited amount of time left in the game, what techniques can you use in this situation?**

Thigh, Hip, and Pelvis

CASE STUDY

Near the end of the first period, Robert Greene, a defenseman on the Davis Junior College hockey team, is pushed into the goal by an opponent while attempting to gain control of the puck. His right anterior thigh strikes the right goal post. Following stoppage of play, Julie Knox, ATC, comes onto the ice to evaluate Robert. From the bench, Julie observed the mechanism of injury and begins to gather information from Robert about the play. Following the on-ice evaluation, Robert is helped to the locker room, where the team physician is waiting.

In the locker room, Julie continues to question Robert about his previous injury to his right thigh, while the team physician begins an evaluation. Robert tells Julie he has suffered two previous contusions to his right anterior thigh during the last year and a half. The team physician completes the evaluation and determines that Robert has sustained a third degree right anterior quadriceps contusion. Robert is placed on crutches for non–weight-bearing ambulation. Julie begins treatment immediately. What wrapping techniques are appropriate to provide compression to control swelling in this case?

After several follow-up appointments with the team physician and a comprehensive therapeutic exercise program, Robert is allowed to return to sport- and position-specific practice activities on the ice. The team physician and Julie agree that protective padding of the right thigh during these activities is warranted. Which padding techniques can you use to provide shock absorption for Robert's right quadriceps?

Robert has progressed with his activities on the ice but recently began to notice an increase in the amount of soreness in the anterior thigh after practice. Julie performs an evaluation in the athletic training room and finds mild swelling and point tenderness over the anterior quadriceps. Robert demonstrates bilateral strength and flexibility. Julie refers Robert to the team physician. The team physician performs an evaluation and obtains radiographs, which are negative. He is concerned about Robert's past history of injury and the possible development of myositis ossificans. The team physician meets with Julie and recommends the following: 1) closely monitor and reduce swelling, 2) maintain strength and flexibility, and 3) consider the use of additional protective padding. The team physician allows Robert to return to practice as tolerated. What are the appropriate wrapping techniques to control the swelling associated with the condition? Lastly, which protective padding techniques could be used to prevent further injury?

WRAP UP

- Acute and chronic injuries and conditions to the thigh, hip, and pelvis can be the result of single or repeated direct forces, structural abnormalities, repetitive stress and tension, and rapid stretch, contraction, or weakness of the musculature.
- The circular thigh and hip pointer taping techniques provide support and anchor protective padding to the thigh, hip, and pelvis.
- Compression wrap techniques provide compression to control mild, moderate, and severe swelling following injury.
- The quadriceps strain wrapping techniques can be used to provide compression and support and to anchor protective padding.
- The hamstrings, adductor, hip flexor, and gluteal strain wrapping techniques provide compression and support.
- The hip pointer wrapping techniques anchor protective padding to the iliac crest.
- Neoprene sleeves and shorts, and thigh, hip, and pelvis combination braces are used to provide compression and mild support.
- Soft, semirigid, and rigid orthotics provide support, absorb shock, and correct structural abnormalities.

- Various high-density open- and closed-cell foams, and plastic and thermoplastic materials absorb shock and provide protection when preventing and treating injuries and conditions.
- The NCAA and NFHS require the use of mandatory protective equipment for the thigh, hip, and pelvis in football.

■ WEB REFERENCES

About
http://about.com/
· This Web site allows you to search for information about a variety of thigh, hip, and pelvis injuries and conditions.

SportsInjuryClinic.net
http://www.sportsinjuryclinic.net/
· This Web site has an injury index that can be searched for treatment and rehabilitation information about a variety of thigh, hip, and pelvis injuries and conditions.

The American Orthopaedic Society for Sports Medicine
http://www.aossm.org/
· This site provides access to The American Journal of Sports Medicine.

WorldOrtho
http://www.worldortho.com/
· This site provides access to full online textbooks, pictures, and other educational materials.

REFERENCES

1. Ackerman, LV: Extra-osseous localized non-neoplastic bone and cartilage formation (so-called myositis ossificans): Clinical and pathological confusion with malignant neoplasms. J Bone Joint Surg Am 40:279–298, 1958.
2. Anderson, K, Strickland, SM, and Warren, R: Hip and groin injuries in athletes. Am J Sports Med 29:521–533, 2001.
3. Clanton, TO, and Coupe, KJ: Hamstring strains in athletes: Diagnosis and treatment. J Am Acad Orthop Surg 6:237–248, 1998.
4. Ekstrand, J, and Gillquist, J: Soccer injuries and their mechanisms: A prospective study. Med Sci Sports Exerc 15:267–270, 1983.
5. Estwanik, JJ, and McAlister, JA, Jr: Contusions and the formation of myositis ossificans. Phys Sportsmed 18:52–64, 1990.
6. Jackson, DW, and Feagin, JA: Quadriceps contusions in young athletes. J Bone Joint Surg Am 55:95–105, 1973.
7. Kaeding, CC, Sanko, WA, and Fischer, RA: Myositis ossificans: Minimizing downtime. Phys Sportsmed 23:77–82, 1995.
8. Larson, CM, Almekinders, LC, Karas, SG, and Garrett, WE: Evaluating and managing muscle contusion and myositis ossificans. Phys Sportsmed 30:41–50, 2002.
9. Michelsson, JE, Granroth, G, and Andersson, LC: Myositis ossificans following forcible manipulation of the leg: A rabbit model for the study of heterotopic bone formation. J Bone Joint Surg Am 62:811–815, 1980.
10. Morris, AF: Sports Medicine: Prevention of Athletic Injuries. Wm. C. Brown Publishers, Dubuque 1984.
11. National Collegiate Athletic Association, http://www.ncaa.org/library/sports_sciences/sports_med_handbook/2003-04/index.html, Sports medicine handbook, 2003–2004.
12. National Federation of State High School Associations. 2004 Football Rules Book. Indianapolis, IN: National Federation of State High School Associations;2004.
13. Ryan, JB, Wheeler, JH, Hopkinson, WJ, Arciero, RA, and Kolakowski, KR: Quadriceps contusions: West Point update. Am J Sports Med 19:299–304, 1991.
14. Starkey, C, and Ryan, JL: Evaluation of Orthopedic and Athletic Injuries, ed 2. FA Davis, Philadelphia, 2002.

Shoulder and Upper Arm

LEARNING OBJECTIVES

1. Discuss common injuries and conditions that occur to the shoulder and upper arm.
2. Demonstrate taping, wrapping, bracing, and padding techniques for the shoulder and upper arm when preventing, treating, and rehabilitating injuries.
3. Explain and demonstrate appropriate taping, wrapping, bracing, and padding techniques for the shoulder and upper arm within a therapeutic exercise program.

INJURIES AND CONDITIONS

Acute and chronic injuries and conditions to the shoulder and upper arm can result from direct and indirect compressive forces, excessive range of motion, and repetitive stress. The structure of the shoulder allows for a considerable amount of range of motion; the surrounding musculature provides the shoulder's main stabilization. The available range of motion and lack of stability provided by bony, ligamentous, and tendinous structures place the joint at risk for injury. A contusion, sprain, dislocation/subluxation, or fracture can result when a runner stumbles and falls to the ground on the tip of her shoulder or on the outstretched arm. Repetitive overhead movements experienced in throwing sports can cause strains and overuse injuries and conditions. Common injuries to the shoulder and upper arm include:

• Contusions
• Sprains
• Dislocations/subluxations
• Fractures
• Strains
• Ruptures
• Overuse injuries and conditions

Contusions

Contusions to the shoulder and upper arm are caused by compressive forces and are common in athletic activities. Falling on the tip of the shoulder or experiencing a direct force to this area can cause a contusion to the distal end of the clavicle (**shoulder pointer**) (Illustration 8–1). An acute or series of repeated direct forces to the musculature of the upper arm can result in swelling, pain, and loss of range of motion. Commonly, the anterolateral aspect of the upper arm is involved, affecting the deltoid, brachialis, biceps brachii, and triceps brachii muscles, and the humerus (Illustrations 8–2 and 8–3). For example, a contusion to the proximal upper arm can occur when a football player cuts the sleeves off his practice jersey,

allowing movement of the shoulder pad cups while running, and exposing the area to a direct blow. Repeated forces can lead to the development of myositis ossificans in a muscle or **exostosis (tackler's exostosis)** on the humerus.

Sprains

Shoulder sprains are caused by compression and shear forces, excessive range of motion, and overuse. Forceful abduction, excessive external rotation and extension, or a direct force that translates the humerus posteriorly can result in a **glenohumeral (GH) joint** sprain (Illustration 8–4). A sprain, for instance, could result from a football linebacker tackling a running back, using only the right arm and causing violent abduction, external rotation, and extension of the arm. Sprains to the **sternoclavicular (SC) joint** are caused by indirect forces placed on the clavicle, which may occur with a fall on the outstretched arm, direct compression on the lateral shoulder, or traction and torsion forces. Acromioclavicular (AC) joint sprains are the result of the acromion process being forced away from the clavicle or the clavicle being forced away from the acromion. This mechanism can occur with a fall on the outstretched hand, flexed elbow, or tip of the shoulder; direct force to the acromion; or repetitive forces and overhead activities. AC joint sprains are common in collision and contact sports, as a result of being tackled or falling on the playing surface.

Dislocations/Subluxations

Dislocations and subluxations of the GH joint are common in athletic and work activities because of the vast range of motion and minimal ligamentous support present at the joint. Both acute and chronic mechanisms are associated with these injuries. **Anterior dislocations** and **subluxations,** caused by excessive abduction, external rotation, and extension of the humerus, account for the majority of GH dislocations.[8] This mechanism of injury is identical to the GH joint sprain mechanism. A direct

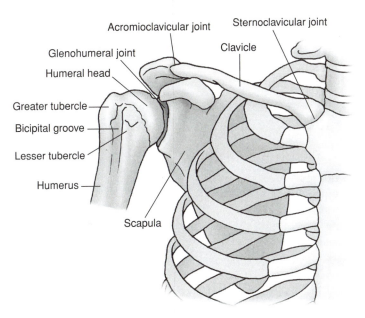

Illustration 8-1 Anterior view of the bones and joints of the shoulder.

force to the posterior or posterolateral shoulder can also result in an anterior dislocation and/or subluxation.

A direct force to the anterior shoulder, excessive adduction and internal rotation of the humerus, or a fall on the outstretched, internally rotated arm can result in a **posterior dislocation** and/or **subluxation.** For example, a posterior dislocation/subluxation can occur as a right-handed baseball outfielder chases a fly ball to his left, near the warning track, reaches the ball with a backhanded

catch, then collides with the wall, causing a longitudinal anterior force on the GH joint and excessive internal rotation of the right humerus. **Inferior dislocations** and **subluxations** are rare.

Following acute dislocations and/or subluxations, **anterior, posterior, inferior,** and **multidirectional instability** of the GH joint can develop. Due to the high occurrence of anterior dislocations/subluxations, anterior instability is more common. Instability can also be

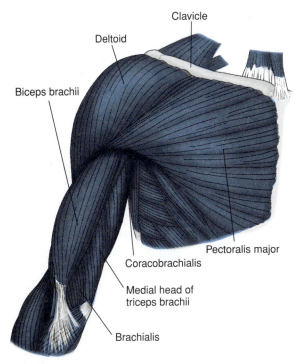

Illustration 8-2 Superficial muscles of the anterior shoulder and upper arm.

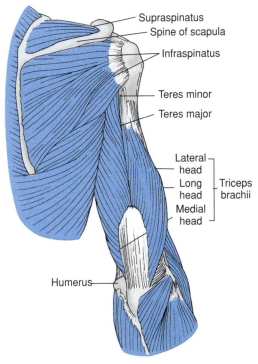

Illustration 8-3 Deep muscles of the posterior shoulder and upper arm.

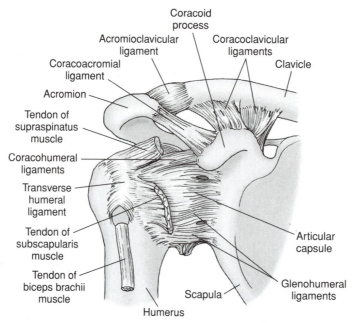

Illustration 8-4 Anterior view of the glenohumeral and acromioclavicular joints.

the result of chronic, repetitive forces placed on the GH joint. Repetitive forces from overhead activities, such as throwing in baseball and softball, serving in tennis, and swimming, can cause instability. Acute anterior dislocations or chronic anterior instability of the GH joint can result in a **Bankart lesion** on the anterior labrum, a **Hill-Sachs lesion** on the posterior humeral head, or a **superior labrum anteroposterior (SLAP) lesion** on the anterior and posterior superior labrum. Posterior instability is most often associated with repetitive microtrauma and can cause a **reverse Hill-Sachs lesion** on the anterior humeral head.[16] Inferior and superior instabilities are rare and limited by the bony structure of the shoulder. Acute and chronic dislocations and subluxations can also result in multidirectional instability, which is instability in more than one plane of motion at the GH joint.

Fractures

Fractures can occur to the clavicle, scapula, and humerus. A fall on the outstretched arm or tip of the shoulder can cause a clavicular fracture, as can a direct force. The most common fracture site occurs at the middle third of the clavicle.[13] A clavicular fracture can result, for example, when a cyclist is thrown from his bike and falls to the ground on the outstretched arm. Scapular fractures are the result of a direct force, a fall on the outstretched arm, violent muscular contractions, and shoulder dislocations and subluxations. A direct force, a fall on the outstretched arm or upper arm, and shoulder dislocations can also result in a humeral fracture.

Strains

Strains to the shoulder commonly affect the **rotator cuff** musculature, teres minor, infraspinatus, supraspinatus, and subscapularis (Illustration 8–5). Injury can be caused by repetitive microtrauma and overload; shoulder impingement syndrome, with associated mechanical compression and chronic inflammation; glenohumeral instability; and falls on the outstretched arm.[9] For example, a strain can occur in a youth league baseball pitcher as a result of repetitive throwing without appropriate recovery periods.

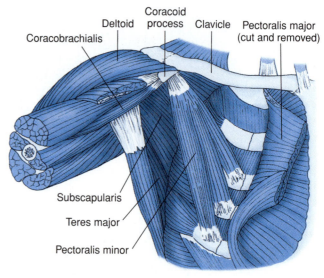

Illustration 8-5 Deep muscles of the anterior shoulder and upper arm.

Ruptures

A rupture of the biceps brachii is caused by a forceful concentric or eccentric contraction against resistance. The proximal portion of the tendon located near the bicipital groove is injured most frequently. A rupture can result, for instance, when a gymnast performs a movement on the rings with his elbows in flexion, then loses grip of the left hand, and attempts to regrip the ring as he is falling, causing a violent eccentric contraction of the left biceps brachii.

Overuse

Overuse injuries and conditions come from repetitive stress, rotator cuff pathology, and impingement. Rotator cuff or bicipital tendinitis may result from repetitive overload and stress, muscle imbalance and weakness of the rotator cuff, and shoulder impingement syndrome.

Taping Techniques

Several taping techniques may be used to prevent and treat injuries and conditions of the shoulder and upper arm. All of the techniques are also used to anchor off-the-shelf and custom-made pads to the upper arm and/or shoulder. Protective padding techniques are illustrated in the Padding section.

CIRCULAR UPPER ARM Figure 8–1

▸ **Purpose:** Use the circular upper arm technique to provide mild support and anchor protective padding (Fig. 8–1). The technique is used with off-the-shelf and custom-made pads to absorb shock when preventing and treating upper arm contusions, myositis ossificans, and exostosis.

▸ **Materials:**
  • Pre-tape material or self-adherent wrap, 2 inch or 3 inch elastic tape, adherent tape spray, taping scissors

  Option:
  • 1½ inch non-elastic tape

▸ **Position of the individual:** Sitting on a taping table or bench or standing with the involved arm at the side of the body and the elbow placed in 90° of flexion with moderate isometric contraction of the biceps and triceps muscles.

▸ **Preparation:** Apply adherent tape spray to the upper arm.

▸ **Application:**

  STEP 1: Apply pre-tape material or self-adherent wrap in a circular pattern around the upper arm ◀▬▶ .

  STEP 2: Place the pad over the injured area. Anchor 2 inch or 3 inch elastic tape directly to the distal pad (Fig. 8–1A).

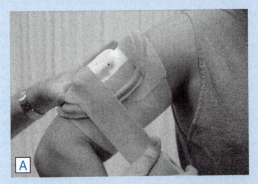

  STEP 3: Continue around the upper arm in a circular, distal-to-proximal pattern with moderate roll tension, overlapping the tape by ½ of its width ◀▬▶ (Fig. 8–1B). Cover the entire pad and anchor on the anterolateral area to prevent irritation. Avoid gaps, wrinkles, or inconsistent roll tension.

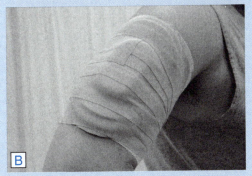

Figure 8-1

STEP 4: To prevent migration of the pad, apply a distal circular strip of elastic tape with distal-to-proximal tension (Fig. 8–1C) or apply the proximal circular tape strips to the skin. No additional anchors are required.

Option: *Loosely apply one to two circular strips of 1½ inch non-elastic tape around the pad for additional anchors* ◀▬▶ .

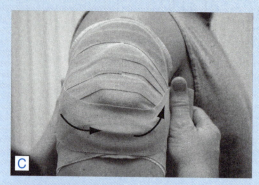

Figure 8-1 *continued*

SHOULDER POINTER/AC JOINT SPRAIN TAPE Figure 8–2

▸ **Purpose:** The shoulder pointer/AC joint sprain technique anchors off-the-shelf and custom-made pads to the shoulder to absorb shock when preventing and treating contusions and AC joint sprains (Fig. 8–2).

▸ **Materials:**
  • 2 inch or 3 inch heavyweight elastic tape, adherent tape spray, taping scissors

▸ **Position of the individual:** Standing with the hand of the involved arm placed on the lateral hip in a relaxed position.

▸ **Preparation:** Apply the shoulder pointer/AC joint sprain technique directly to the skin.

▸ **Application:**

STEP 1: Apply adherent tape spray over the pad area and 4–6 inches beyond over the anterior and posterior shoulder. Allow the spray to dry.

STEP 2: Cut several strips of 2 inch or 3 inch heavyweight elastic tape in lengths that will cover the pad and extend 4–6 inches beyond the pad on the two sides. Place the pad over the injured area. Anchor the first tape strip on the posterior shoulder, 4–6 inches from the edge of the pad, and pat down (Fig. 8–2A). Do not stretch the tape as the anchor is applied.

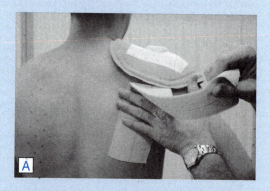

STEP 3: Continue to apply the strip to the edge of the pad. At the edge, hold the strip on the posterior shoulder with one hand and pull the strip over the pad with tension on the tape (Fig. 8–2B).

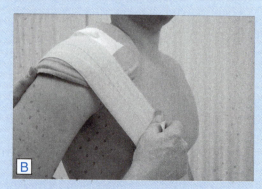

Figure 8-2

STEP 4: When the strip completely covers the pad, release the tension in the tape, anchor it to the anterior shoulder, and pat down (Fig. 8–2C). This technique is the release-stretch-release sequence illustrated in Figures 1–13A–G.

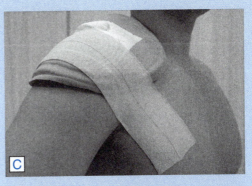

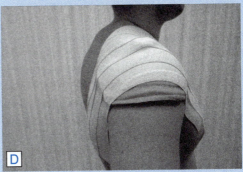

STEP 5: Continue with additional strips in the same manner, overlapping each by ½ the width of the tape (Fig. 8–2D). Apply enough strips to cover the majority of the pad .

Figure 8-2 *continued*

> **Helpful Hint:** To prevent skin damage from the tape adhesive, apply tape removal solvent to the skin before removing the shoulder pointer/AC joint sprain taping technique.

Wrapping Techniques

Wrapping techniques provide compression, support, and immobilization in order to prevent and treat upper arm contusions; myositis ossificans; exostosis; shoulder pointers; GH, SC, and AC joint sprains; dislocations and subluxations; clavicular, scapular, and humeral fractures; rotator cuff strains; ruptures; and tendinitis. Wrapping techniques also attach protective pads to the shoulder and upper arm.

COMPRESSION WRAP TECHNIQUE ONE Figure 8–3

- **Purpose:** Compression wrap technique one for the upper arm aids in reducing mild to moderate swelling following contusions and ruptures (Fig. 8–3).

- **Materials:**
  - 3 inch or 4 inch width by 5 yard length elastic wrap determined by the size of the upper arm, metal clips, 1½ inch non-elastic or 2 inch or 3 inch elastic tape, taping scissors

  Options:
  - ¼ inch or ½ inch foam or felt
  - 3 inch or 4 inch width self-adherent wrap

- **Position of the individual:** Sitting on a taping table or bench, or standing with the involved arm at the side of the body and the elbow placed in a pain-free, flexed position.

- **Preparation:** To lessen migration, apply adherent tape spray, tape strips, or anchors directly to the skin (see Fig. 1–7).

  Option: *Cut a ¼ inch or ½ inch foam or felt pad and place it over the inflamed area directly to the skin to assist in controlling swelling.*

▶ **Application:**

STEP 1: Anchor the extended end of the wrap around the distal upper arm directly to the skin and encircle the anchor ◀▶ (Fig. 8–3A).

Option: *If an elastic wrap is not available, 3 inch or 4 inch self-adherent wrap may be used.*

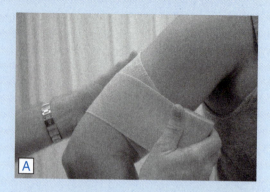

A

STEP 2: Continue to apply the wrap in a spiral pattern, overlapping the wrap by ½ of its width, and moving in a distal-to-proximal direction (see Fig. 8–3B). Apply the greatest amount of roll tension distally and over the inflamed area and lessen the amount of roll tension as the wrap continues proximally.

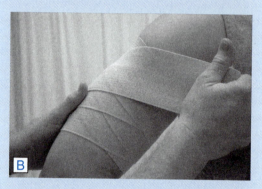

B

STEP 3: Finish the wrap over the proximal upper arm. Anchor with Velcro, metal clips, or loosely applied 1½ inch non-elastic or 2 inch or 3 inch elastic tape ◀▶ (Fig. 8–3C). End the tape on the anterolateral area to prevent irritation.

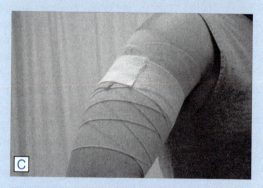

C

Figure 8-3

COMPRESSION WRAP TECHNIQUE TWO Figure 8–4

▶ **Purpose:** Use this compression wrap technique to control moderate to severe swelling when treating second and third degree upper arm contusions and ruptures. This technique prevents distal migration of postinjury swelling (Fig. 8–4).

▶ **Materials:**
   • 4 inch or 6 inch width by 10 yard length elastic wrap, metal clips, 1½ inch non-elastic or 2 inch or 3 inch elastic tape, taping scissors

   Option:
   • ¼ inch or ½ inch foam or felt

▶ **Position of the individual:** Sitting on a taping table or bench, or standing with the involved arm at the side of the body and the elbow placed in a pain-free, flexed position.

▶ **Preparation:** To lessen migration, apply adherent tape spray, tape strips, or anchors directly to the skin.

Option: *Cut a ¼ inch or ½ inch foam or felt pad and place it over the inflamed area directly to the skin to assist in venous return.*

▶ **Application:**

STEP 1: Anchor the elastic wrap around the wrist directly to the skin and encircle the anchor ◀ (Fig. 8–4A).

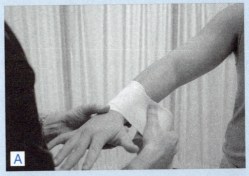

STEP 2: In a spiral pattern, continue to apply the wrap in a distal-to-proximal direction, overlapping the wrap by ½ of its width (Fig. 8–4B).

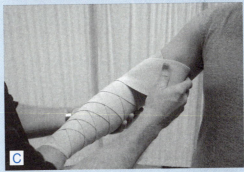

STEP 3: Continue to apply the wrap over the elbow to the distal upper arm (Fig. 8–4C) ʃ .

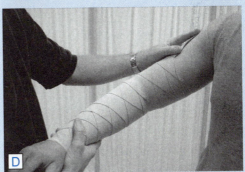

STEP 4: At the distal upper arm, finish this technique with compression wrap one (Fig. 8–4D). Apply the greatest amount of roll tension distally and over the inflamed area and lessen tension as the wrap continues proximally.

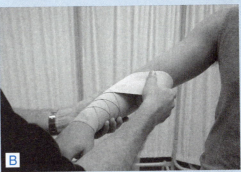

STEP 5: Anchor the wrap over the proximal upper arm with Velcro, metal clips, or loosely applied 1½ inch non-elastic or 2 inch or 3 inch elastic tape ◀ (Fig. 8–4E). Finish the tape on the anterolateral upper arm.

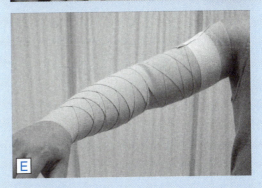

Figure 8-4

Helpful Hint: Extended wear of the compression wrap may cause irritation of the skin over the cubital fossa. To prevent this irritation, place a thin foam pad over the cubital fossa underneath the wrap.

COMPRESSION WRAP TECHNIQUE THREE Figure 8–5

▶ **Purpose:** An elastic sleeve may also be used over the upper arm to control mild to moderate swelling with contusions and ruptures (Fig. 8–5). This technique differs from compression wrap techniques one and two in that, after receiving instruction, the individual can apply and remove this wrap without assistance.

▶ **Materials:**
- 3 inch or 5 inch width elastic sleeve determined by the size of the upper arm, taping scissors
- **Option:**
- ¼ inch or ½ inch foam or felt

▶ **Position of the individual:** Sitting on a taping table or bench, or standing with the involved arm at the side of the body and the elbow placed in a pain-free, flexed position.

▶ **Preparation:** Cut a sleeve from a roll to extend from the elbow to the proximal upper arm area or from the wrist to the proximal upper arm. Cut and use a double length sleeve to provide additional compression.

Option: Cut a ¼ inch or ½ inch foam or felt pad and place it over the inflamed area to assist in controlling swelling.

▶ **Application:**

STEP 1: Place the hand through the sleeve and pull onto the upper arm or arm in a distal-to-proximal pattern. If using a double length sleeve, pull the distal end over the first layer to provide an additional layer (Fig. 8–5). No anchors are required. The elastic sleeve can be cleaned and reused.

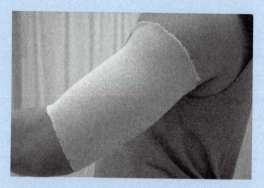

Figure 8-5

CIRCULAR UPPER ARM WRAP Figure 8–6

▶ **Purpose:** The circular upper arm technique is used to provide compression and mild support and to anchor off-the-shelf and custom-made pads to absorb shock when preventing and treating upper arm contusions, myositis ossificans, and exostosis (Fig. 8–6).

▶ **Materials:**
- 3 inch, 4 inch, or 6 inch width by 5 yard length elastic wrap, 2 inch or 3 inch elastic tape, taping scissors
- **Options:**
- 3 inch or 4 inch width self-adherent wrap
- 1½ inch non-elastic tape

▶ **Position of the individual:** Sitting on a taping table or bench, or standing with the involved arm at the side of the body and the elbow placed in 90° of flexion with moderate isometric contraction of the biceps and triceps muscles.

▶ **Preparation:** To lessen migration, apply adherent tape spray, tape strips, or anchors directly to the skin.

▶ **Application:**

STEP 1: Place the pad over the injured area. Anchor the wrap directly to the skin below the distal pad and encircle the anchor ◀▶ (Fig. 8–6A).

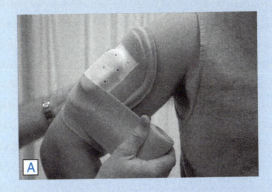

STEP 2: Continue to apply the wrap in a circular pattern with moderate roll tension, overlapping the wrap by ½ of its width, in a distal-to-proximal pattern (Fig. 8–6B). Avoid gaps, wrinkles, or inconsistent roll tension.

Option: *Three inch or 4 inch self-adherent wrap may be used if an elastic wrap is not available.*

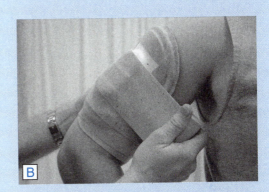

STEP 3: Completely cover the pad and finish the wrap above the proximal pad. To anchor, place 2 inch or 3 inch elastic tape on the distal pad and apply two to three continuous circular patterns, with moderate roll tension, finishing on the tape pattern on the lateral upper arm to ensure adherence and prevent irritation ◀▶ (Fig. 8–6C). To lessen migration, apply a distal circular strip of elastic tape with distal-to-proximal tension and anchor the loose end on the circular tape pattern. The proximal portion of the elastic tape may also be applied partially on the skin.

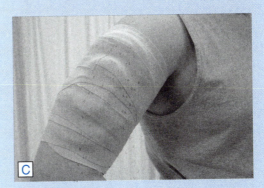

Figure 8-6

Option: *Additional 1½ inch non-elastic circular strips may be applied loosely around the upper arm to anchor the pad* ◀▶ .

SHOULDER SPICA Figure 8–7

▶ **Purpose:** The shoulder spica technique provides mild support and anchors off-the-shelf and custom-made pads to absorb shock when preventing and treating shoulder pointers and AC joint sprains (Fig. 8–7).

▶ **Materials:**
• 4 inch or 6 inch width by 10 yard length elastic wrap, 2 inch or 3 inch elastic tape, taping scissors

▶ **Position of the individual:** Standing with the hand of the involved arm placed on the lateral hip in a relaxed position.

▶ **Preparation:** Apply the off-the-shelf or custom-made pad over the injured area directly to the skin.

▶ Application:

STEP 1: Anchor the extended end of the wrap on the mid-to-proximal lateral upper arm directly to the skin and proceed around the upper arm in a medial direction to encircle the anchor (see Fig. 8–7A).

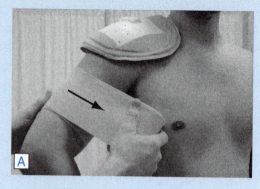

STEP 2: At the posterior upper arm, continue the wrap in a medial direction over the lateral shoulder and pad, across the chest, under the axilla of the noninvolved arm, then across the upper back (Fig. 8–7B). Next, continue over the lateral involved shoulder, under the axilla, and encircle the upper arm (Fig. 8–7C). Apply the wrap with moderate roll tension.

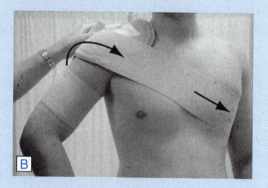

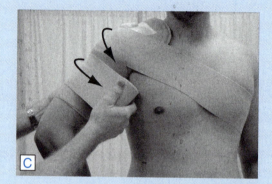

STEP 3: Repeat this pattern two to four times with the wrap, overlapping slightly, leaving a small area in the middle of the pad exposed (Fig. 8–7D) 🦴. Monitor roll tension to prevent constriction and irritation of the **axilla** areas.

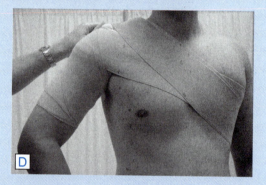

STEP 4: Finish the wrap over the involved shoulder, upper back, or thorax. Anchor 2 inch or 3 inch elastic tape directly on the exposed portion of the pad (Fig. 8–7E) and apply one to two spica patterns over the wrap and pad with moderate roll tension (Fig. 8–7F).

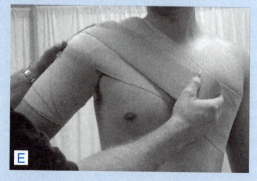

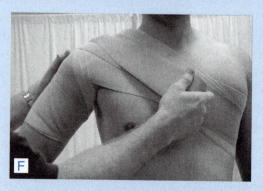

Figure 8-7

STEP 5: Anchor the tape on the circular tape pattern over the pad (Fig. 8–7G). No additional anchors are needed.

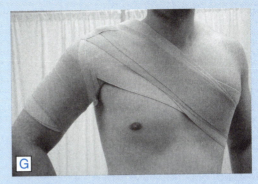

Figure 8-7 *continued*

 Helpful Hint: Make sure you leave an exposed area in the middle of the pad because the exposed area in the spica technique will allow for the elastic tape anchor(s) to adhere directly to the pad, lessening migration.

Critical Thinking Question 1

During the first week of preseason practice, an attackman on the lacrosse team suffers a left shoulder pointer. After several days of treatment, the athlete returns to practice with an off-the-shelf pad anchored directly to the skin with elastic tape. Practice and application of the pad continue twice daily, and the adherent tape spray and tape adhesive begin to cause irritation of the skin.

▶ **Question: What techniques can you use in this situation?**

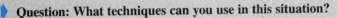

4 S (SPICA, SLING, SWATHE, AND SUPPORT) WRAP Figure 8–8

▶ **Purpose:** Use the 4 S technique to provide mild to moderate support and immobilization when treating sprains, strains, dislocations, subluxations, ruptures, and stable fractures (Fig. 8–8). The 4 S wrap can replace a sling and swathe in the immediate treatment of shoulder and upper arm injuries and conditions.

▶ **Materials:**
• 4 inch or 6 inch width by 10 yard length elastic wrap, 2 inch or 3 inch elastic tape, taping scissors

▶ **Position of the individual:** Sitting or standing with the involved arm in a pain-free position next to the body with the elbow placed in flexion.

▶ **Preparation:** Apply the 4 S wrap directly to the skin or over tight-fitting clothing.

▶ **Application:**
STEP 1: Anchor the wrap around the mid-to-proximal lateral upper arm and apply one to two shoulder *spica* patterns with moderate roll tension (Fig. 8–8A).

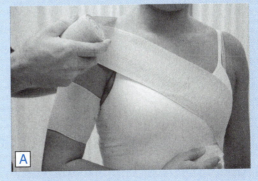

Figure 8-8

STEP 2: At the involved posterior upper arm, continue the wrap over the involved shoulder, down the upper arm, under the elbow, then up the upper arm, and finish over the shoulder (Fig. 8–8B). Repeat this pattern one to two times with moderate roll tension, moving distally on the forearm with each pattern to form a *sling* (Fig. 8–8C).

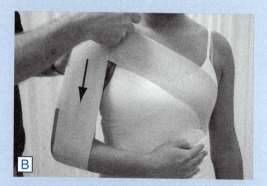

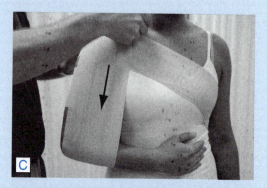

STEP 3: Next, continue the wrap from the involved shoulder across the chest toward the involved hand, around the mid-to-low back, and across the distal upper arm (Fig. 8–8D). Continue to apply the wrap over the forearm, wrist, and hand, then encircle the trunk again with moderate roll tension (Fig. 8–8E).

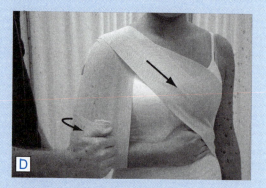

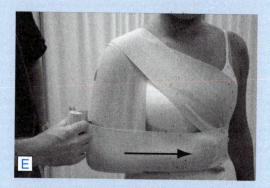

STEP 4: Finish over the forearm to form a *swathe* (Fig. 8–8F). Leave the fingertips exposed to monitor circulation.

STEP 5: Anchor 2 inch or 3 inch elastic tape over the involved shoulder and apply the spica, sling, and swathe patterns with moderate roll tension, finishing on the forearm or wrist (Fig. 8–8G). No additional anchors are required.

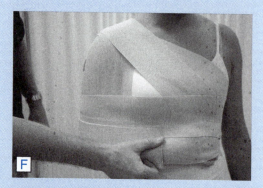

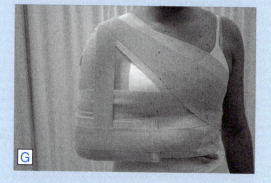

Figure 8-8 *continued*

FIGURE-OF-EIGHT WRAP Figure 8–9

▶ **Purpose:** The figure-of-eight technique provides mild to moderate support and immobilization when treating SC joint sprains and stable clavicular fractures (Fig. 8–9). The wrap is used in the immediate treatment of these injuries to retract the scapulae.

▶ **Materials:**
- 4 inch or 6 inch width by 10 yard length elastic wrap, 2 inch or 3 inch elastic tape, taping scissors

▶ **Position of the individual:** Sitting or standing with the hands of the involved and noninvolved arms placed in a pain-free position on the hips with elbow flexion.

▶ **Preparation:** Apply the figure-of-eight wrap directly to the skin or over tight-fitting clothing.

▶ **Application:**
> **STEP 1:** Anchor the extended end of the wrap over the noninvolved shoulder and continue in a posterior direction, under the axilla, and encircle the anchor (Fig. 8–9A).

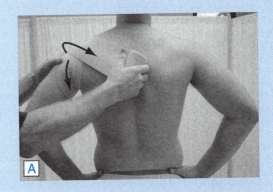

> **STEP 2:** Continue the wrap across the upper back with moderate roll tension, under the axilla of the involved shoulder, then up and across the shoulder with a moderate posterior pull (Fig. 8–9B).

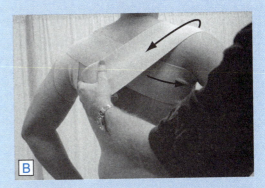

> **STEP 3:** Next, proceed from the involved shoulder across the upper back, under the axilla of the noninvolved shoulder, then up and across the shoulder with a moderate posterior pull (Fig. 8–9C).

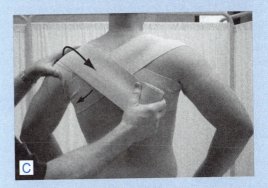

Figure 8-9

STEP 4: Repeat the figure-of-eight pattern two to four times. The wrap should resemble an "X" pattern over the upper back. Monitor roll tension to prevent constriction and irritation of the axilla areas.

STEP 5: Anchor 2 inch or 3 inch elastic tape over the noninvolved shoulder and apply one figure-of-eight pattern with moderate roll tension, again supporting retraction of the scapulae. Anchor the tape on the tape pattern on the upper back. No additional anchors are needed (Fig. 8–9D).

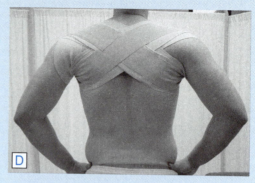

Figure 8-9 *continued*

...IF/THEN...

IF an individual with a stable clavicular fracture requires support and immobilization prior to transportation to an emergency facility for further evaluation, **THEN** consider using the figure-of-eight wrap rather than a brace technique; the wrap can be applied in less time and is cost effective in this situation, as most facilities will cut off the immobilization technique to perform an evaluation.

SWATHE WRAP Figure 8–10

▶ **Purpose:** Use the swathe wrap technique with slings to provide mild to moderate support and immobilization by anchoring the arm to the trunk when treating sprains, dislocations, subluxations, instabilities, lesions, fractures, strains, ruptures, and overuse injuries and conditions (Fig. 8–10).

▶ **Materials:**
  • 4 inch or 6 inch width by 10 yard length elastic wrap, metal clips, 2 inch or 3 inch elastic tape, taping scissors

▶ **Position of the individual:** Sitting or standing with the involved arm in a pain-free position next to the body with the elbow placed in flexion.

▶ **Preparation:** Place the hand, wrist, forearm, and elbow in a sling (see Figs. 8–11B and C). Apply the swathe wrap over the sling.

▶ **Application:**
STEP 1: Anchor the extended end of the wrap over the elbow of the involved arm (Fig. 8–10A).

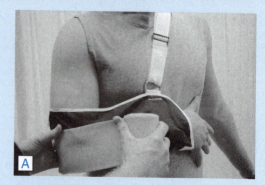

Figure 8-10

STEP 2: Apply the wrap in a lateral-to-medial pattern over the forearm, hand, and fingers with moderate roll tension. Continue around the back and return to the elbow (Fig. 8–10B).

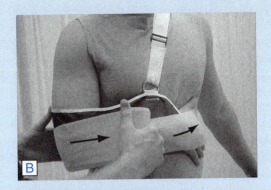

STEP 3: Next, overlap the wrap by ⅓ of its width in a proximal direction and encircle the distal upper arm and trunk (Fig. 8–10C).

STEP 4: Continue to encircle the upper arm and trunk two to three times with moderate roll tension. Leave the fingertips exposed to monitor circulation.

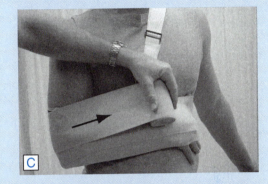

STEP 5: Anchor with Velcro, metal clips, or one lateral-to-medial circular pattern on the wrap, with 2 inch or 3 inch elastic tape and moderate roll tension (Fig. 8–10D). No additional anchors are required.

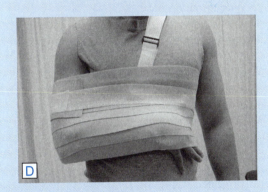

Figure 8-10 *continued*

Bracing Techniques

Bracing techniques for the shoulder and upper arm provide support, stability, compression, and immobilization, and limit range of motion. The designs are available off-the-shelf and custom-made, and are used to prevent and treat contusions, sprains, dislocations/subluxations, fractures, strains, ruptures, and overuse injuries and conditions.

SLINGS Figures 8–11, 8–12

▸ **Purpose:** Slings are designed to provide complete support and to immobilize the shoulder and arm following injury and surgery. Slings are used to treat contusions, sprains, dislocations, subluxations, instabilities, lesions, fractures, strains, ruptures, and overuse injuries and conditions. Two sling techniques are illustrated to accommodate for the intended purposes of support and immobilization following injury and/or surgery.

Sling Technique One

▸ **Purpose:** This sling technique provides complete support and immobilization of the shoulder, upper arm, elbow, forearm, wrist, and hand, and is used for varying periods of time following injury and/or surgery (Fig. 8–11). Typically, these slings are less expensive than those used in sling technique two.

○ **DETAILS**

Consider applying the swathe wrap technique over the sling for additional support and immobilization of the shoulder and arm.

▸ **Design:**
- The universal fit designs are purchased in predetermined sizes according to the length of the forearm, commonly measured from the olecranon to the fifth metacarpophalangeal joint.
- The slings are constructed of a cotton, poplin, or polyester material pouch with a closed end at the elbow and an open or closed end at the fingers. Adjustable nylon or cotton straps incorporated into the pouch through metal or plastic rings attach the sling to the body (Fig. 8–11A).
- Some designs are available with padded straps for additional comfort.
- Many designs have a loop or strap incorporated into the distal end of the pouch to provide support for the wrist, hand, and/or thumb.

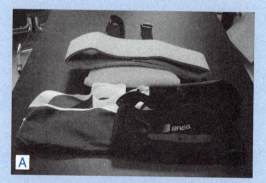

Figure 8-11A Slings. (Top) Sling with swathe. (Bottom) Universal fit slings.

- Another design uses two straps to support the proximal and distal forearm to provide immobilization.
- When properly applied, this sling technique immobilizes the shoulder in internal rotation against the trunk.
- With some designs, a swathe is available to provide additional support of the shoulder and arm.

▸ **Position of the individual:** Sitting or standing with the involved arm in a pain-free position next to the body with the elbow placed in flexion.

▸ **Preparation:** Apply the sling directly to the skin or over clothing.

Instructions for application are included with each sling. The following guidelines pertain to most designs.

▸ **Application:**

(**STEP 1:**) Begin by loosening the strap on the anterior pouch.

(**STEP 2:**) Place the hand, wrist, forearm, and elbow into the pouch by applying the closed end over the fingers and hand, and continue pulling the pouch toward the elbow. Assistance may be required to prevent movement of the injured area (Fig. 8–11B).

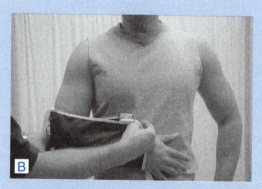

Figure 8-11

STEP 3: Position the elbow against the closed end of the pouch.

STEP 4: Apply the strap located at the elbow upward across the back, over the opposite shoulder and neck, then down across the chest and through the ring on the anterior pouch (Fig. 8–11C). Adjust the tightness of the strap to achieve the desired position of the arm as indicated by a physician. Anchor the strap with Velcro or a buckle. Prevent irritation of the shoulder and/or neck with padding .

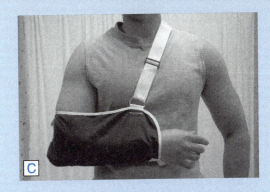

Helpful Hint: Cut a ½ inch foam or felt pad slightly wider than the strap, approximately 6–8 inches in length. Place the pad under the strap as it crosses the shoulder/neck area. A pad may also be cut and attached to the strap. First, cut the pad. Then, make two vertical cuts in the pad with taping scissors the width of the strap (Fig. 8–11D). Insert the strap through the pad and position over the shoulder/neck area (Fig. 8–11E). The pad can also be attached to the strap with self-adherent wrap.

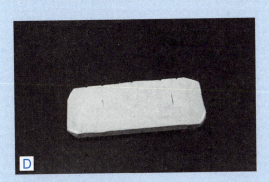

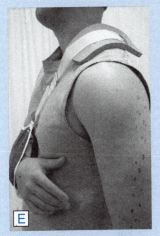

Figure 8-11 *continued*

Sling Technique Two

▸ **Purpose:** Sling technique two also provides complete support and immobilization of the shoulder, upper arm, elbow, forearm, wrist, and hand (Fig. 8–12). This technique is used when treating dislocations, subluxations, and postoperative procedures of the shoulder that require extended periods of immobilization in varying degrees of motion.

▸ **Design:**
- The universal fit designs are manufactured in predetermined sizes corresponding to chest circumference measurements or forearm length from the olecranon to the fifth metacarpophalangeal joint.
- The pouch and straps are constructed of soft cotton and nylon materials; most designs are available with padded straps.
- When using these designs, a pad or inflatable air pillow is used to immobilize the shoulder in varying degrees of abduction based on the injury and/or surgical procedure (Fig. 8–12A).

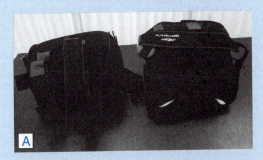

Figure 8-12A Slings. (Left) Inflatable pillow. (Right) Padded pillow with exercise ball.

- Some designs are constructed with the pouch attached to the pad or pillow with Velcro. Other designs use straps to attach the forearm to the pad or pillow.
- Adjustable straps incorporated into the pouch, pad, and/or pillow attach the sling to the shoulder and waist.
- Some designs have a loop or strap incorporated into the distal end of the pouch to provide support for the wrist, hand, and/or thumb. Several designs have a strap to limit posterior movement of the shoulder.

‣ **Position of the individual:** Sitting or standing with the involved arm in a pain-free position next to the body with the elbow placed in flexion.

‣ **Preparation:** Set the pad or inflatable pillow to the desired range of abduction as indicated by a physician and/or therapeutic exercise program. Apply the sling directly to the skin or over clothing.

Application of these sling designs should follow manufacturers' instructions, which are included with the slings when purchased. The following general application guidelines apply to most designs.

‣ **Application:**

STEP 1: Begin application by loosening the straps and unfolding the sling.

STEP 2: The application of the straps will depend on the specific design. Apply the shoulder straps of some designs by placing the harness over the noninvolved shoulder (Fig. 8–12B).

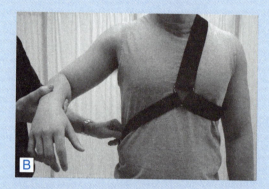

STEP 3: Position the pad or pillow under the involved shoulder and arm and attach to the harness (Fig. 8–12C).

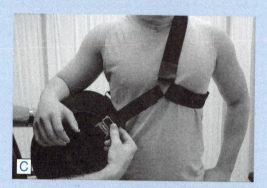

STEP 4: Attach the forearm and wrist to the pad or pillow with Velcro straps (Fig. 8–12D).

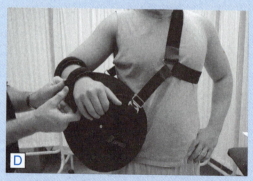

Figure 8-12 *continued*

STEP 5: Next, apply the strap around the waist (Fig. 8–12E). Readjust the straps if needed.

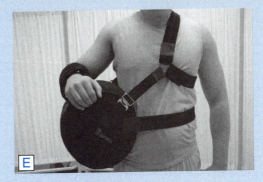

E

Figure 8-12 *continued*

...**IF/THEN**...

IF support and immobilization of the shoulder and arm in 35° of abduction is required for 2 weeks following a surgical rotator cuff repair, **THEN** use sling technique two, rather than technique one, because sling technique two is designed to be worn for extended periods and to immobilize the shoulder and arm in specific ranges of abduction.

Critical Thinking Question 2

The CEO of a local architectural firm is allowed by the surgeon to begin cardiovascular activity as tolerated following a procedure to the right shoulder. An avid runner and tennis player, the CEO is currently in a postoperative sling and swathe. The surgeon will continue its use for an additional 2 weeks. The CEO plans to ride a stationary bike during the lunch hour and return to work, but is concerned about soiling the postoperative sling and swathe during the workout.

▶ **Question: What type of brace can you use for support and immobilization during the cardiovascular activity?**

OFF-THE-SHELF SHOULDER STABILIZERS Figure 8–13

▶ **Purpose:** Off-the-shelf shoulder stabilizer braces are used to provide moderate to maximal support and limit range of motion when preventing and treating sprains, dislocations, subluxations, instabilities, strains, and overuse injuries and conditions (Fig. 8–13). These braces commonly limit GH joint abduction and external rotation while allowing normal flexion, extension, and horizontal adduction. Some designs can be applied to limit several ranges of motion based on the specific needs of the individual's injury or condition.

▶ **Design:**
  • The off-the-shelf braces are available in two basic designs: a torso vest with an arm cuff and an individual arm cuff.
  • The torso vest braces are constructed of neoprene, canvas, leather, or polyester materials and are available in individual fit designs corresponding to chest and upper arm circumference measurements (Fig. 8–13A).
  • Some vest designs attach over the torso and involved shoulder while others attach over the upper abdomen and shoulders using various straps. Adjustable straps or laces are used to achieve proper fit.

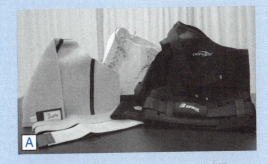

A

Figure 8-13A Torso vest shoulder stabilizers.

  • The arm cuffs of several designs are incorporated into the vest. Other designs use a plastic or metal ring to attach the arm cuff to the vest.
  • Some vest designs use neoprene straps that are applied in various patterns based on the specific injury or condition.
  • Torso vest braces can be worn underneath protective athletic equipment and uniforms.

- The individual arm cuff braces are manufactured in universal fit designs from neoprene, leather, or nylon in predetermined sizes according to upper arm circumference measurements (Fig. 8–13B).
- The adjustable cuff attaches to the upper arm and is anchored to the breast plate of football shoulder pads with laces, screws, or buckles .

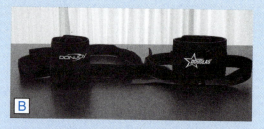

Figure 8-13B Individual arm cuff shoulder stabilizers.

Helpful Hint: When an adjustable off-the-shelf shoulder stabilizer cuff requires permanent attachment to the breast plate of football shoulder pads, first contact the manufacturer; drilling holes in the breast plate may lessen the protection provided and void the pads' warranty.

▶ **Position of the individual:** Standing with the involved arm placed at the side of the body.

▶ **Preparation:** Apply the torso vest design directly to the skin or over a shirt to lessen irritation. When using the individual cuff brace, anchor the cuff to the breast plate of football shoulder pads. Apply the cuff design directly to the skin or over a shirt.

Follow manufacturers' instructions, which are included with the braces when purchased, during application of these designs. The following guidelines pertain to most braces.

▶ **Application:**

STEP 1: Begin application of torso vest braces by loosening all the straps.

STEP 2: When using some designs, place the involved arm into the cuff and wrap the vest around the shoulder and torso (Fig. 8–13C).

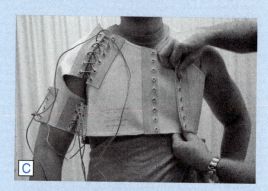

STEP 3: Adjust the vest and cuff with straps, buckles, or laces to limit the desired range of motion as indicated by a physician, then anchor (Fig. 8–13D). If using a multiple strap design, apply the appropriate straps to limit the range of motion based on the specific injury or condition (Fig. 8–13E).

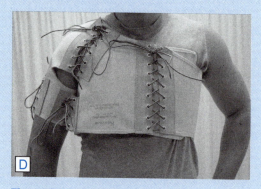

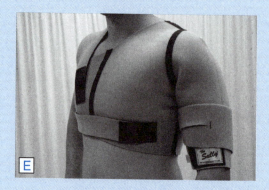

Figure 8-13 *continued*

STEP 4: Apply other vest designs by placing the vest over the shoulders and around the torso, then anchor (Fig. 8–13F). Next, place the cuff around the upper arm and anchor (Fig. 8–13G).

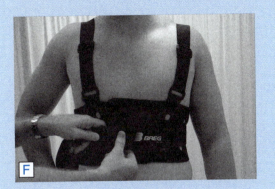

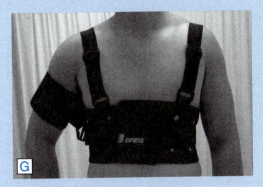

STEP 5: When using the individual cuff designs, apply and anchor the shoulder pads. Next, apply the cuff around the proximal upper arm, superior to the belly of the biceps brachii (Fig. 8–13H).

STEP 6: Adjust the cuff and strap to limit the desired range of motion and anchor with Velcro or buckles (Fig. 8–13I).

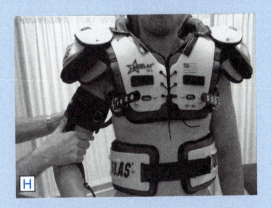

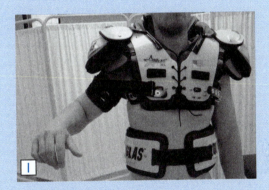

Figure 8-13 *continued*

> **Helpful Hint:** Daily use of the cuff may cause irritation and pinching of the skin. To prevent this irritation, apply 3 inch or 4 inch self-adherent wrap loosely in a circular pattern around the proximal upper arm ◀▬▶ . Apply enough wrap to cover an area slightly larger than the cuff. Anchor the cuff over the wrap.

...IF/THEN...

IF limits in range of motion are required when treating GH joint instability for a football athlete, **THEN** consider using an individual cuff design; a torso vest brace can be effective, but a cuff design may be more comfortable to wear in hot and humid weather because the cuff design eliminates the need to wear a vest.

CUSTOM-MADE SHOULDER STABILIZER   Figure 8–14

▶ **Purpose:** Use the custom-made shoulder stabilizer brace to prevent and treat sprains, dislocations, subluxations, instabilities, strains, and overuse injuries and conditions, and to provide moderate to maximal support and limit range of motion (Fig. 8–14). The brace can be used when off-the-shelf designs are not available.

▶ **Materials:**
- 1 inch width by 60 inch length nylon belt with a D-ring fastener (commonly used with football pants), ¼ inch or ½ inch foam, 3 inch or 4 inch self-adherent wrap, 2 inch or 3 inch elastic tape, taping scissors

▶ **Position of the individual:** Standing with the involved arm placed at the side of the body and the elbow placed in 90° of flexion with moderate isometric contraction of the biceps and triceps muscles.

▶ **Preparation:** Cut a ¼ inch or ½ inch foam pad to cover a 4 inch area completely around the proximal upper arm. Thread the belt through the anterior shoulder pad laces and anchor around the breast plate of the noninvolved side with the D-ring (Fig. 8–14A). Determine painful range(s) of motion, commonly abduction and external rotation at the GH joint. To determine painful abduction, stabilize the scapula and thorax. Place a hand on the distal forearm and slowly move the arm into abduction until pain occurs. For external rotation, place the involved shoulder in 90° of abduction and the elbow in 90° of flexion.

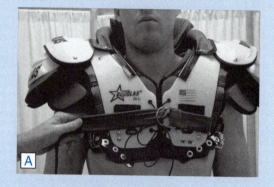

Stabilize the scapula and thorax and grasp the arm at the elbow and distal forearm. Slowly move the arm into external rotation until pain occurs. Once painful range of motion is determined, place the shoulder in a pain-free range and maintain this position during application.

▶ **Application:**

(**STEP 1:**) Apply and anchor the shoulder pads.

(**STEP 2:**) Place the foam pad directly on the skin over the proximal upper arm. Using 3 inch or 4 inch self-adherent wrap, anchor the pad with mild roll tension in a circular pattern ◀▬▶ (Fig. 8–14B). The pad will prevent skin irritation.

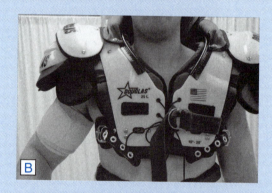

(**STEP 3:**) Pull the belt tight and wrap the remaining portion of the belt around the proximal upper arm, over the foam pad, with moderate tension ◀▬▶ (Fig. 8–14C). Monitor the pain-free position of the shoulder.

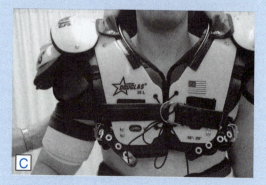

Figure 8-14

STEP 4: Anchor 2 inch or 3 inch elastic tape over the end of the belt and apply three to four continuous circular patterns with moderate roll tension ◀▬▶ (Fig. 8–14D). Finish the tape on the lateral aspect of the upper arm to prevent irritation. No additional anchors are needed.

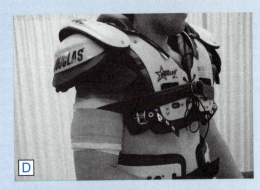

Figure 8-14 *continued*

RESEARCH BRIEF

Shoulder stabilizer braces are designed to limit range of motion at the GH joint in attempts to prevent further injury. Research efforts to examine the indications for and effectiveness of shoulder stabilizer braces are limited in the literature[3]; the few studies examining shoulder stabilizer designs have produced mixed results. Among 11 major league amateur hockey athletes, using a torso vest shoulder stabilizer brace within a therapy program consisting of rest, muscle stimulation, and weight-training resulted in no recurrence of injury.[14] All subjects had a history of shoulder dislocation or subluxation; the duration of the therapy program to return the subjects back to activity ranged from 3 to 7 weeks.

The ability of three torso vest stabilizer designs to limit forward flexion, abduction, and external rotation at the GH joint following isokinetic exercise has been examined.[3] The researchers found that all three braces experienced loosening and allowed a significant increase in postexercise forward flexion, compared to predetermined motion limitations. The findings also revealed that postexercise external rotation in allowed abduction did not significantly increase among the three braces. These researchers[3] suggested several factors that should be considered by health-care professionals when selecting shoulder stabilizer braces. First, determining the mechanism of injury will assist in identifying the specific range(s) of motion to restrict. Second, knowledge of the individual's sport or work activities will identify essential movements required for participation, such as an overhead motion. Third, familiarity with brace designs will provide the health-care professional the information needed to choose and apply the most appropriate brace to fit the needs of the individual.

Although a large amount of research examines the effects of taping and bracing techniques on joint-reposition sense in the lower extremities, studies examining the effects on the upper extremities are lacking. Many researchers have shown that shoulder injury and instability negatively affect passive joint-reposition sense.[7,15,17] Focusing on the shoulder, researchers have examined the effects of a neoprene torso vest on active joint-reposition sense.[2] The data revealed that brace wear significantly improved active joint-reposition sense at 10° from full external rotation among subjects with unstable shoulders. Shoulder external rotation was limited with brace wear in subjects with stable shoulders, but no effect was found among the unstable group. The researchers[2] proposed that an increase in cutaneous input at the shoulder from the brace may have caused the improvement in active joint-reposition sense. This increase in stimulation may enhance proprioception and lessen the recurrence of dislocations or subluxations. Other researchers have also demonstrated that applying elastic wraps and braces enhanced cutaneous stimulation.[5,6] Further research is needed to examine the effects of shoulder stabilizer braces on proprioception.

FIGURE-OF-EIGHT BRACE Figure 8–15

▸ **Purpose:** The figure-of-eight brace is designed to provide moderate to maximal support and longitudinal traction to the clavicle (Fig. 8–15). Use this technique to retract the scapulae when treating SC joint sprains and clavicular fractures.

Shoulder and Upper Arm

RESEARCH BRIEF

Researchers have demonstrated no difference between using a sling or a figure-of-eight brace in the healing and functional outcome of clavicular fractures.[1]

▸ **Design:**
- The braces are available in universal fit designs in predetermined sizes according to chest circumference measurements.
- The braces consist of two foam and nylon straps covered with stockinet, attached over the upper back with buckles, plastic rings, or Velcro closures to allow for tension adjustments.

▸ **Position of the individual:** Standing with the hands of the involved and noninvolved arms placed on the hips with elbow flexion.

▸ **Preparation:** Apply the figure-of-eight brace directly to the skin or over clothing.
   Specific instructions for application are included with each brace. The following guidelines apply to most designs.

▸ **Application:**

STEP 1: Position the brace on the upper back (Fig. 8–15A).

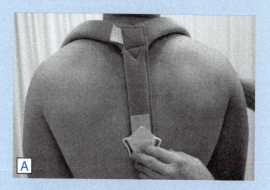

STEP 2: Apply the straps across the anterior shoulders, under the axillae, and anchor on the upper back through the buckles, rings, or closures (Fig. 8–15B).

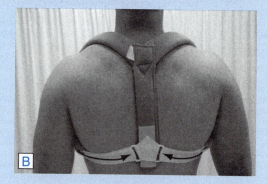

STEP 3: Adjust the straps to the desired tension, as indicated by a physician, to promote scapular retraction (Fig. 8–15C). Monitor strap tension to prevent brachial artery or nerve impingement.

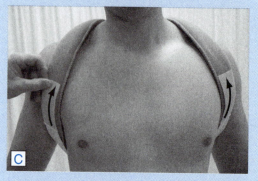

Figure 8-15

ACROMIOCLAVICULAR JOINT BRACE Figure 8–16

▶ **Purpose:** The acromioclavicular joint brace provides moderate to maximal support, compression, and immobilization when treating AC joint sprains (Fig. 8–16).

▶ **Design:**
- The braces are manufactured in universal fit designs and are similar to sling technique one.
- The designs are constructed of a cotton, poplin, or polyester material pouch with adjustable nylon or cotton straps.
- The straps of some braces are designed to cross the noninvolved shoulder and AC joint of the involved shoulder.
- Other designs use a multiple strap pattern over the AC joint of the involved shoulder and across the chest.
- The strap positioned over the involved AC joint is lined with felt and is designed to provide mild to moderate compression to the joint.

▶ **Position of the individual:** Sitting or standing with the involved arm in a pain-free position next to the body with the elbow placed in flexion.

▶ **Preparation:** Apply the acromioclavicular joint brace directly to the skin or over clothing.
   Instructions for application are included with each brace when purchased. The following guidelines pertain to most designs.

▶ **Application:**

STEP 1: Begin application by loosening all the straps.

STEP 2: The application of straps will depend on the specific brace design. With some designs, apply the short strap and pad over the involved AC joint. Next, attach the long strap and pad to the short strap at the anterior involved shoulder. Continue to apply the longer strap across the chest, under the axilla of the noninvolved shoulder, and attach to the short strap over the posterior involved shoulder (Fig. 8–16A).

STEP 3: Continue application by placing the hand, wrist, forearm, and elbow into the pouch as illustrated in Figure 8-11B. Next, attach the pouch to the short and long straps with buckles (Fig. 8–16B). Adjust the short strap that crosses the involved AC joint for proper compression as indicated by a physician.

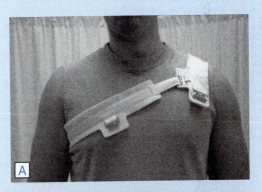
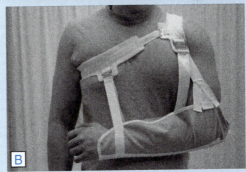

Figure 8-16

NEOPRENE SLEEVE Figure 8–17

▶ **Purpose:** Neoprene sleeves provide compression and mild support when treating sprains, strains, and overuse injuries and conditions (Fig. 8–17).

> ○ DETAILS
> The sleeves may be used during rehabilitative, athletic, work, and casual activities.

▶ **Design:**
- Off-the-shelf sleeves are available in individual fit designs in predetermined sizes, corresponding to chest circumference measurements.
- The sleeves extend from the mid upper arm, cover the shoulder, and encircle the chest. Velcro closures anchor the sleeve around the upper arm and chest.

▶ **Position of the individual:** Standing with the involved arm placed next to the body with the elbow placed in flexion.

▶ **Preparation:** Apply the neoprene sleeve directly to the skin.

▶ **Application:**

STEP 1: To apply, place the sleeve over the shoulder and chest. Anchor the ends of the sleeve around the upper arm and chest with Velcro closures (Fig. 8–17). Adjust the sleeve if needed.

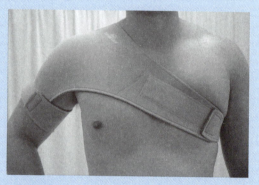

Figure 8-17

Padding Techniques

Use off-the-shelf and custom-made padding techniques to absorb shock and provide protection when preventing and treating shoulder and upper arm injuries and conditions. Several high school and intercollegiate sports require mandatory padding of the shoulder and upper arm. The mandatory padding techniques will be discussed in Chapter 13.

RESEARCH BRIEF

Athletes participating in collision and contact sports should return to activity following an AC joint sprain with protective padding.[4,12] An off-the-shelf or custom-made design worn over the AC joint will lessen the chance of reinjury.

OFF-THE-SHELF Figure 8–18

▶ **Purpose:** Use off-the-shelf padding techniques to absorb shock and provide protection when preventing and treating AC joint sprains, shoulder pointers, and upper arm contusions, myositis ossificans, and exostosis (Fig. 8–18).

○ DETAILS—————————————

Each of these off-the-shelf padding techniques can be used with mandatory protective equipment or worn alone .

Helpful Hint: When working with athletes in collision and contact sports, such as field hockey, football, ice hockey, lacrosse, or soccer, purchase several off-the-shelf pad designs for the shoulder and upper arm. These pads can be fitted and applied in less time than custom-made pads and can also be reused.

Design:

- Several padding techniques are available in individual and universal fit designs and are manufactured in predetermined sizes.
- Many AC joint designs are constructed of a thermoplastic material outer shell lined with open- and closed-cell foams with a raised area over the joint (Fig. 8–18A).
- Some of these designs can be molded to the shoulder by hand while others require immersion in water to mold.
- Most designs use neoprene straps to attach the pads to the shoulder.
- Other designs are constructed of viscoelastic polymer or gel materials covered with cotton or nylon and are available in predetermined sizes (Fig. 8–18B).
- These pads are designed to be used in combination with football shoulder pads. The designs are attached to the inner lining of shoulder pads with Velcro.
- Other designs, used primarily underneath football shoulder pads, are constructed of vinyl-coated foam in a skeleton pattern or closed-cell foam that covers the shoulders and upper chest and back (Fig. 8–18C).
- The skeleton pad has anterior and posterior laces and is anchored under the axilla with elastic straps. The closed-cell foam design attaches around the chest with Velcro straps.
- Upper arm designs are manufactured with high-density plastics covered by open- and closed-cell foams (Fig. 8–18D). These pads are contoured to the upper arm; some are designed to be used in combination with football shoulder pads.
- Another upper arm design consists of a high-density shell lined with foam incorporated into neoprene straps.

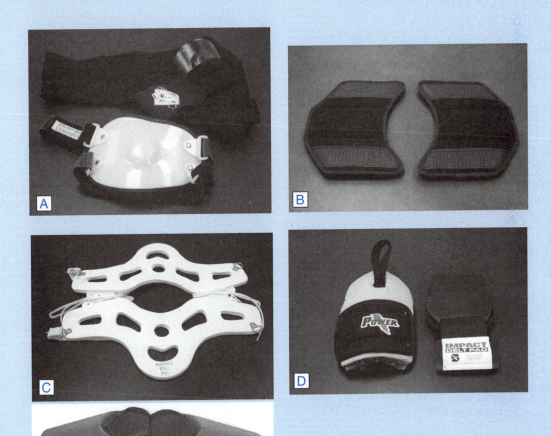

Figure 8-18 A AC joint pads. (Top) Pad in a neoprene sleeve. (Bottom) Pad with straps. **B** Viscoelastic polymer pad. **C** (Top) Skeleton pad. (Bottom) Closed-cell foam pad. (Courtesy of Riddell, Elyria, OH). **D** Upper arm pads. (Left) Pad that can be attached to football shoulder pads. (Right) Pad with straps.

▶ **Position of the individual:** Standing with the hand of the involved arm placed on the lateral hip in a relaxed position.

▶ **Preparation:** Apply the off-the-shelf designs directly to the skin or over tight-fitting clothing.

▶ **Application:**

STEP 1: Begin application of neoprene strap designs by placing the pad over the injured area. When using most designs, wrap the straps around the chest and under the axilla (Fig. 8–18E). Anchor the straps with Velcro.

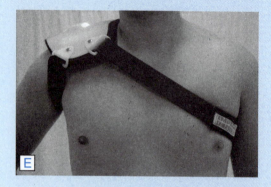

STEP 2: Apply the viscoelastic polymer and gel material pads directly to the existing inner padding of the football shoulder pads. Determine placement of the pad and anchor with Velcro (Fig. 8–18F).

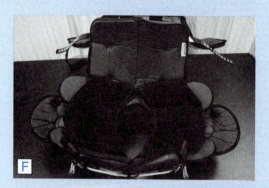

STEP 3: Place the skeleton pad over the head and insert the arms through the openings. Pull the pad onto the shoulders, chest, and back (Fig. 8–18G).

STEP 4: When using the closed-cell foam pad, place the pad onto the shoulders and wrap around the chest. Anchor with Velcro.

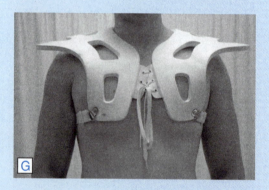

STEP 5: When using the upper arm pad designs, attach the pad to the cup of the football shoulder pad using the incorporated strap. Anchor the pad around the upper arm with the Velcro strap (Fig. 8–18H).

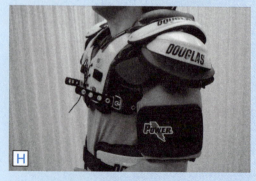

Figure 8-18 *continued*

STEP 6: When using other designs, apply the pad over the injured area and wrap the neoprene straps around the upper arm. Anchor with Velcro (Fig. 8–18I).

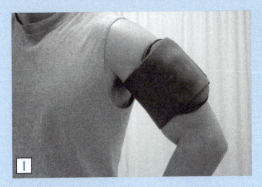

Figure 8-18 *continued*

Critical Thinking Question 3

Since the ninth grade, a senior linebacker on the high school football team has sustained five mild contusions to the anterolateral aspect of the left upper arm. You and the team physician have followed the athlete during this time; he has worn several different pads over the area for protection. The pad design that provides the most effective protection and is the most comfortable migrates during activity. This particular design attaches to the cup of the shoulder pad and to the upper arm with a strap.

▶ **Question: How can you manage this situation?**

CUSTOM-MADE Figure 8–19

▶ **Purpose:** Absorb shock and provide protection when preventing and treating AC joint sprains, shoulder pointers, and upper arm contusions, myositis ossificans, and exostosis with thermoplastic material and foam (Fig. 8–19). Use these pads when off-the-shelf designs are not available.

▶ **Materials:**
  • Paper, felt tip pen, thermoplastic material, ⅛ inch or ¼ inch foam or felt, a heating source, 2 inch or 3 inch elastic tape, an elastic wrap, soft, low-density foam, rubber cement, taping scissors

▶ **Position of the individual:** Standing with the hand of the involved arm placed on the lateral hip in a relaxed position.

▶ **Preparation:** Design the pad with a paper pattern (see Fig. 1–14), then cut, mold, and shape the thermoplastic material on the shoulder or upper arm over the injured area. Attach soft, low-density foam to the inside surface of the material (see Fig. 1–15).

▶ **Application:**
  STEP 1: Attach the pad to the AC joint or tip of the shoulder with the shoulder pointer/AC joint sprain taping technique (see Figs. 8–2A–D) or the shoulder spica wrapping technique (see Figs. 8–7A–G; Fig. 8–19).

  STEP 2: For the upper arm, attach the pad with the circular upper arm taping (see Figs. 8–1A–C) or wrapping (see Figs. 8–6A–C) technique.

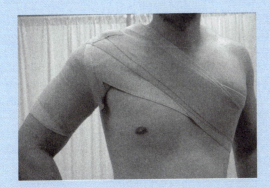

Figure 8-19

Critical Thinking Question 4

An intercollegiate baseball shortstop is struck on the acromion process of his throwing shoulder by a base runner during a double play. In the athletic training room, you and the team physician complete an evaluation and determine that the athlete sustained a first degree AC joint sprain. The team physician will allow a return to activity when the athlete can demonstrate full, bilateral strength and range of motion and a preinjury throwing motion. The team physician also requests that protective padding be applied upon the athlete's return, to prevent further injury.

▶ **Question: What padding technique(s) are appropriate to provide protection?**

MANDATORY PADDING

▶ Protective equipment is required in several high school and intercollegiate sports. The NCAA[10] and the NFHS[11] require that athletes participating in fencing, football, ice hockey, and lacrosse wear protective padding on the shoulder and/or upper arm during all practices and competitions. These pads are normally purchased off-the-shelf; many designs are constructed for specific sports and positions. Chapter 13 will provide a more in-depth discussion of these padding techniques.

CASE STUDY

Midway through the racing schedule, Tanner Compton suffers a first-time, right glenohumeral (GH) joint dislocation while in the pits. Tanner is the rear tire carrier for the RN Racing Team and was injured during a pit stop. As he lifted the tire off the pit wall, Tanner did not notice that the air hose for the air impact wrench had become wrapped around the tire and his right wrist. As the rear tire changer quickly moved away from the pit wall and across the back of the race car, the air hose was violently pulled, placing an abduction, external rotation force on Tanner's right shoulder. Tanner was moved behind the pit wall and evaluated by Jordon Young, the ATC with the Race Team. The evaluation showed an acute anterior GH joint dislocation. Jordon immobilized the shoulder and took Tanner to the in-field care center for further evaluation by a physician. What wrapping and/or bracing techniques could you apply to support and immobilize the GH joint in the immediate management of this case?

The orthopedist at the in-field care center obtained radiographs and reduced the shoulder. Tanner returned home with the Race Team and was scheduled for a follow-up evaluation with an orthopedic surgeon. The surgeon performed an evaluation and ordered additional radiographs and magnetic resonance imaging. The imaging studies were negative; the surgeon decided on a nonsurgical rehabilitation approach for Tanner and continued immobilization of his shoulder for 3 weeks. What wrapping and/or bracing techniques could be used to support and immobilize the GH joint during this period?

Tanner progresses with the rehabilitation program without any delays and begins functional activities around postinjury week 20. A follow-up evaluation with the surgeon demonstrates mild anterior instability of the right shoulder. Jordon designs a functional activity program, which includes lifting, carrying, and setting a 75 lb racing tire onto the rear lug nuts of a race car. These activities are performed in standing and kneeling positions, and require flexion, extension, abduction, adduction, and internal and external rotation at the GH joint. The surgeon and Jordon decide that using a brace may lessen the possibility of reinjury in this phase of rehabilitation and upon his return to full activity with the Race Team. What bracing technique would help to support and limit range of motion in this case?

Tanner returns to full activity during week 23. Jordon designs a maintenance strengthening and flexibility program for Tanner to follow throughout the remainder of the racing season. Which bracing techniques can you use to allow Tanner to continue his activities with the Race Team?

WRAP UP

- Shoulder and upper arm contusions, sprains, dislocations, subluxations, fractures, strains, ruptures, and overuse injuries and conditions can be caused by compressive and shear forces, excessive range of motion, forceful muscular contractions, and repetitive stresses.
- The circular upper arm and shoulder pointer/AC joint sprain taping techniques provide support and anchor protective padding.
- Elastic wraps and sleeves and self-adherent wrap provide compression and assist in reducing swelling.
- The circular upper arm and shoulder spica wrapping techniques can be used to provide support and anchor padding.
- The 4 S, figure-of-eight, and swathe wrapping techniques are used to support and immobilize the shoulder and upper arm.

- Sling, figure-of-eight, and acromioclavicular joint bracing techniques provide support and immobilization following injury and surgery.
- Shoulder stabilizer bracing techniques are used to provide support and limit range of motion of the glenohumeral joint.
- Neoprene sleeves can be used to provide compression and mild support.
- Off-the-shelf and custom-made padding techniques constructed of open- and closed-cell foams and hard, high-density, viscoelastic polymer and gel materials absorb shock and provide protection.
- Protective padding is required for the shoulder and/or upper arm in several sports by the NCAA and NFHS.

■ WEB REFERENCES

American Academy of Orthopaedic Surgeons
http://www.aaos.org/
- This site provides access to information regarding the treatment and rehabilitation of shoulder and upper arm injuries and conditions.

The Hughston Clinic
http://www.hughston.com/
- This site allows access to the Hughston Health Alert newsletter and online articles about a variety of injuries and conditions.

United States National Library of Medicine
http://www.nlm.nih.gov/
- This Web site provides access to shoulder and upper arm injury prevention, treatment, and rehabilitation information among a variety of populations.

Virtual Hospital
http://www.vh.org/index.html
- This Web site is a digital health sciences library that allows you to search for information about shoulder and upper injuries and conditions.

■ REFERENCES

1. Andersen, K, Jensen, PO, and Lauritzen, J: Treatment of clavicular fractures: Figure-of-eight bandage versus a simple sling. Acta Orthop Scand 58:71–74, 1987.
2. Chu, JC, Kane, EJ, Arnold, BL, and Gansneder, BM: The effect of a neoprene shoulder stabilizer on active joint-reposition sense in subjects with stable and unstable shoulders. J Athl Train 37:141–145, 2002.
3. DeCarlo, M, Malone, K, Gerig, B, and Hunker, M: Evaluation of shoulder instability braces. J Sport Rehabil 4:143–150, 1996.
4. Johnson, RJ: Acromioclavicular joint injuries: Identifying and treating "separated shoulder" and other conditions. The Physician and Sportsmedicine 29:31–35, 2001.
5. Khabie, V, Schwartz, MC, Rokito, AS, Gallagher, MA, Cuomo, F, and Zuckerman, JD: The effect of intraarticular anesthesia and elastic bandaging on elbow proprioception. J Shoulder Elbow Surg 7:501–504, 1998.
6. Lephart, SM, Kocher, MS, Fu, FH, Borsa, PA, and Harner, CD: Proprioception following anterior cruciate ligament reconstruction. J Sport Rehabil 1:188–196, 1992.
7. Lephart, SM, Warner, JP, Borsa, PA, and Fu, FH: Proprioception of the shoulder joint in healthy, unstable, and surgically repaired shoulders. J Shoulder Elbow Surg 3:371–380, 1994.
8. Magee, DJ, and Reid, DC: Shoulder injuries. In Zachazewski, JE, Magee, DJ, Quillen, WS (eds): Athletic Injuries and Rehabilitation. WB Saunders, Philadelphia, 1996.
9. Meister, K, and Andrews, JR: Classification and treatment of rotator cuff injuries in the overhead athlete. J Orthop Sports Phys Ther 18:413–421, 1993.
10. National Collegiate Athletic Association, http://www.ncaa.org/library/sports_sciences/sports_med_handbook/2003-04/2003-04_sports_med_handbook.pdf, Sports medicine handbook, 2003–2004.
11. National Federation of State High School Associations. 2004-05 Ice Hockey Rules Book. Indianapolis, IN: National Federation of State High School Associations, 2004.
12. Prentice, WE: Rehabilitation Techniques for Sports Medicine and Athletic Training, ed 4. McGraw-Hill, Boston, 2004.
13. Prentice, WE: Arnheim's Principles of Athletic Training, ed 11. McGraw-Hill, Boston, 2003.
14. Sawa, TM: An alternate conservative management of shoulder dislocations and subluxations. J Athl Train 4:366–369, 1992.
15. Smith, RL, and Brunolli, J: Shoulder kinesthesia after anterior glenohumeral joint dislocation. Phys Ther 69:106–112, 1989.
16. Starkey, C, and Ryan, JL: Evaluation of Orthopedic and Athletic Injuries, ed 2. FA Davis, Philadelphia, 2002.
17. Warner, JJ, Lephart, S, and Fu, FH: Role of proprioception in pathoetiology of shoulder instability. Clin Orthop 330:35–29, 1996.

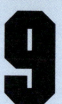
Elbow and Forearm

LEARNING OBJECTIVES

1. Discuss common injuries and conditions that occur to the elbow and forearm.
2. Demonstrate the application of taping, wrapping, bracing, and padding techniques for the elbow and forearm when preventing, treating, and rehabilitating injuries.
3. Explain and demonstrate the application of taping, wrapping, bracing, and padding techniques for the elbow and forearm within a therapeutic exercise program.

INJURIES AND CONDITIONS

Direct forces, excessive range of motion, and repetitive and overload stresses can result in acute and chronic injuries and conditions to the elbow and forearm. Contusions, fractures, and bursitis can be caused by a direct blow or fall. Valgus, varus, and/or rotary forces can be produced during many athletic and work activities and result in a sprain, dislocation, or fracture. Overload and repetitive contractions of the musculature can lead to strains, ruptures, and overuse injuries and conditions. Common injuries to the elbow and forearm include:

• Contusions
• Sprains
• Strains
• Ruptures
• Dislocations
• Fractures
• Bursitis
• Overuse injuries and conditions
• Abrasions

Contusions

Contusions to the elbow and forearm are caused by direct forces and commonly occur over bony prominences. The **olecranon** is frequently involved because of its exposure and lack of protection by soft tissue (Illustration 9–1). In collision and contact sports, direct blows can lead to contusions of the forearm. The ulnar side of the forearm, because of its location, is susceptible to injury as a result of contact with opponents and equipment. A contusion to the olecranon and/or ulnar forearm can occur, for instance, as a football tight end catches a pass, runs down field with the ball in his right arm, and is tackled, receiving a blow to the right elbow and forearm from the helmet of a defensive back.

Sprains

Sprains to the elbow are caused by acute and chronic forces. An acute valgus, varus, or rotary force or a fall on the outstretched arm causing hyperextension at the elbow can result in injury to the **ulnar collateral, radial collateral,** or **annular ligaments** (Illustration 9–2). Hyperextension of an elbow can take place, for instance, if the arms are extended to lessen the impact during a backward fall to the ground. More commonly, sprains to the ulnar collateral ligament are caused by repetitive valgus forces, which occur during the overhead throwing motion.[17] For example, a baseball, softball, or tennis player with a history of medial elbow pain, indicating possible overuse, can be injured during the late cocking and early acceleration phases of the throwing motion, when valgus forces at the medial elbow are extreme. The position of the arm against the trunk protects the elbow from varus forces; injury to the radial collateral ligament is uncommon.

Strains

Strains of the elbow and forearm are caused by a variety of mechanisms during athletic and work activities. Brachialis, biceps brachii, and brachioradialis strains can be caused by repetitive microtrauma and overload, a fall on the outstretched arm, or a violent concentric or eccentric contraction (Illustration 9–3). A strain to the brachialis or brachioradialis can result as a construction worker attempts to catch a large box of nails, thrown from a height, with his elbows in a flexed position. This may cause a violent eccentric contraction. A strain to the triceps brachii can also result from a violent concentric or eccentric contraction (Illustration 9–4).

Ruptures

A forceful eccentric contraction against resistance can cause a rupture of the biceps brachii. The proximal portion of the tendon is typically injured.

Dislocations

A fall on the outstretched arm with the elbow in hyperextension, as well as valgus and rotary forces, can cause an elbow dislocation. With a dislocation, the ulna and/or radius can be positioned in an anterior, posterior, or lateral direction. Dislocations are often accompanied by fractures and ligamentous and muscular trauma. For example, a dislocation can occur as a pole vaulter misses

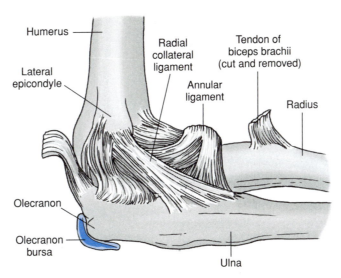

Illustration 9-1   Ligaments of the lateral elbow.

the plant of the pole, is thrown to the side of the landing pit, and lands on his right outstretched arm, causing hyperextension and rotary stress.

Fractures

Fractures to the elbow and forearm may involve the radius, ulna, and olecranon. A fall on the outstretched arm or on a flexed elbow, direct forces, and valgus, varus, or tensile stresses can result in a fracture.

Bursitis

The **olecranon bursa** can become inflamed through acute or chronic trauma. A fall on the flexed elbow or a direct force to the olecranon can cause acute olecranon bursitis. Repetitive compression and friction or infection can result in the development of chronic olecranon bursitis. Bursitis can be caused by activities, such as wrestling without proper padding or leaning on a desktop while writing or reading.

Overuse

Overload and repetitive stresses and faulty mechanics can cause elbow and forearm overuse injuries and conditions. **Lateral epicondylitis (tennis elbow)** can result from repetitive, eccentric overload of the wrist extensor musculature, faulty mechanics, and ill fitting equipment. The extensor carpi radialis brevis is most commonly involved. For example, lateral epicondylitis can occur as a racquetball player participates in daily practices for several weeks without adequate rest to improve her backhand. Repetitive wrist flexion, forearm pronation, and valgus stress at the elbow; training errors, and improper technique can cause **medial epicondylitis (golfer's elbow).** The origins of the pronator teres and flexor carpi radialis are common sites of involvement.[16] Medial epicondylitis can be caused by a youth league pitcher learning how to throw a curveball, resulting in repetitive wrist flexion and valgus stress at the elbow. Repetitive muscular contractions, commonly

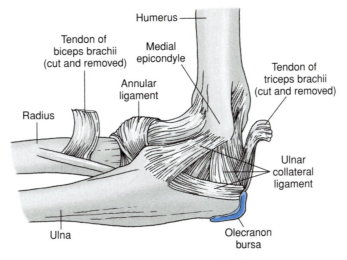

Illustration 9-2   Ligaments of the medial elbow.

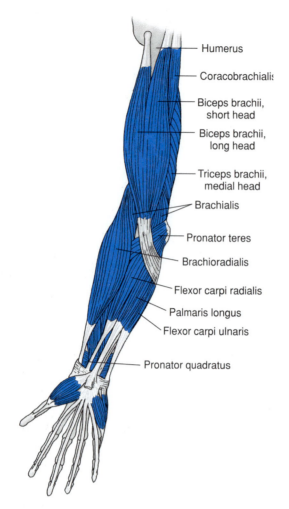

Illustration 9-3 Superficial muscles of the anterior upper arm, elbow, and forearm.

Labels: Humerus; Coracobrachialis; Biceps brachii, short head; Biceps brachii, long head; Triceps brachii, medial head; Brachialis; Pronator teres; Brachioradialis; Flexor carpi radialis; Palmaris longus; Flexor carpi ulnaris; Pronator quadratus

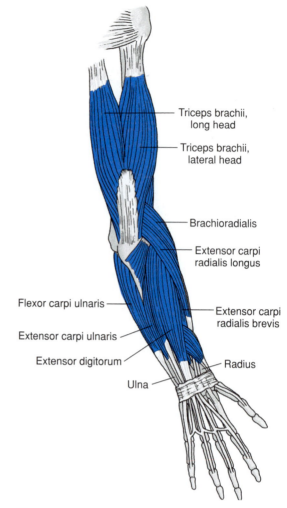

Illustration 9-4 Superficial muscles of the posterior upper arm, elbow, and forearm.

Labels: Triceps brachii, long head; Triceps brachii, lateral head; Brachioradialis; Extensor carpi radialis longus; Flexor carpi ulnaris; Extensor carpi radialis brevis; Extensor carpi ulnaris; Extensor digitorum; Radius; Ulna

static, can cause inflammation within the compartments of the forearm (**forearm splints**).

Abrasions

Abrasions to the elbow and forearm are common in athletic activities. Rubbing and friction forces on the posterior elbow and ulnar side of the forearm during contact with athletic surfaces can result in abrasions (**turf burn**).

DETAILS

Commonly referred to as epicondylitis, the condition involves degeneration rather than the traditional inflammatory process.[9,10] As a result, the term tendinosis, instead of tendinitis or epicondylitis, is often used to describe the condition.[17]

Taping Techniques

Use taping techniques to provide support and reduce stress to the musculature and soft tissue, limit excessive range of motion, and immobilize the elbow and forearm when preventing and treating injuries and conditions. Following sprains, use several techniques to lessen excessive range of motion and immobilize the elbow and forearm. Use other techniques with overuse injuries and conditions to reduce the tension of the wrist extensor or flexor musculature during contractions. Techniques are also available to anchor protective padding to the elbow and forearm to prevent and treat contusions.

HYPEREXTENSION Figures 9–1, 9–2, 9–3

▶ **Purpose:** Use the hyperextension technique when treating sprains to limit hyperextension of the elbow and stretch on the soft tissues. Three interchangeable methods are illustrated in the application of the technique. Choose according to individual preferences.

Hyperextension Technique One

▶ **Materials:**
- Pre-tape material, thin foam pads, 2 inch or 3 inch heavyweight elastic tape, adherent tape spray, skin lubricant, taping scissors

Option:
- 4 inch or 6 inch width by 5 yard length elastic wrap

▶ **Position of the individual:** Sitting on a taping table or bench or standing with the involved arm at the side of the body. Determine the range of extension that produces pain. Stabilize the involved shoulder and place the forearm in supination. Support the posterior elbow and place a hand on the wrist. Slowly move the elbow into extension until pain occurs. Once painful range of motion is determined, place the involved elbow in a pain-free range and maintain this position during application. Also, maintain a moderate isometric contraction of the upper arm and forearm musculature.

▶ **Preparation:** Shave the arm from the proximal upper arm to mid forearm. Apply this technique directly to the skin or over one layer of pre-tape material. Place thin foam pads over the cubital fossa to prevent irritation. A skin lubricant may also be used. Apply adherent tape spray from the proximal upper arm to the mid forearm.

▶ **Application:**

STEP 1: Apply two anchors of 2 inch or 3 inch heavyweight elastic tape around the proximal upper arm and the mid forearm with a mild amount of roll tension ◀▬▶ (Fig. 9–1A).

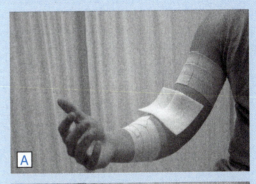

STEP 2: Using 2 inch or 3 inch heavyweight elastic tape, anchor on the proximal lateral upper arm, continue distally across the cubital fossa, and anchor the strip on the medial mid forearm (Fig. 9–1B). Monitor the pain-free position of the elbow and apply the tape with moderate roll tension.

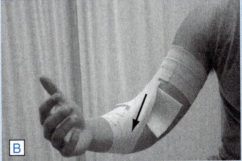

STEP 3: Apply another strip of 2 inch or 3 inch heavyweight elastic tape from the proximal medial upper arm, across the cubital fossa, and anchor on the lateral mid forearm (Fig. 9–1C). These strips should form an "X" over the cubital fossa.

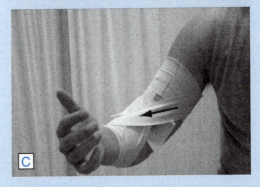

Figure 9-1

STEP 4: Begin the next strip on the anterior proximal upper arm, across the cubital fossa, and anchor on the anterior mid forearm (Fig. 9–1D). These strips can be repeated, overlapping by ⅓ of the tape width to provide additional support.

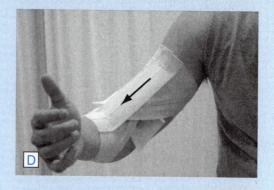

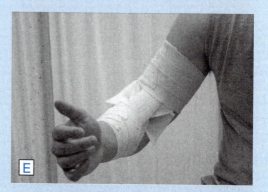

STEP 5: At the proximal upper arm and mid forearm, apply three to four circular closure patterns with 2 inch or 3 inch heavyweight elastic tape, overlapping each by ½ of the tape width with mild tension ◀▶ (Fig. 9–1E). The closure patterns should not enclose or cause constriction of the cubital fossa ∫. Non-elastic tape anchors are not necessary.

Option: *Apply a 4 inch or 6 inch width by 5 yard length elastic wrap in a circular pattern with moderate roll tension in a proximal-to-distal direction over the technique to lessen migration and unraveling of the tape ◀▶. Anchor with 2 inch or 3 inch elastic tape in a circular pattern with mild roll tension. Finish the anchor on the mid anterolateral forearm to prevent irritation from the tape ◀▶ (Fig. 9–1F).*

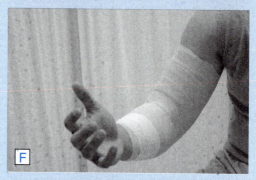

Figure 9-1 *continued*

 Helpful Hint: Improper application of elbow and/or forearm taping, wrapping, bracing, and/or padding techniques can compress soft tissues and the radial, median, and ulnar nerves as they superficially cross the elbow. This will affect the sensory distribution of the nerves. If numbness occurs in the hand, fingers, and/or thumb following application, immediately remove the technique and monitor the condition.

Hyperextension Technique Two

▶ **Materials:**
- Pre-tape material, thin foam pads, 2 inch or 3 inch heavyweight elastic tape, adherent tape spray, skin lubricant, taping scissors

Option:
- 4 inch or 6 inch width by 5 yard length elastic wrap

▶ **Position of the individual:** Sitting on a taping table or bench or standing with the involved arm at the side of the body. Determine the range of extension that produces pain. Once determined, place the involved elbow in a pain-free range and maintain this position during application. Maintain a moderate isometric contraction of the upper arm and forearm musculature.

▶ **Preparation:** Shave the arm from the proximal upper arm to mid forearm. Apply the technique directly to the skin or over one layer of pre-tape material. Place thin foam pads over the cubital fossa to prevent irritation. A skin lubricant may also be used. Apply adherent tape spray from the proximal upper arm to the mid forearm.

▶ **Application:**

STEP 1: Apply anchors as illustrated in Figure 9–1A.

STEP 2: Anchor a strip of 2 inch or 3 inch heavyweight elastic tape on the medial anterior proximal upper arm, continue across the cubital fossa, and anchor on the medial anterior mid forearm (Fig. 9–2A). Apply the strip with a moderate amount of roll tension. Monitor the pain-free position of the elbow.

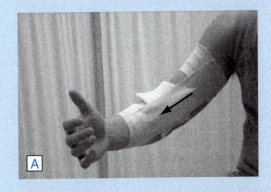

STEP 3: Place the next strip of 2 inch or 3 inch heavyweight elastic tape on the anterior proximal upper arm, overlapping the first by ½ of the tape width, across the cubital fossa, and anchor on the anterior mid forearm (Fig. 9–2B).

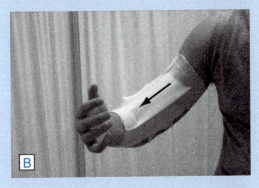

STEP 4: Apply a strip, overlapping the second strip by ½ of its width, from the lateral anterior proximal upper arm, continue across the cubital fossa, and anchor on the lateral anterior mid forearm (Fig. 9–2C).

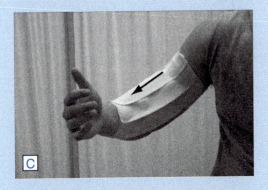

STEP 5: Apply three to four circular closure patterns with mild tension around the proximal upper arm and mid forearm with 2 inch or 3 inch heavyweight elastic tape 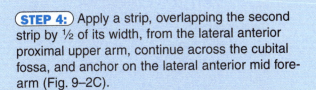 (Fig. 9–2D). Anchors of non-elastic tape are not required. Monitor the cubital fossa for constriction.

Options: *Consider applying a 4 inch or 6 inch width by 5 yard length elastic wrap with moderate roll tension in a circular pattern in a proximal-to-distal direction over the technique to prevent migration and unraveling of the tape. Anchor with elastic tape and finish on the mid anterolateral forearm* 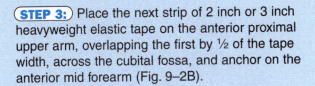 *.*

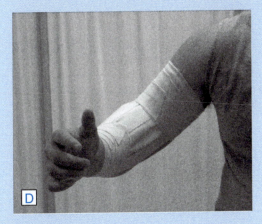

Figure 9-2

Hyperextension Technique Three

▶ **Materials:**
- Pre-tape material, thin foam pads, 4 inch or 6 inch width heavy resistance exercise band, 2 inch or 3 inch heavyweight elastic tape, adherent tape spray, skin lubricant, taping scissors

Option:
- 4 inch or 6 inch width by 5 yard length elastic wrap

▶ **Position of the individual:** Sitting on a taping table or bench or standing with the involved arm at the side of the body. Determine the range of extension that produces pain. Once determined, place the involved elbow in a pain-free range and maintain this position during application. Maintain a moderate isometric contraction of the upper arm and forearm musculature.

▶ **Preparation:** Shave the arm from the proximal upper arm to mid forearm. Apply this technique directly to the skin or over one layer of pre-tape material. Place thin foam pads over the cubital fossa to prevent irritation. A skin lubricant may also be used. Apply adherent tape spray from the proximal upper arm to the mid forearm.

▶ **Application:**

STEP 1: Apply anchors as illustrated in Figure 9–1A.

STEP 2: Place a piece of 4 inch or 6 inch width heavy resistance exercise band over the anterior proximal upper arm and anchor with 2 inch or 3 inch heavyweight elastic tape with a mild amount of roll tension in a circular pattern, leaving approximately 2–3 inches of the band extending proximally beyond the anchor ◀▬▶ (Fig. 9–3A).

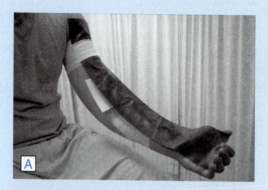

STEP 3: Pull the band distally with moderate tension across the cubital fossa and anchor on the anterior mid forearm with 2 inch or 3 inch heavyweight elastic tape with mild roll tension ◀▬▶ (Fig. 9–3B). Monitor the pain-free position of the elbow. Cut the band approximately 2–3 inches below the anchor. A second piece of elastic exercise band may be applied directly over the first for additional support.

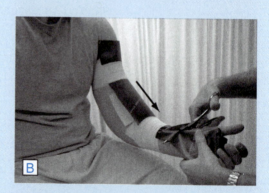

STEP 4: At the upper arm, fold the excess of the band over the tape anchor and apply three to four circular closure patterns with mild roll tension with 2 inch or 3 inch heavyweight elastic tape, covering the band ◀▬▶ (Fig. 9–3C).

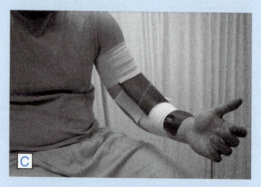

Figure 9-3

STEP 5: Fold the excess band over onto the forearm anchor and apply three to four circular closure patterns with 2 inch or 3 inch heavyweight elastic tape with mild roll tension, also covering the band (Fig. 9–3D). Monitor the cubital fossa. Anchors of non-elastic tape are not required.

Option: *Apply a 4 inch or 6 inch width by 5 yard length elastic wrap in a circular pattern over the technique in a proximal-to-distal direction with moderate roll tension to lessen migration and unraveling of the tape* ◀━━ . *Anchor with elastic tape and end on the mid anterolateral forearm* ◀━━ .

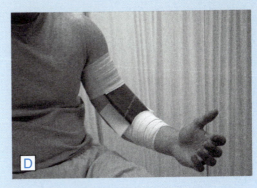

Figure 9-3 *continued*

Critical Thinking Question 1

A high school wrestler suffered a hyperextension injury to his right elbow several weeks ago. He has completed rehabilitation and returned to practice with a hyperextension taping technique on the elbow to prevent further injury. After 45 minutes of practice, the "X" and longitudinal elastic tape strips that cross the cubital fossa begin to tear from the edges, decreasing the effectiveness of the technique.

▶ **Question: What options are available in this situation?**

COLLATERAL "X" Figure 9–4

▶ **Purpose:** The collateral "X" technique is used when treating radial collateral ligament sprains to provide support and protection against mild to moderate varus forces at the elbow (Fig. 9–4).

▶ **Materials:**
  • Pre-tape material, 2 inch or 3 inch heavyweight elastic tape, adherent tape spray, taping scissors

  Option:
  • 4 inch or 6 inch width by 5 yard length elastic wrap

▶ **Position of the individual:** Sitting on a taping table or bench or standing with the involved arm at the side of the body and the involved elbow placed in slight flexion. Maintain a moderate isometric contraction of the upper arm and forearm musculature.

▶ **Preparation:** Shave the arm from the proximal upper arm to mid forearm. Apply the technique directly to the skin or over one layer of pre-tape material. Apply adherent tape spray from the proximal upper arm to the mid forearm.

▶ **Application:**
  STEP 1: Apply an anchor of 2 inch or 3 inch heavyweight elastic tape around the proximal upper arm and mid forearm with mild tension ◀━━ (Fig. 9–4A).

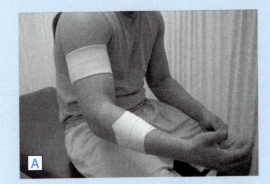

Figure 9-4

STEP 2: Anchor the first strip of 2 inch or 3 inch heavyweight elastic tape on the lateral proximal upper arm. Continue distally over the elbow joint with moderate roll tension, and anchor on the posterior mid forearm (Fig. 9–4B).

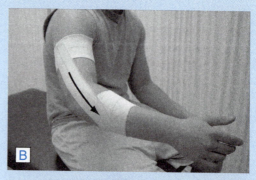

STEP 3: Anchor the second strip on the posterior proximal upper arm, proceed distally across the joint with moderate roll tension, and finish on the anterior mid forearm, forming an "X" over the radial collateral ligament (Fig. 9–4C).

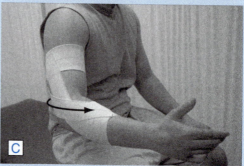

STEP 4: Begin the third strip on the lateral proximal upper arm, continue over the joint with moderate roll tension, and anchor on the lateral mid forearm (Fig. 9–4D).

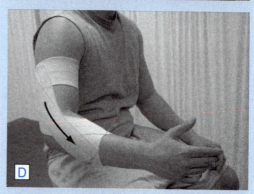

STEP 5: Repeat the strips, overlapping the tape by ⅓ of its width (Fig. 9–4E).

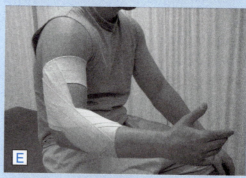

STEP 6: At the proximal upper arm and mid forearm, apply three to four circular closure patterns with 2 inch or 3 inch heavyweight elastic tape, overlapping by ½ of the tape width with mild tension ◄ (Fig. 9–4F). The closure patterns should not enclose or cause constriction of the cubital fossa. Anchors of non-elastic tape are not required.

Option: *Apply a 4 inch or 6 inch width by 5 yard length elastic wrap in a proximal-to-distal direction with moderate roll tension in a circular pattern over the technique to lessen migration and unraveling of the tape ◄. Anchor with elastic tape and finish on the mid anterolateral forearm ◄.*

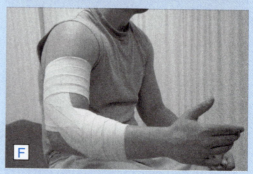

Figure 9-4 *continued*

LATERAL EPICONDYLITIS STRAP   Figures 9–5, 9–6

▶ **Purpose:** The strap technique is used when treating lateral epicondylitis to reduce the tension or pull of the wrist extensor musculature at its origin on the lateral epicondyle of the humerus. These straps can be made from taping materials or purchased off-the-shelf. The off-the-shelf designs are illustrated in the Bracing section. Two interchangeable methods are illustrated in the application of the technique; the different methods accommodate individual preferences and available supplies.

Lateral Epicondylitis Strap Technique One

▶ **Materials:**
  • Pre-tape material or self-adherent wrap, 1 inch or 2 inch heavyweight elastic tape, taping scissors

▶ **Position of the individual:** Sitting on a taping table or bench or standing with the involved arm at the side of the body, the involved elbow placed in slight flexion, and the forearm in a neutral position.

▶ **Preparation:** Apply the technique directly to the skin or over pre-tape material or self-adherent wrap.

▶ **Application:**
  STEP 1: Anchor 1 inch or 2 inch heavyweight elastic tape on the lateral forearm approximately ¾ of an inch distal from the lateral epicondyle of the humerus (Fig. 9–5A). Continue around the forearm in a circular, lateral-to-medial pattern and return to the anchor position (Fig. 9–5B).

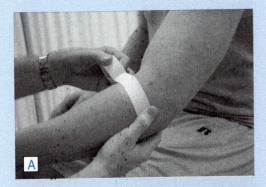

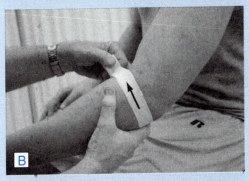

  STEP 2: Without overlapping, continue to apply the tape around the forearm with three to four continuous circular patterns and finish on the lateral forearm (Fig. 9–5C) ✂. Additional non-elastic tape strips are not necessary.

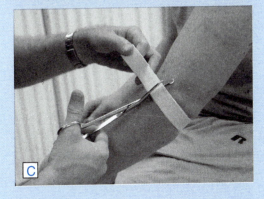

Figure 9-5

 Helpful Hint: The roll tension of the elastic tape to achieve proper tension and relief of pain will vary among individuals. Check the tension of the tape by allowing the individual to perform a previously painful activity. Readjust the tension of the tape if necessary.

RESEARCH BRIEF

The exact positioning of a taping material strap or off-the-shelf brace on the proximal forearm is critical, but not adequately addressed in the literature.[11]

Several studies suggest a position ¾ of an inch distal to the lateral epicondyle of the humerus.[19,21]

Lateral Epicondylitis Strap Technique Two

▶ **Materials:**
- Pre-tape material or self-adherent wrap, 1 inch non-elastic tape

▶ **Position of the individual:** Sitting on a taping table or bench or standing with the involved arm at the side of the body, the involved elbow placed in slight flexion, and the forearm in a neutral position.

▶ **Preparation:** Apply the technique directly to the skin or over pre-tape material or self-adherent wrap.

▶ **Application:**

STEP 1: Place 1 inch non-elastic tape on the lateral forearm approximately ¾ of an inch distal from the lateral epicondyle of the humerus and continue around the forearm in a circular, lateral-to-medial pattern, returning to the anchor position (Fig. 9–6A). Roll tension will vary among individuals.

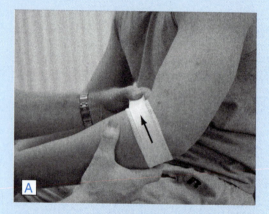

STEP 2: Continue with three to four continuous circular patterns around the forearm, without overlapping, and anchor on the lateral forearm (Fig. 9–6B). Additional anchors are not necessary. Readjust the tension of the tape if necessary.

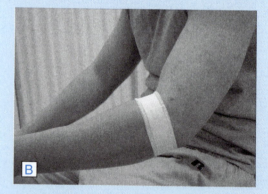

Figure 9-6

FIGURE-OF-EIGHT ELBOW TAPE Figure 9–7

▶ **Purpose:** Use the figure-of-eight elbow technique to provide mild support and anchor protective padding (Fig. 9–7). Use the technique with off-the-shelf and custom-made padding to absorb shock when preventing or treating elbow contusions and olecranon bursitis. Protective padding techniques are illustrated in the Padding section.

▶ **Materials:**
- Pre-tape material or self-adherent wrap, 2 inch or 3 inch elastic tape, adherent tape spray, taping scissors

Option:
- 1½ inch non-elastic tape

• **Position of the individual:** Sitting on a taping table or bench or standing with the involved arm at the side of the body and the involved elbow placed in slight flexion. Maintain a moderate isometric contraction of the upper arm and forearm musculature.

• **Preparation:** Apply the technique directly to the skin or over pre-tape material or self-adherent wrap. Apply adherent tape spray to the distal upper arm and proximal forearm.

• **Application:**

STEP 1: Anchor 2 inch or 3 inch elastic tape to the proximal lateral forearm, continue around in a lateral-to-medial pattern with mild to moderate roll tension, and encircle the anchor (Fig. 9–7A). Place the pad over the injured area.

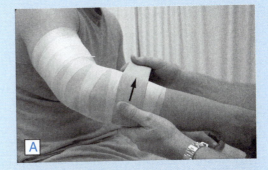

STEP 2: Continue around to the medial forearm, then pull the tape proximally, with moderate roll tension, across the pad, to the distal lateral upper arm (Fig. 9–7B).

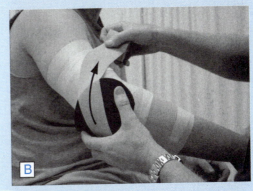

STEP 3: Encircle the distal upper arm in a lateral-to-medial pattern with mild to moderate roll tension (Fig. 9–7C).

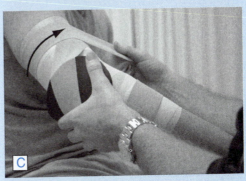

STEP 4: Continue around to the medial distal upper arm, then pull the tape distally, with moderate roll tension, across the pad to the lateral forearm (Fig. 9–7D). The tape should form an "X" over the pad and posterior elbow.

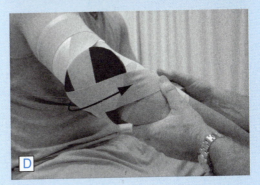

Figure 9-7

STEP 5: Repeat the figure-of-eight pattern, overlapping by 1/3–1/2 of the tape width (Fig. 9–7E). Finish and anchor on the tape pattern on the proximal anterior forearm. The pattern should not enclose or cause constriction of the cubital fossa.

Option: Apply one to two circular strips of 1½ inch non-elastic tape loosely around the proximal forearm for additional anchors 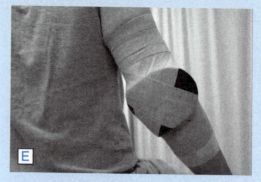.

Figure 9-7 *continued*

CIRCULAR FOREARM Figure 9–8

▶ **Purpose:** The circular forearm technique provides mild support and anchors off-the-shelf and custom-made pads to absorb shock when preventing and treating forearm contusions (Fig. 9–8).

▶ **Materials:**
- Pre-tape material or self-adherent wrap, 2 inch or 3 inch elastic tape, adherent tape spray, taping scissors

Option:
- 1½ inch non-elastic tape

▶ **Position of the individual:** Sitting on a taping table or bench or standing with the involved arm at the side of the body and the involved elbow placed in slight flexion. Maintain a moderate isometric contraction of the forearm musculature.

▶ **Preparation:** Apply adherent tape spray to the forearm.

▶ **Application:**

STEP 1: Apply pre-tape material or self-adherent wrap in a circular pattern around the forearm.

STEP 2: Place the pad over the injured area. Anchor 2 inch or 3 inch elastic tape directly to the distal lateral pad and encircle the anchor (Fig. 9–8A).

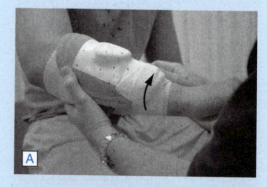

STEP 3: Continue to apply the tape in a circular, lateral-to-medial direction around the forearm with moderate roll tension, overlapping the tape by ½ of its width (Fig. 9–8B). Apply the tape in a distal-to-proximal pattern and cover the entire pad.

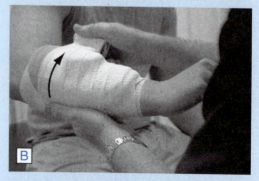

Figure 9-8

STEP 4: Anchor the tape on top of the pad on the circular pattern (Fig. 9–8C). Avoid gaps, wrinkles, or inconsistent roll tension. To lessen migration of the pad, apply the proximal circular tape strips to the skin.

Option: *Loosely apply one to two circular anchors of 1½ inch non-elastic tape around the pad, ending on top of the pad* ◀▬▶ *(Fig. 9–8D).*

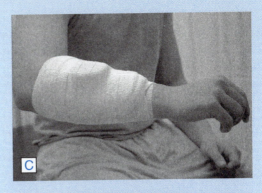

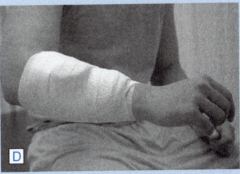

Figure 9-8 *continued*

SPIRAL FOREARM   Figure 9–9

▸ **Purpose:** Use the spiral forearm technique to provide mild to moderate compression when treating forearm splints (Fig. 9–9). Anecdotally, compression over inflamed areas may lessen pain levels. However, with some individuals, this technique may increase pain. Following application, monitor for an increase in pain levels during activity.

▸ **Materials:**
  • 2 inch or 3 inch elastic tape, adherent tape spray, taping scissors
  Option:
  • 2 inch, 3 inch, or 4 inch width by 5 yard length elastic wrap

▸ **Position of the individual:** Sitting on a taping table or bench or standing with the involved arm at the side of the body, the involved elbow placed in slight flexion, and the forearm in a neutral position with a moderate isometric contraction.

▸ **Preparation:** Shave the forearm and apply adherent tape spray to the forearm. Apply the technique directly to the skin.

▸ **Application:**
  STEP 1: Anchor the 2 inch or 3 inch elastic tape on the distal lateral forearm and proceed around to encircle the anchor in a lateral-to-medial pattern (Fig. 9–9A).

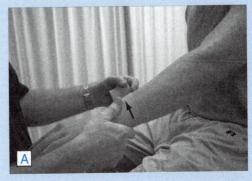

Figure 9-9

STEP 2: Continue to apply the 2 inch or 3 inch elastic tape in a distal-to-proximal spiral pattern with moderate roll tension (Fig. 9–9B). Overlap the tape by ½ of its width.

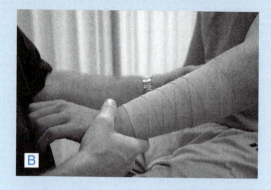

STEP 3: Anchor the tape on the pattern over the proximal anterior forearm (Fig. 9–9C). No additional anchors are needed. Avoid inconsistent roll tension or constriction of the cubital fossa.

Option: *Apply a 2 inch, 3 inch, or 4 inch width by 5 yard length elastic wrap in a circular pattern with moderate roll tension in a distal-to-proximal pattern over the technique to lessen migration and unraveling of the tape* ◄═►. *Anchor with elastic tape over the proximal anterior forearm* ◄═►.

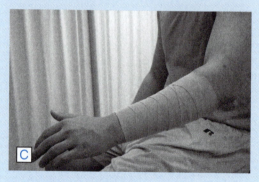

Figure 9-9 *continued*

ELASTIC MATERIAL Figure 9–10

▶ **Purpose:** Use elastic materials to cover the posterior elbow and ulnar side of the forearm when preventing and treating abrasions (Fig. 9–10).

▶ **Materials:**
• Adhesive gauze material (pre-cut strips or from roll), taping scissors
Option:
• Adherent tape spray

▶ **Position of the individual:** Sitting on a taping table or bench or standing with the involved arm at the side of the body and the involved elbow placed in flexion.

▶ **Preparation:** To make a strip, cut a piece of adhesive gauze material to cover the posterior elbow and/or ulnar side of the forearm. Apply adhesive gauze material directly to the skin or over a sterile wound dressing. Round all corners of the material to prevent the edges from rolling upon contact with clothing and surfaces.
Option: *Apply adherent tape spray over the area for additional adherence.*

▶ **Application:**
STEP 1: Remove the backing and place the piece of adhesive gauze material directly on the skin (Fig. 9–10A).

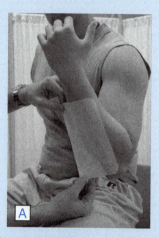

Figure 9-10

STEP 2: Smooth the material to the elbow and/or forearm (Fig. 9–10B). No additional anchors are required.

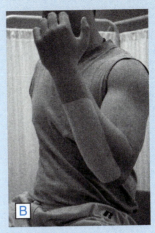

B

Figure 9-10 *continued*

POSTERIOR SPLINT Figure 9–11

▶ **Purpose:** The posterior splint technique is used to immobilize the elbow when treating dislocations, following a reduction and postoperative procedures (Fig. 9–11). This technique is identical to the posterior splint illustrated in Chapter 4 (see Fig. 4–9), with regard to the materials used. Two interchangeable methods are illustrated for the application of the technique to accommodate available supplies.

○ **DETAILS**

Periods of immobilization are normally determined by a physician following evaluation of the individual. Complete immobilization can be provided by cast technicians and physicians using rigid cast tape applied over stockinet.

▶ **Design:**
  • Off-the-shelf rigid splints are available in pre-cut and padded designs. The splints are constructed of several layers of rigid fiberglass material, covered with fabric and foam padding in 2, 3, 4, and 5 inch widths by 10, 12, 15, 30, 35, and 45 inch lengths.

Posterior Splint Technique One

▶ **Materials:**
  • Off-the-shelf rigid, padded splint, water, towel, two 4 inch width by 10 yard length elastic wraps, metal clips, 1½ inch non-elastic tape

▶ **Position of the individual:** Sitting on a taping table or bench with the involved arm at the side of the body and the forearm in a neutral position or prone on a taping table or bench with the involved arm extended off the edge and the forearm in a neutral position. Place the elbow in the desired range of flexion as indicated by a physician. Maintain this position during application.

▶ **Preparation:** Mold and apply the padded splint directly to the skin.

▶ **Application:**
  STEP 1: Remove the splint from the package and immerse in water of 70° to 75° F to begin the chemical reaction. Remove the splint and place lengthwise on a towel.

STEP 2: Quickly roll the splint and towel together to remove excess water (Fig. 9–11A).

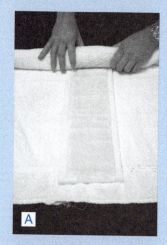

A

STEP 3: Apply the splint from the proximal posterior upper arm to the wrist (Fig. 9–11B).

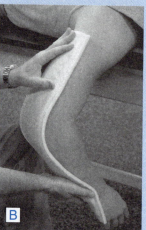

B

STEP 4: Mold the splint to the body contours with the application of a 4 inch width by 10 yard length elastic wrap in a spiral pattern with moderate roll tension ◄► (Fig. 9–11C). Continue to mold and shape the splint with the hands. Monitor the position of elbow flexion. After 10–15 minutes, the fiberglass should be cured; remove the elastic wrap.

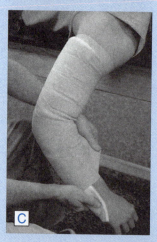

C

STEP 5: Using another 4 inch width by 10 yard length elastic wrap, attach the splint to the upper arm, elbow, forearm, and wrist in a spiral, distal-to-proximal pattern with moderate roll tension ◄► (Fig. 9–11D). Anchor the wrap with metal clips or loosely applied 1½ inch non-elastic tape. The individual may need a sling for daily activities.

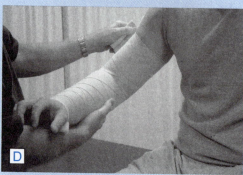

D

Figure 9-11

Posterior Splint Technique Two

▶ **Materials:**
  • 3 inch, 4 inch, or 5 inch width rigid cast tape, stockinet, gloves, 4 inch width by 10 yard length elastic wrap, metal clips, 1½ inch non-elastic tape, taping scissors

▶ **Position of the individual:** Prone on a taping table or bench with the involved arm extended off the edge with the forearm in a neutral position or sitting on a taping table or bench with the involved arm at the side of the body and the forearm in a neutral position. Place the elbow in the desired range of elbow flexion as indicated by a physician. Maintain this position during application.

▶ **Preparation:** Apply one layer of stockinet from the proximal upper arm to the wrist.

▶ **Application:**
  STEP 1: Remove the cast tape from the pouch and immerse in water of 70° to 75° F. Apply the tape on the proximal posterior upper arm, continue distally over the elbow and forearm, and finish at the wrist (Fig. 9–11E).

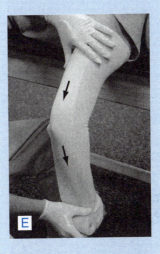

  STEP 2: At the wrist, reverse the tape and continue over the previous strip toward the proximal upper arm (Fig. 9–11F). Continue with this sequence until four to five layers have been applied. Use additional rolls of cast tape if needed. Mold the tape with gloved hands. Monitor the position of elbow flexion. Curing should be complete in 10–15 minutes.

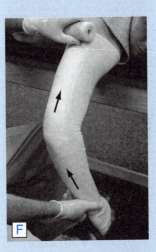

  STEP 3: Cut the stockinet lengthwise down the anterior wrist, forearm, elbow, and upper arm, and fold the stockinet over the splint to protect against skin irritation (Fig. 9–11G).

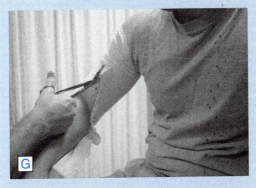

Figure 9-11 *continued*

STEP 4: Attach the splint with a 4 inch width by 10 yard length elastic wrap in a spiral, distal-to-proximal pattern with moderate roll tension ◀▬▶ (Fig. 9–11H). Anchor the wrap with metal clips or loosely applied 1½ inch non-elastic tape. A sling may be required for daily activities.

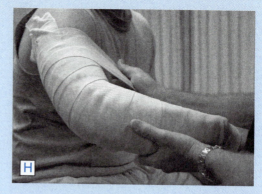

Figure 9-11 *continued*

Wrapping Techniques

Use wrapping techniques to provide compression and support and to anchor protective padding to the elbow and forearm when preventing and treating contusions, sprains, strains, ruptures, dislocations, and olecranon bursitis. There are five compression wrapping techniques that provide mechanical pressure over the upper arm, elbow, forearm, and hand following injury. Choose a technique based on the amount of swelling and effusion present.

COMPRESSION WRAP TECHNIQUE ONE Figure 9–12

▶ **Purpose:** Apply compression wrap technique one when treating contusions, sprains, strains, ruptures, dislocations, and olecranon bursitis of the elbow to control mild to moderate swelling and effusion (Fig. 9–12).

▶ **Materials:**
- 4 inch or 6 inch width by 5 yard length elastic wrap, metal clips, 1½ inch non-elastic or 2 inch or 3 inch elastic tape, taping scissors

Options:
- ¼ inch or ½ inch foam or felt
- 3 inch or 4 inch width self-adherent wrap
- ¼ inch or ½ inch open-cell foam

▶ **Position of the individual:** Sitting on a taping table or bench or standing with the involved arm at the side of the body and the involved elbow placed in a pain-free, flexed position.

▶ **Preparation:** To lessen migration, apply adherent tape spray, tape strips, or anchors directly to the skin (see Fig. 1–7).

Option: *Cut a ¼ inch or ½ inch foam or felt pad and place it over the inflamed area directly to the skin to assist in venous return.*

▶ **Application:**

STEP 1: Apply the extended end of the wrap around the mid forearm directly to the skin and encircle the anchor ◀▬▶ (Fig. 9–12A).

Option: *Three inch or 4 inch self-adherent wrap may be used when an elastic wrap is not available.*

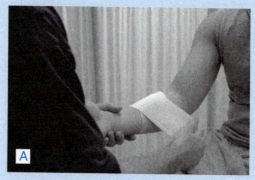

Figure 9-12

STEP 2: Continue to apply the wrap in a spiral pattern, moving in a distal-to-proximal direction, and overlapping the wrap by ½ of its width (Fig. 9–12B). Apply the greatest amount of roll tension distally and over the inflamed area and lessen roll tension as the wrap continues proximally.

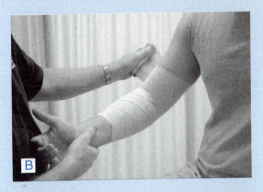

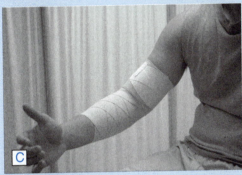

STEP 3: Finish the spiral pattern over the mid upper arm and anchor with Velcro, metal clips, or loosely applied 1½ inch non-elastic or 2 inch or 3 inch elastic tape ◀▬▶ (Fig. 9–12C). Finish the tape on the anterolateral upper arm to prevent irritation.

Option: A ¼ inch or ½ inch open-cell foam pad may be placed over the posterior elbow, extending from the lateral humeral epicondyle to the medial humeral epicondyle, for additional compression around the olecranon process (see Fig. 9–28A). The pad is particularly useful when treating olecranon bursitis. Apply the pad directly on the skin and cover with the compression wrap (Fig. 9–12D).

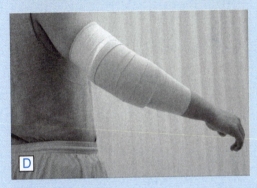

Figure 9-12 *continued*

COMPRESSION WRAP TECHNIQUE TWO Figure 9–13

▸ **Purpose:** Use this compression wrap technique to control mild to moderate swelling when treating forearm contusions and strains (Fig. 9–13).

▸ **Materials:**
- 3 inch or 4 inch width by 5 yard length elastic wrap, metal clips, 1½ inch non-elastic or 2 inch or 3 inch elastic tape, taping scissors

Options:
- ¼ inch or ½ inch foam or felt
- 3 inch or 4 inch width self-adherent wrap

▸ **Position of the individual:** Sitting on a taping table or bench or standing with the involved arm at the side of the body and the involved elbow placed in a pain-free, flexed position.

▸ **Preparation:** To lessen migration, apply adherent tape spray, tape strips, or anchors directly to the skin.

Option: Cut a ¼ inch or ½ inch foam or felt pad and place it over the inflamed area directly to the skin to assist in controlling swelling.

▶ **Application:**

STEP 1: Anchor the extended end of the wrap around the wrist directly to the skin and encircle the anchor ◀ (Fig. 9–13A).

Option: *If an elastic wrap is not available, 3 inch or 4 inch self-adherent wrap may be used.*

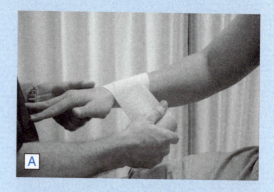

STEP 2: Using a spiral pattern, apply the wrap in a distal-to-proximal direction (Fig. 9–13B). Overlap the wrap by ½ of its width; apply the greatest amount of roll tension distally and over the inflamed area.

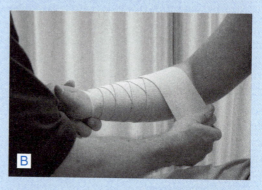

STEP 3: Finish the wrap at the proximal forearm (Fig. 9–13C).

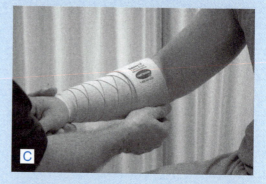

STEP 4: Anchor the wrap over the proximal forearm with Velcro, metal clips, or loosely applied 1½ inch non-elastic or 2 inch or 3 inch elastic tape, finishing on the anterolateral proximal forearm ◀ (Fig. 9–13D).

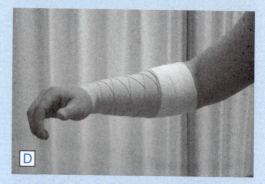

Figure 9-13

COMPRESSION WRAP TECHNIQUE THREE Figure 9–14

▶ **Purpose:** Use compression wrap technique three to control moderate to severe swelling when treating second and third degree forearm contusions and strains. The technique prevents distal migration of postinjury swelling (Fig. 9–14).

♦ **Materials:**
  • 3 inch or 4 inch width by 5 yard length elastic wrap, metal clips, 1½ inch non-elastic or 2 inch or 3 inch elastic tape, taping scissors

  Option:
  • ¼ inch or ½ inch foam or felt

♦ **Position of the individual:** Sitting on a taping table or bench or standing with the involved arm at the side of the body and the involved elbow placed in a pain-free, flexed position.

♦ **Preparation:** To lessen migration, apply adherent tape spray, tape strips, or anchors directly to the skin.

  Option: *Cut a ¼ inch or ½ inch foam or felt pad and place it over the inflamed area directly to the skin to assist in venous return.*

♦ **Application:**

  (STEP 1:) Anchor the wrap in a circular pattern on the dorsal surface of the hand just distal to the MCP joints of fingers two through five and apply the hand compression wrap technique (see Figs. 10–11 and 9–14A).

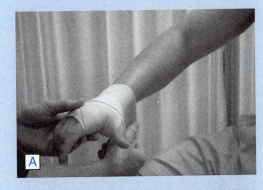

  (STEP 2:) At the wrist, finish the technique with compression wrap two (see Figs. 9–13 and 9–14B).

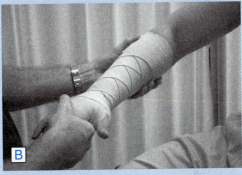

  (STEP 3:) Anchor over the proximal forearm with Velcro, metal clips, or loosely applied 1½ inch non-elastic or 2 inch or 3 inch elastic tape (Fig. 9–14C). End the tape on the anterolateral proximal forearm.

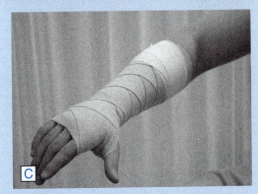

Figure 9-14

COMPRESSION WRAP TECHNIQUE FOUR Figure 9–15

♦ **Purpose:** Use this compression wrap technique when treating second and third degree elbow contusions, sprains, strains, ruptures, dislocations, and olecranon bursitis. The technique controls moderate to severe swelling and prevents distal migration of postinjury swelling (Fig. 9–15).

▶ **Materials:**
- 4 inch or 6 inch width by 10 yard length elastic wrap, metal clips, 1½ inch non-elastic or 2 inch or 3 inch elastic tape, taping scissors

Options:
- ¼ inch or ½ inch foam or felt
- ¼ inch or ½ inch open-cell foam

▶ **Position of the individual:** Sitting on a taping table or bench or standing with the involved arm at the side of the body and the involved elbow placed in a pain-free, flexed position.

▶ **Preparation:** To lessen migration, apply adherent tape spray, tape strips, or anchors directly to the skin.

Option: *Cut a ¼ inch or ½ inch foam or felt pad and place it over the inflamed area directly to the skin to assist in controlling swelling.*

▶ **Application:**

STEP 1: This wrap technique for the elbow and forearm is identical to the compression technique for the upper arm illustrated in Figure 8–4 (Fig. 9–15A). Apply the greatest amount of roll tension distally and lessen tension as the wrap continues proximally. This technique may be started with a circular pattern just distal to the MCP joints of the fingers; apply the hand compression wrap technique (Fig. 9–15B).

Option: *Consider using a ¼ inch or ½ inch open-cell foam pad over the posterior elbow for additional compression to assist in venous return.*

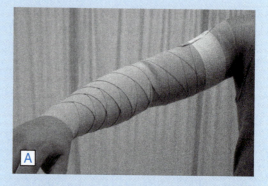

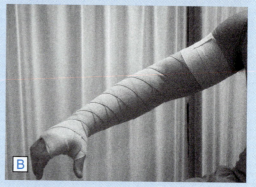

Figure 9-15

COMPRESSION WRAP TECHNIQUE FIVE Figure 9–16

▶ **Purpose:** Use an elastic sleeve to control mild to moderate swelling and effusion when treating elbow and forearm contusions, sprains, strains, ruptures, dislocations, and olecranon bursitis (Fig. 9–16). Following proper instruction, this compression wrap can be applied and removed by the individual without assistance.

▶ **Materials:**
- 3 inch or 5 inch width elastic sleeve determined by the size of the upper arm and forearm, taping scissors

Options:
- ¼ inch or ½ inch foam or felt
- ¼ inch or ½ inch open-cell foam

▶ **Position of the individual:** Sitting on a taping table or bench or standing with the involved arm at the side of the body and the involved elbow placed in a pain-free, flexed position.

▶ **Preparation:** Cut a sleeve from a roll to extend from the mid forearm to the mid upper arm, wrist to the proximal forearm, MCP joints of the hand to the proximal forearm, wrist to the proximal upper arm, or the MCP joints of the hand to the proximal upper arm. Cut and use a double length sleeve to provide additional compression.

Option: *Cut a ¼ inch or ½ inch foam or felt pad and place it over the inflamed area directly to the skin to assist in controlling swelling.*

▶ **Application:**

STEP 1: Apply the sleeve over the fingers and pull onto the forearm, elbow, and/or upper arm in a distal-to-proximal pattern (Fig. 9–16A). If using a technique that includes the hand, cut a small hole in the sleeve with taping scissors for the thumb (Fig. 9–16B). When using a double length sleeve, pull the distal end over the first layer to provide an additional layer. No anchors are required; the sleeve can be cleaned and reused.

Option: *A ¼ inch or ½ inch open-cell foam pad may be cut and placed over the posterior elbow for additional compression.*

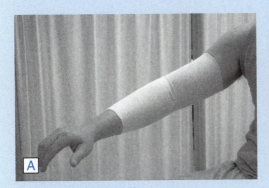 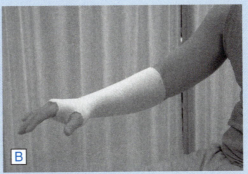

Figure 9-16

Critical Thinking Question 2

A sharpshooter on the SWAT team has been practicing for an upcoming national competition. One of the events requires him to be in a prone position on his elbows for extended periods of time. He begins to develop pain in the right posterior elbow and is evaluated by a physician. The sharpshooter is diagnosed with right elbow olecranon bursitis and allowed to continue practice if the condition does not worsen.

▶ **Question: What techniques can you use to treat the condition?**

CIRCULAR ELBOW WRAP Figure 9–17

▶ **Purpose:** Use the circular elbow technique to provide compression and mild support and to anchor off-the-shelf and custom-made pads that absorb shock when preventing and treating elbow contusions and olecranon bursitis (Fig. 9–17).

▶ **Materials:**
- 3 inch, 4 inch, or 6 inch width by 5 yard length elastic wrap, 2 inch or 3 inch elastic tape, taping scissors

Options:
- 3 inch or 4 inch width self-adherent wrap
- 1½ inch non-elastic tape

▶ **Position of the individual:** Sitting on a taping table or bench or standing with the involved arm at the side of the body and the involved elbow placed in slight flexion. Maintain a moderate isometric contraction of the upper arm and forearm musculature.

▶ **Preparation:** To lessen migration, apply adherent tape spray, tape strips, or anchors directly to the skin.

▶ **Application:**

STEP 1: Place the pad over the injured area. Anchor the extended end of the wrap directly to the skin below the distal pad and encircle the anchor ◀▬▶ (Fig. 9–17A).

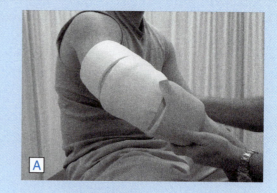

STEP 2: In a circular pattern with moderate roll tension, continue to apply the wrap in a distal-to-proximal pattern, overlapping the wrap by ½ of its width (Fig. 9–17B). Completely cover the pad with the wrap and finish on the upper arm. Avoid gaps, wrinkles, or inconsistent roll tension.

Option: Three inch or 4 inch width self-adherent wrap may be used if an elastic wrap is not available.

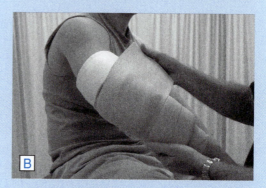

STEP 3: Anchor 2 inch or 3 inch elastic tape on the loose end of the wrap and apply two to three continuous circular patterns, with moderate roll tension, and finish on the tape pattern on the lateral upper arm to prevent irritation ◀▬▶ (Fig. 9–17C). For additional support and to lessen migration of the pad, anchor 2 inch or 3 inch elastic tape on the proximal lateral forearm and apply the figure-of-eight taping technique.

Option: Loosely apply one to two 1½ inch non-elastic tape circular strips over the elastic tape around the upper arm to anchor ◀▬▶. Finish the tape on the lateral upper arm.

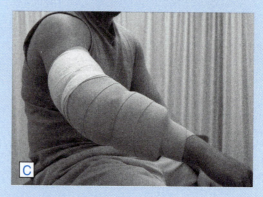

Figure 9-17

CIRCULAR FOREARM WRAP   Figure 9–18

▶ **Purpose:** The circular forearm technique provides compression and mild support and attaches off-the-shelf and custom-made pads to the forearm to absorb shock when treating contusions (Fig. 9–18).

▶ **Materials:**
- 3 inch or 4 inch width by 5 yard length elastic wrap, 2 inch or 3 inch elastic tape, taping scissors

Options:
- 3 inch or 4 inch width self-adherent wrap
- 1½ inch non-elastic tape

▶ **Position of the individual:** Sitting on a taping table or bench or standing with the involved arm at the side of the body and the involved elbow placed in flexion. Maintain a moderate isometric contraction of the fore-arm musculature.

▶ **Preparation:** To lessen migration, apply adherent tape spray, tape strips, or anchors directly to the skin.

♦ **Application:**

STEP 1: Apply the pad over the injured area. Anchor the wrap directly to the skin below the distal pad on the lateral forearm and encircle the anchor in a lateral-to-medial direction (Fig. 9–18A).

Option: *If an elastic wrap is not available, 3 inch or 4 inch width self-adherent wrap may be used.*

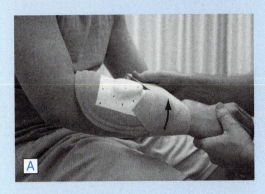

STEP 2: Continue the wrap in a circular, lateral-to-medial pattern, overlapping by ½ of the width with moderate roll tension, in a distal-to-proximal pattern (Fig. 9–18B). Cover the pad with the wrap and finish on the proximal forearm. Avoid gaps, wrinkles, or inconsistent roll tension.

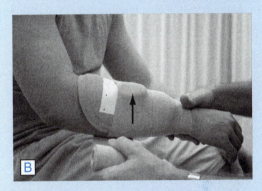

STEP 3: To anchor, apply 2 inch or 3 inch elastic tape on the proximal lateral pad and apply two to three lateral-to-medial continuous circular patterns, with moderate roll tension, finishing on the tape pattern on the proximal lateral forearm to prevent irritation (Fig. 9–18C).

Option: *Apply one to two 1½ inch non-elastic tape circular strips loosely over the elastic tape around the proximal forearm to anchor* 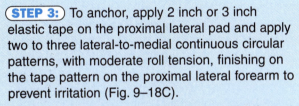 *. End the anchors on the lateral forearm.*

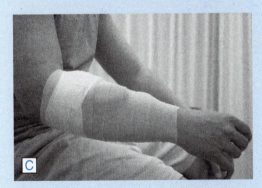

Figure 9-18

...IF/THEN...

IF a compression wrap is needed following an injury to the elbow, **THEN** carefully consider the injury and technique objective(s) prior to application. When treating severe swelling and effusion, using technique one may allow swelling/effusion to migrate distally into the hand, while technique four provides compression from the wrist or distal MCP joints to the proximal upper arm, lessening distal migration.

Bracing Techniques

Several bracing techniques for the elbow and forearm are available in off-the-shelf and custom-made designs. Some bracing techniques are used following sprains, dislocations, and postoperative procedures to provide immobilization, support, and compression, and to limit range of motion. Other bracing techniques can be used to provide compression and correct structural abnormalities when treating overuse injuries and conditions.

REHABILITATIVE Figure 9–19

- **Purpose:** Rehabilitative braces provide immobilization, mild to moderate support, and protected range of motion when treating elbow sprains, dislocations, and postoperative procedures (Fig. 9–19). These designs can replace a plaster or fiberglass cast or splint. The braces are removable, allowing for treatment and rehabilitation, and have adjustable range of motion to control and support early movement.

> **DETAILS**
>
> Consider using this design in combination with several compression wrapping techniques (see Figs. 9–12, 9–15, and 9–16).

- **Design:**
  - The braces are available in universal fit and right or left styles in predetermined sizes, corresponding to mid upper arm circumference measurements or length of the forearm.
  - Most designs are constructed of foam or polyethylene material in upper arm and forearm wraps or cuffs, with unilateral or bilateral aluminum bars.
  - In some designs, the bars are incorporated into plastic materials that are attached directly to the wraps or cuffs; other designs use Velcro straps to attach the bars.
  - The single polycentric hinge on most designs allows for control and locking of range of motion. Easy-to-use dials for quick range of motion settings are available with some designs.
  - Straps incorporated into the aluminum bars anchor the brace to the upper arm and forearm.
  - Some designs are available with a detachable sling.
  - Other designs have a bar incorporated into the distal end of the brace to provide support and immobilization of the wrist and hand.

- **Position of the individual:** Sitting on a taping table or bench with the involved elbow in a pain-free range of motion.

- **Preparation:** Set the brace range of motion at the desired settings of flexion and extension as indicated by a physician and/or therapeutic exercise program ✂. Apply the brace directly to the skin or over a tight-fitting shirt.

> **Helpful Hint:** Following application of the brace, check the actual range of flexion and extension with a goniometer to ensure the correct settings.

Specific instructions for applying the braces are included with each design. The following general application guidelines apply to most designs.

- **Application:**
  STEP 1: Begin application by loosening the straps and unfolding the brace.

STEP 2: Position the brace under the involved upper arm, elbow, and forearm. Align the hinge(s) with the joint line and the bar(s) along the medial and/or lateral upper arm and forearm (Fig. 9–19A). Reposition the wraps or cuffs if necessary. With some designs, position the hand on the attached distal bar.

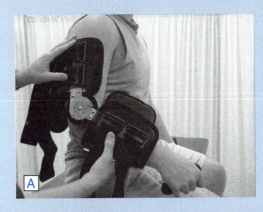

STEP 3: Anchor the wraps or cuffs around the upper arm and forearm. At the distal upper arm, pull the strap tight and anchor. Next, anchor the proximal forearm strap. Continue to anchor the remaining straps in this alternating pattern (Fig. 9–19B).

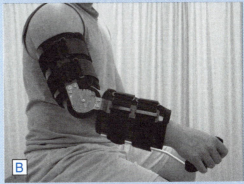

STEP 4: When using sling designs, apply the strap located at the posterior elbow or anterior upper arm upward over the opposite shoulder and neck, then down across the chest to the distal brace or wrist, and anchor (Fig. 9–19C).

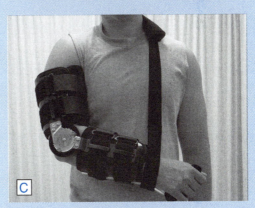

Figure 9-19

FUNCTIONAL Figure 9–20

▸ **Purpose:** Functional braces are designed to provide moderate stability to the elbow when treating sprains, dislocations, and postoperative procedures (Fig. 9–20). The designs are commonly used following injury to the ulnar collateral, radial collateral, or annular ligaments to control valgus, varus, rotary, and hyperextension stresses.

DETAILS

Functional braces are commonly used to provide elbow stability for athletes in sports such as field hockey, football, ice hockey, lacrosse, and wrestling, but can also be useful with work and casual activities. The nonpliable materials of the brace must be padded to meet NCAA[12] and NFHS[13] rules.

▶ **Design:**

- These braces are available in off-the-shelf and custom-made designs in universal and right or left styles.
- Off-the-shelf designs are constructed in predetermined sizes corresponding to mid upper arm circumference measurements. Small size adjustments may be made during wear.
- Some designs consist of a one-piece neoprene sleeve with medial and lateral hinged aluminum bars. Proximal and distal pockets or pouches anchor the bars to the sleeve. Nylon straps with Velcro closures provide additional support to the bars and anchor the brace.
- Many of the sleeve designs are available with an adjustable upper arm portion, an open cubital fossa cut-out, and epicondyle pads located under the hinge(s).
- Other designs consist of an upper arm and forearm cuff with lateral hinged aluminum bars. Nylon straps are used to anchor the cuffs.
- Most off-the-shelf designs have polycentric hinges that allow for range of motion control. A hyperextension block is also available.
- Some designs use additional straps to prevent hyperextension.
- Many off-the-shelf braces are available with posterior elbow padding for additional protection.
- Custom-made designs are manufactured for a specific individual following casting of the upper arm, elbow, and forearm by a manufacturer's representative or orthopedic technician. Following brace construction, adjustments in size are limited.
- These braces are similar to custom-made functional knee designs (see Fig. 6–14) and consist of a frame or shell, epicondyle pads, liners, and straps.
- The frames are manufactured of carbon composite and carbon/graphite laminate materials with monocentric or polycentric hinges that allow for control over range of motion. Most designs contain a hyperextension block.
- Epicondyle pads and liners are constructed of suede or chamois. Some designs have pneumatic pads to enhance fit and comfort. Nylon straps with Velcro closures anchor the brace.

▶ **Position of the individual:** Sitting on a taping table or bench or standing with the involved arm at the side of the body and the involved elbow placed in slight flexion.

▶ **Preparation:** Set the brace range of motion at the desired settings of flexion and extension. Apply functional braces directly to the skin. Loosen all straps.

Instructions for application of functional braces are included with each design. For proper application and use, follow the step-by-step procedure. The following general application guidelines apply to most functional designs.

▶ **Application:**

<u>STEP 1:</u> Apply many sleeve designs by placing the larger end over the fingers and hand. Pull the sleeve in a proximal direction until the hinges are centered over the joint line (Fig. 9–20A). When using upper arm wrap designs, encircle the upper arm and anchor this portion with Velcro.

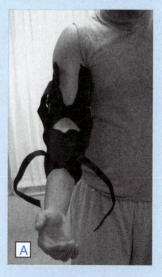

Figure 9-20

STEP 2: The application of straps will depend on the specific sleeve design. Apply most straps by pulling the straps tight and anchoring with Velcro (Fig. 9–20B).

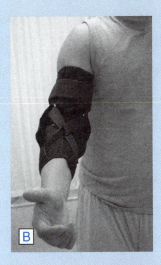

B

STEP 3: Apply other off-the-shelf designs by positioning the cuffs on the upper arm and forearm. Center the hinges over the joint line (Fig. 9–20C).

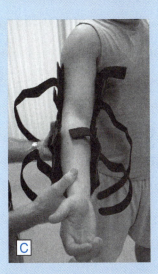

C

STEP 4: Anchor the cuffs and pull the upper arm and forearm straps tight and anchor with Velcro (Fig. 9–20D).

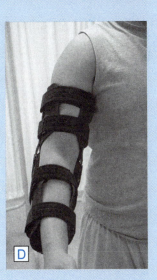

D

Figure 9-20 *continued*

STEP 5: Begin application of custom-made designs by pulling the brace onto the upper arm, elbow, and forearm in a distal-to-proximal direction (Fig. 9–20E). Position the hinges approximately ½ inch superior to the joint line.

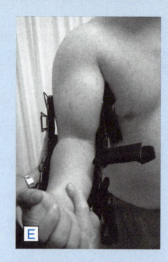

STEP 6: The application of straps will depend on the specific brace design. When using some designs, anchor the proximal, anterior upper arm strap (Fig. 9–20F), then the distal, anterior forearm strap (Fig. 9–20G).

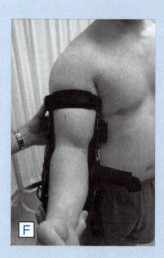

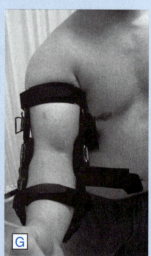

STEP 7: Next, anchor the posterior upper arm strap (Fig. 9–20H). Continue and anchor the posterior forearm strap (Fig. 9–20I).

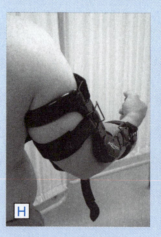

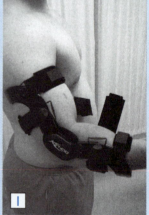

Figure 9-20 *continued*

STEP 8: Anchor the distal, anterior upper arm strap (Fig. 9–20J). Last, anchor the proximal, anterior forearm strap (Fig. 9–20K).

STEP 9: Allow the individual to actively flex and extend the elbow to ensure proper fit. Retighten the straps and/or reposition the brace if necessary.

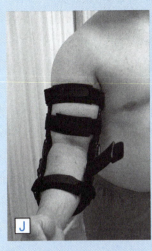
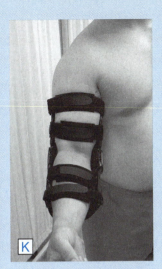

Figure 9-20 *continued*

NEOPRENE SLEEVE WITH HINGED BARS Figures 9–21, 9–22

▸ **Purpose:** Neoprene sleeves with hinged bars designed for the knee (see Fig. 6–17) may be used to provide compression and mild to moderate support when treating elbow sprains, dislocations, and postoperative procedures. Use this technique when off-the-shelf elbow brace designs are not available or resources do not permit the purchase of these designs. Two methods are illustrated for the application of the technique to accommodate individual preferences and available supplies.

○ **DETAILS**

Use the braces during rehabilitative, athletic, work, and casual activities. Apply padding to all nonpliable materials, commonly the hinges, to meet NCAA and NFHS rules.

Neoprene Sleeve with Hinged Bars Technique One

▸ **Materials:**
  • Off-the-shelf neoprene sleeve with hinged bars

  Options:
  • 2 inch or 3 inch elastic tape or self-adherent wrap, taping scissors

▸ **Position of the individual:** Sitting on a taping table or bench or standing with the involved arm at the side of the body and the involved elbow placed in slight flexion.

▸ **Preparation:** Set the brace range of motion at the desired settings of flexion and extension. Apply neoprene sleeves with hinged bars directly to the skin. Loosen the straps.

▶ **Application:**

STEP 1: Apply the larger end of the brace over the fingers and hand. Continue to pull in a proximal direction over the elbow. Position the hinges over the joint line and the patellar cut-out over the olecranon (Fig. 9–21A) ✂.

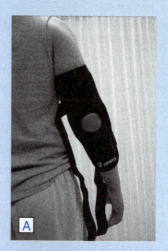

STEP 2: Tighten the straps and anchor with Velcro (Fig. 9–21B).

Option: *Apply additional anchors with 2 inch or 3 inch elastic tape or self-adherent wrap in a circular pattern with moderate roll tension around the upper arm and forearm* ◀━ *(Fig. 9–21C).*

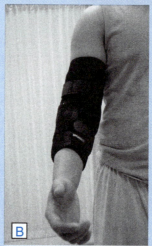
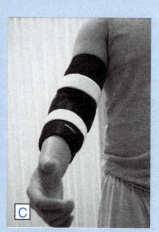

Figure 9-21

Helpful Hint: Neoprene sleeves with hinged bar braces for the knee are manufactured in predetermined sizes corresponding to thigh and knee circumference measurements. Because of the difference in girth measurements with the upper arm and forearm, off-the-shelf knee braces in sizes of XS, S, and M are typically required for use on the elbow.

Neoprene Sleeve with Hinged Bars Technique Two

▶ **Materials:**
- Off-the-shelf neoprene sleeve with hinged bars, 2 inch or 3 inch heavyweight elastic tape, ¼ inch or ½ inch foam, adherent tape spray, taping scissors

Options:
- Pre-tape material, self-adherent wrap, or neoprene elbow sleeve
- 1½ inch non-elastic tape

▶ **Position of the individual:** Sitting on a taping table or bench or standing with the involved arm at the side of the body and the involved elbow placed in flexion. Maintain a moderate isometric contraction of the upper arm and forearm musculature.

▶ **Preparation:** Remove the medial hinged aluminum bar from the brace pockets or pouches of a right knee brace for use on the right lateral elbow and the lateral bar for use on the left lateral elbow. Set the brace range of motion at the desired settings of flexion and extension. Apply adherent tape spray on the upper arm and forearm. Apply the aluminum bar directly to the skin.

Option: *Apply pre-tape material, self-adherent wrap, or a neoprene sleeve over the upper arm and forearm to lessen irritation.*

▶ **Application:**

STEP 1: Pad the inside surface of the aluminum bars with ¼ inch or ½ inch foam (Fig. 9–22A). If condyle pads are attached to the hinge, leave them in place.

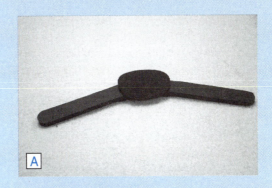

A

STEP 2: For this example, apply one layer of self-adherent wrap around the upper arm and forearm ◀▶ (Fig. 9–22B).

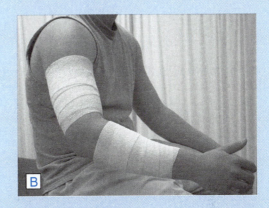

B

STEP 3: Center the hinge over the lateral joint line of the elbow with the bars extending proximally over the lateral upper arm and distally over the lateral forearm (Fig. 9–22C). A hinged bar may be applied over the medial joint line with the bars extending over the medial upper arm and forearm for additional support.

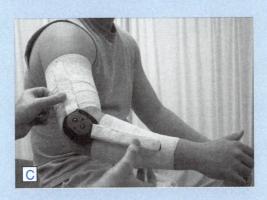

C

STEP 4: Anchor 2 inch or 3 inch heavyweight elastic tape directly on the distal end of the brace bar and continue around the upper arm in a circular, lateral-to-medial pattern with moderate roll tension. Overlap the tape by ½ of its width, cover the entire bar, and anchor on the tape pattern proximal to the bar on the lateral upper arm (Fig. 9–22D). Avoid gaps, wrinkles, or inconsistent roll tension.

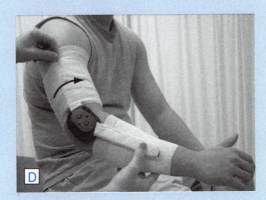

D

Figure 9-22

STEP 5: Anchor 2 inch or 3 inch heavyweight elastic tape on the proximal brace bar and proceed around the forearm in a circular, lateral-to-medial pattern with moderate roll tension (Fig. 9–22E). Anchor on the tape pattern distal to the end of the bar on the lateral forearm.

Option: *Apply one to two additional anchors with 1½ inch non-elastic tape in circular strips loosely around the upper arm and forearm* ◀▬▶ *.*

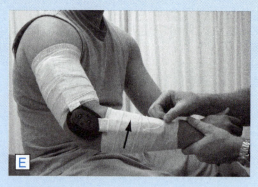

Figure 9-22 *continued*

...IF/THEN...

If using the neoprene sleeve with hinged bars technique one and the distal end is not snugly fitted on the forearm, allowing migration, *THEN* consider the application of technique two. The heavyweight elastic tape will conform to the upper arm and forearm and securely anchor the bars.

...IF/THEN...

If application of hyperextension taping technique one, two, or three is not effective in limiting hyperextension during a return to activity following a sprain, *THEN* consider using a functional brace or neoprene sleeve with hinged bars technique one or two to provide greater support and limits in hyperextension.

Critical Thinking Question 3

At the end of a busy day, a window cleaner stepped off the scaffolding and caught his foot on several safety straps. The cleaner fell to the ground and landed on the right outstretched arm, sustaining a posterior elbow dislocation and third degree ulnar collateral ligament sprain. Following surgery and rehabilitation, he returns to work. The surgeon recommends bracing for the elbow for the next 5 months to provide support.

▶ **Question: What bracing techniques are appropriate in this situation?**

EPICONDYLITIS STRAP Figure 9–23

▶ **Purpose:** Many epicondylitis strap brace designs are available to lessen tension on the wrist extensor or flexor musculature when treating lateral or medial epicondylitis (Fig. 9–23). These designs are commonly referred to as counterforce braces.[15] Use the straps with athletic, work, or casual activities.

▶ **Design:**
  • Purchase the straps off-the-shelf in universal styles and predetermined sizes corresponding to proximal forearm circumference measurements. Several designs are available in universal sizes.
  • Most designs are manufactured of neoprene or foam composite materials with a D-ring Velcro closure.
  • Some designs are constructed of a non-elastic foam material.
  • The straps contain a conformed neoprene, foam, air cell, viscoelastic, gel, padded plastic, or padded plastic/metal buttress incorporated into the strap.
  • Some braces are designed specifically for lateral or medial epicondylitis, while other braces can be positioned for both conditions.

▶ **Position of the individual:** Sitting on a taping table or bench or standing with the involved arm at the side of the body, the involved elbow placed in slight flexion, and the forearm in a neutral position.

▶ **Preparation:** Apply epicondylitis straps directly to the skin. No anchors are required.

▶ **Application:**

STEP 1: Apply lateral epicondylitis designs by placing the buttress on the lateral forearm approximately ¾ of an inch distal from the lateral epicondyle of the humerus (Fig. 9–23A).

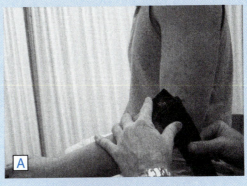

STEP 2: Wrap the strap snugly around the proximal forearm and/or through the D-ring and anchor (Fig. 9–23B).

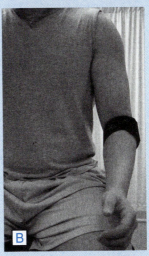

STEP 3: Apply medial epicondylitis designs by positioning the buttress on the medial forearm just distal from the medial epicondyle of the humerus (Fig. 9–23C).

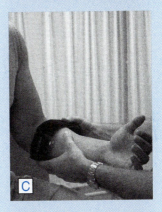

STEP 4: Wrap and anchor the strap (Fig. 9–23D).

STEP 5: Allow the individual to perform a previously painful activity. Readjust the tension of the strap if necessary.

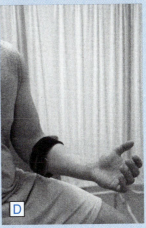

Figure 9-23

Critical Thinking Question 4

A javelin thrower on the track and field team has been receiving treatment for lateral epicondylitis over the past 3 weeks. He has returned to activity with the use of a counterforce brace to lessen the pain associated with the throwing motion. After a few days of wearing the brace during practice, the brace loosens and the pain returns to the lateral forearm. He has worn taping material straps, but they were not effective in lessening the symptoms.

▶ **Question: What can be done in this situation?**

RESEARCH BRIEF

A bracing technique for the forearm was first introduced in 1971[3]; many techniques are currently used in combination with other modalities in various treatment and rehabilitation programs for lateral epicondylitis. Many studies have been conducted to investigate the effects of counterforce braces[15] on electromyographic activity, strength, and pain of the forearm musculature. These studies have resulted in contradictory findings.

Several theoretical mechanisms of action for the braces are presented in the literature. Many researchers[4,5,7,19] have suggested that braces lessen tension at the proximal musculotendinous junction by reducing muscular expansion and decreasing the force of muscular contractions. Other researchers[8,14,16,21] believe the braces broaden the area for the common extensor tendon origin, artificially creating a second, wider muscle origin. This broadening may direct stress to healthy tissues or the band, decreasing stress on the lateral epicondyle.

Electromyographic investigations of the forearm musculature with brace wear have produced positive findings. Examining a group of tennis players without symptoms of lateral epicondylitis, researchers demonstrated lower electromyographic activity of the extensor carpi ulnaris and extensor carpi radialis among the brace group than among the unbraced group during backhand and serve strokes.[6] Brace wear has also been shown to significantly reduce electromyographic activity of the extensor carpi radialis brevis and extensor digitorum communis in normal subjects, as compared with controls.[19] Despite these findings, reductions in electromyographic activity associated with counterforce bracing have not been shown to correlate with clinical improvement of lateral epicondylitis.[11]

The effects of counterforce braces and a taping technique on pain associated with lateral epicondylitis have produced mixed results. Researchers have demonstrated no significant effects on visual analogue scales of pain perception during a gripping motion in a group of subjects with lateral epicondylitis with the use of two braces and a placebo compared with a no-brace situation.[22] With brace wear, pain perception levels among the subjects increased. Other researchers have also found no significant changes in visual analogue scales of pain perception with brace use among a group of subjects with lateral epicondylitis.[21] In combination with injection therapy, the braces reportedly relieved pain in 10 out of 12 subjects with lateral epicondylitis, although the extent was not described.[3] The application of a diamond shape taping technique has been shown to reduce pressure pain threshold scores in subjects with lateral epicondylitis compared to a placebo or no-tape situation.[20] However, the results were not statistically significant. The taping technique consisted of four strips of non-elastic tape anchored directly on the skin in a diamond pattern around the lateral epicondyle. As each strip was applied, the soft tissue was pushed perpendicular to the tape, toward the epicondyle.

Several studies have examined the effects of bracing and taping on pain-free grip strength. Changes in grip strength with brace wear have been shown to increase 4% to 5% in subjects with lateral epicondylitis compared to nonbrace wear.[2,21,22] When a diamond taping technique was used, an increase in grip strength of 24% was found immediately and 30 minutes after application.[20] Note that counterforce braces applied pressure around the proximal forearm circumferentially, and the taping technique concentrated pressure on the dorsolateral elbow and proximal forearm. Further research is needed to examine the differences in pressure and force on the soft tissue and extensor muscle mass.

Recommendations on when and how to apply counterforce braces when treating lateral epicondylitis vary in the literature. Several investigators suggest using the braces in the acute phase of treatment[3,5]; only during painful activities[3]; during all activities if moderate symptoms are present, and all the time (excluding sleep) if severe symptoms are present[18]; and when symptoms have resolved[4] for a 1-year period.[3] Most researchers agree that counterforce bracing is an adjunct to a comprehensive treatment program.[11]

The amount of tension with which the brace should be applied on the forearm remains unknown. In previous studies, application tension has been described with the terms comfortably[3,21] and snugly[18,19] in regard to the fit on the proximal forearm. Some researchers have suggested that an application pressure of 40 mm Hg to 50 mm Hg may provide the optimal mechanical effect.[11] Note that excessive tension of the brace can cause edema and anterior interosseous nerve syndrome, affecting intraneural blood flow and causing deep forearm pain and weakness of the hand musculature.[1] As previously mentioned in the Taping section of this chapter, positioning of the brace ¾ of an inch distal to the lateral epicondyle appears to be the preferred placement on the forearm for treating lateral epicondylitis.[19,21] No specific application recommendations for medial epicondylitis were found in the literature.

While the research has shown mixed results with regard to the effectiveness of counterforce bracing when treating lateral epicondylitis, counterforce bracing continues to be used. The braces should be used within a comprehensive therapeutic exercise program, and individuals should be educated on the braces' proper application and use. Further investigations are necessary to examine application tension and position, optimal periods of application, and the long-term clinical effects of the braces.

NEOPRENE SLEEVE Figure 9–24

- **Purpose:** Neoprene sleeves provide compression and mild support when preventing and treating contusions, sprains, strains, ruptures, dislocations, bursitis, abrasions, and overuse injuries and conditions (Fig. 9–24). Use the sleeves during rehabilitative, athletic, work, and casual activities.

- **Design:**
  - The off-the-shelf sleeves are manufactured in universal fit designs in predetermined sizes corresponding to elbow joint circumference measurements.
  - Most designs extend from the mid upper arm to the mid forearm. Some designs extend to the distal forearm for additional support and protection.
  - Many designs are constructed with protective padding incorporated into the posterior elbow, while other designs use silicone inserts to provide additional compression.
  - Some designs have a lateral and/or medial epicondylitis strap incorporated with a Velcro closure.
  - Several designs are available with an open cubital fossa space.

- **Position of the individual:** Sitting on a taping table or bench or standing with the involved arm at the side of the body and the involved elbow placed in slight flexion.

- **Preparation:** Apply neoprene sleeves directly to the skin. No anchors are required.

- **Application:**
  STEP 1: Hold each side of the sleeve and apply the larger end over the fingers and hand. Pull in a proximal direction until the sleeve is positioned on the elbow (Fig. 9–24A).

  STEP 2: Apply epicondylitis sleeve designs by positioning the buttress, then wrap and anchor the straps.

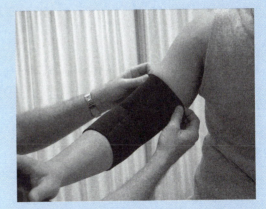

Figure 9-24

SLINGS

▸ **Purpose:** Use slings to provide support and immobilization when treating elbow and forearm injuries and conditions.
  • Use sling technique one (see Fig. 8–11) to treat sprains, strains, ruptures, dislocations, fractures, bursitis, and overuse injuries and conditions; this technique can be used postoperatively as well.

Padding Techniques

Off-the-shelf and custom-made padding techniques provide shock absorption and protection when preventing and treating elbow and forearm injuries and conditions. Padding for the elbow and/or forearm is mandatory with several interscholastic and intercollegiate sports. These mandatory techniques will be discussed further in Chapter 13.

OFF-THE-SHELF Figures 9–25, 9–26

▸ **Purpose:** Off-the-shelf padding techniques are available in a variety of designs to provide shock absorption and protection. Use these techniques when preventing and treating contusions, bursitis, abrasions, and overuse injuries and conditions. Many of these padding designs are similar to the techniques illustrated in Chapter 6 (see Figs. 6–21 and 6–22). Following is a description of two basic designs.

Soft, Low-Density

> ◯ DETAILS
>
> Soft, low-density pads are commonly used to provide shock absorption to the elbow and forearm of athletes in sports such as baseball, basketball, field hockey, football, ice hockey, lacrosse, softball, volleyball, and wrestling. The pads may also be used in work and casual activities.

▸ **Design:**
  • The pads are available in universal fit designs in predetermined sizes based on upper arm, forearm, or elbow joint circumference measurements or weight of the individual (Fig. 9–25A).
  • Many designs are manufactured of high impact open- and closed-cell foams, covered with polyester/spandex or woven fabric materials with Velcro closure elastic straps.
  • Some pads are constructed of woven fabric and neoprene materials, with the neoprene located on the medial aspect of the elbow and forearm to provide an adherent surface for athletic equipment.
  • Other designs incorporate high-impact foam over the posterior elbow in a neoprene or cloth sleeve.
  • Some designs have an open cubital fossa space, while others have a closed space.

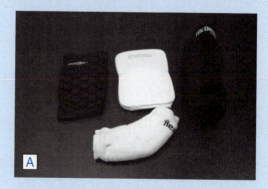

Figure 9-25A Variety of soft, low-density pads.

▸ **Position of the individual:** Sitting on a taping table or bench or standing with the involved arm at the side of the body and the involved elbow placed in slight flexion.

▶ **Preparation:** Apply the soft, low-density designs directly to the skin or over tight-fitting clothing.

▶ **Application:**

STEP 1: Place the larger end of the pad over the fingers and hand. Pull in a proximal direction onto the elbow and/or forearm (Fig. 9–25B). When using some designs, anchor the straps.

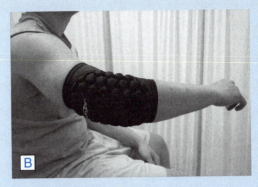

Figure 9-25 *continued*

Hard, High-Density

⬭ **DETAILS**

Hard, high-density pads are commonly used to provide shock absorption to the elbow and forearm of athletes in sports such as baseball, basketball, field hockey, football, ice hockey, lacrosse, skiing, softball, volleyball, and wrestling. The pads may also be used in work and casual activities.

▶ **Design:**
- These pads are available in universal and right or left styles corresponding to upper arm, forearm, or elbow joint circumference measurements or age of the individual (Fig. 9–26A).
- Many designs consist of a polycarbonate or plastic outer shell lined with open- and closed-cell foams incorporated into vinyl or woven fabric materials. These pads are pre-molded to the contours of the upper arm, elbow, and forearm.
- Most pads are designed with protective materials covering the medial and lateral upper arm, elbow, and forearm to provide additional protection.
- Some pads are one-piece designs, while other pads are three-piece to allow for maximum range of motion and comfort.
- The designs are available in a variety of lengths depending on the technique objective.
- Hard, high-density pads are attached to the upper arm, elbow, and forearm with various adjustable nylon straps with Velcro or buckle closures.

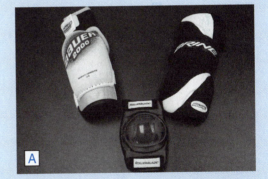

Figure 9-26A Variety of hard, high-density pads. (Left) Ice hockey. (Middle) In-line skating. (Right) Lacrosse.

▶ **Position of the individual:** Sitting on a taping table or bench or standing with the involved arm at the side of the body and the involved elbow placed in slight flexion.

▶ **Preparation:** Apply the hard, high-density designs directly to the skin or over tight-fitting clothing.

▶ **Application:**

STEP 1: Apply the pad over the posterior elbow. The application of straps will depend on the specific design. Normally, pull the straps across the anterior upper arm and forearm and anchor on the pad with Velcro or buckle closures (Fig. 9–26B). Readjust the straps if necessary for proper fit.

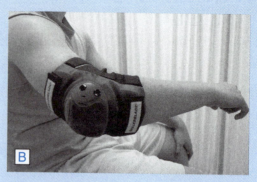

Figure 9-26 *continued*

CUSTOM-MADE Figure 9–27

▶ **Purpose:** Use thermoplastic material to construct custom-made pads to absorb shock and provide protection when preventing and treating elbow and forearm contusions (Fig. 9–27).

▶ **Materials:**
• Paper, felt tip pen, thermoplastic material, ⅛ inch or ¼ inch foam or felt, a heating source, 2 inch or 3 inch elastic tape, an elastic wrap, soft, low-density foam, rubber cement, taping scissors

▶ **Position of the individual:** Sitting on a taping table or bench or standing with the involved arm at the side of the body and the involved elbow placed in a functional position.

▶ **Preparation:** Design the pad with a paper pattern (see Fig. 1–14). Cut, mold, and shape the thermoplastic material on the elbow and/or forearm over the injured area. Attach soft, low-density foam to the inside surface of the material (see Fig. 1–15).

▶ **Application:**

STEP 1: Place the pad over the injured area and attach with the figure-of-eight or circular forearm taping techniques or circular elbow or circular forearm wrapping techniques (Fig. 9–27A). Pad all nonpliable materials to meet NCAA and NFHS rules.

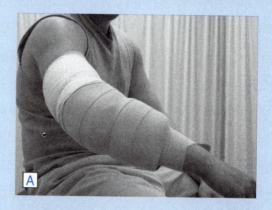

STEP 2: A piece of thermoplastic material may also be molded and attached with cement or elastic tape to an off-the-shelf elbow/forearm pad to provide additional protection for a contusion (Fig. 9–27B).

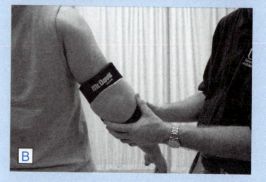

Figure 9-27

COMPRESSION WRAP PAD   Figure 9–28

▶ **Purpose:** Use the compression wrap pad to reduce mild, moderate, or severe swelling and effusion when treating elbow contusions, sprains, strains, ruptures, dislocations, and bursitis (Fig. 9–28).

▶ **Materials:**
  • ¼ inch or ½ inch open-cell foam, taping scissors

▶ **Position of the individual:** Sitting on a taping table or bench or standing with the involved arm at the side of the body and the involved elbow placed in a pain-free, flexed position.

▶ **Preparation:** To lessen migration, apply adherent tape spray, tape strips, or anchors directly to the skin.

▶ **Application:**
  (**STEP 1:**) Extend the pad across the posterior elbow, from the lateral humeral epicondyle to the medial humeral epicondyle, and approximately 3 inches proximally and distally from the olecranon (Fig. 9–28A).

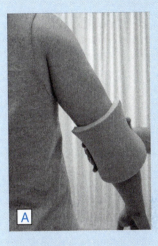

  (**STEP 2:**) Place the pad over the posterior elbow and apply the compression wrap technique to anchor (Fig. 9–28B).

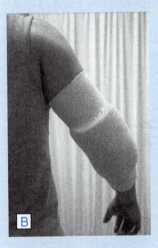

Figure 9-28

MANDATORY PADDING

The NCAA[12] and NFHS[13] require athletes to use protective padding for the elbow and/or forearm during all field hockey, ice hockey, and lacrosse practices and competitions. These padding techniques are available in a variety of off-the-shelf designs. A further discussion of these techniques can be found in Chapter 13.

Critical Thinking Question 5

During rehabilitation of the left knee at the local outpatient orthopedic clinic, a landscape supervisor discusses the problems she is experiencing with her elbow pads. Each weekend when she is rollerblading, the pads slide down onto her forearms. She exchanged the pads and was fitted with another pair at the sporting goods store. The next weekend, these pads also slid down onto her forearms. She is annoyed about the pads and is considering not using any protective equipment for her elbows.

▶ **Question: How can you manage this situation?**

...IF/THEN...

IF a hard, high-density padding technique is required for an individual with an abnormally large olecranon or bursa, ***THEN*** consider constructing a custom-made design; off-the-shelf pads are constructed in universal fit designs in predetermined sizes and may not provide the proper protection.

CASE STUDY

In the second competition of the season, Leo Reagan, a veteran bull rider on the circuit, is thrown from a bull during his first-round ride. Leo was able to release his right hand from the bullrope around the bull, but fell to the ground on the left outstretched arm, sustaining a left posterolateral elbow dislocation. Jay Patrick, the ATC traveling with the circuit, evaluated Leo. Jay immobilized the left elbow, and Leo was transported to a local hospital by EMS. In the emergency room, an orthopedic surgeon performed an evaluation, including imaging studies, and then successfully reduced the elbow. The studies revealed no fractures, but showed a second degree sprain to the ulnar collateral ligament. The surgeon immobilized Leo's left elbow in 90° of flexion and allowed him to return home for a follow-up evaluation with a local orthopedic surgeon. What taping, wrapping, and bracing techniques can you use to provide compression, support, and immobilization at this time?

The next day, Leo is evaluated by the orthopedic surgeon in his hometown. The surgeon reviewed the previous imaging studies, conducted a clinical evaluation, and agreed with the initial diagnosis. The surgeon believed Leo could return to his previous activities, following a nonsurgical rehabilitation approach. Leo remained immobilized in 90° of elbow flexion for three additional days and began rehabilitation at Power Orthopedic Clinic. Five days postinjury, the immobilization was discontinued. The surgeon was concerned about moderate ulnar collateral ligament laxity and recommended that Leo be protected against valgus and hyperextension stress at the elbow during this phase of rehabilitation. Which bracing techniques are appropriate to support and limit excessive range of motion of the elbow during this phase?

Leo tolerates the rehabilitation without problems and has increased flexibility, strength, and dynamic stability of the elbow and surrounding joints. The surgeon is satisfied with Leo's healing and progress and allows a progression into bull riding activities around 11 weeks postinjury. What bracing technique would provide stability to the elbow during these activities?

Leo returns to competitive bull riding using the bracing technique selected for him. During his first week back, he falls several times on his left elbow. Each time, the left elbow was in a flexed position in the brace. Pain and swelling are present over the posterior elbow. Leo is evaluated by a physician and diagnosed with acute olecranon bursitis. The physician allows Leo to continue bull riding activities if protected from further injury. What wrapping techniques can you use to control swelling and which taping and padding techniques are appropriate to provide shock absorption in the management of this case?

WRAP UP

- Acute and chronic injuries and conditions to the elbow and forearm are caused by direct forces, abnormal ranges of motion, forceful muscular contractions, and overload and repetitive stresses.
- The hyperextension and collateral "X" taping techniques provide support and reduce range of motion of the elbow.
- The lateral epicondylitis strap taping and epicondylitis bracing techniques lessen tension of the wrist extensors and/or flexors on the humeral epicondyles.
- The figure-of-eight and circular forearm taping techniques provide support and anchor protective padding.
- The spiral forearm taping technique provides compression.
- Posterior splints and slings provide immobilization following injury/surgery.
- Elastic wraps and sleeves provide compression to control swelling and effusion.
- The circular elbow and forearm wrapping techniques can be used to support and anchor protective padding.
- Rehabilitative braces provide support, immobilization, and protective range of motion, while functional braces provide stability following injury/surgery.
- The neoprene sleeve and sleeve with hinged bars bracing techniques provide compression and support to the elbow.
- Soft, low-density and hard, high-density off-the-shelf and custom-made padding techniques provide shock absorption, protection, and compression.
- The NCAA and NFHS require the use of mandatory protective equipment for the elbow and/or forearm in several sports.

WEB REFERENCES

CCHA Digital Library
http://cchs-dl.slis.ua.edu/index.html
- This site provides you access to the University of Alabama CCHA Health Sciences Digital Libraries Program to search for information about elbow and forearm injuries and conditions.

emedicine
http://www.emedicine.com/
- This site allows you to search for information about acute and chronic injuries and conditions of the elbow and forearm.

The Hughston Clinic
http://www.hughston.com/
- This site allows access to the Hughston Health Alert newsletter and online articles about a variety of elbow and forearm injuries and conditions.

The Physician and Sportsmedicine Online
http://www.physsportsmed.com/index.html
- This Web site provides access to The Physician and Sportsmedicine, which contains a variety of clinical sports medicine manuscripts.

REFERENCES

1. Enzenauer, RJ, and Nordstrom, DM: Anterior interosseous nerve syndrome associated with forearm band treatment of lateral epicondylitis. Orthopedics 14:788–790, 1991.
2. Forbes, A, and Hopper, D: The effect of counterforce bracing on grip strength in tennis players with painful elbows. Aust J Physiother 36:4, 1990.
3. Froimson, AI: Treatment of tennis elbow with forearm support band. J Bone Joint Surg 53:183–184, 1971.
4. Galloway, M, DeMaio, M, and Mangine, R: Rehabilitative techniques in the treatment of medial and lateral epicondylitis. Orthopedics 15:1089–1096, 1992.
5. Gellman, H: Tennis elbow (lateral epicondylitis). Orthop Clin North Am 23:75–82, 1992.
6. Groppel, JL, and Nirschl, RP: A mechanical and electromyographical analysis of the effects of various joint counterforce braces on the tennis player. Am J Sports Med 14:195–200, 1986.
7. Jansen, CW, Olson, SL, and Hasson, SM: The effect of use of a wrist orthosis during functional activities on surface electromyography of the wrist extensors in normal subjects. J Hand Ther 10:283–289, 1997.
8. Kivi, P: The etiology and conservative treatment of humeral epicondylitis. Scand J Rehabil Med 15:37–41, 1982.
9. Kraushaar, BS, and Nirschl, RP: Tendinosis of the elbow (tennis elbow): Clinical features and findings of histological, immunohistochemical, and electron microscopy studies. J Bone Joint Surg Am 81:259–278, 1999.
10. Ljung, BO, Forsgren, S, and Friden, J: Substance P and calcitonin gene-related peptide expression at the extensor carpi radialis brevis muscle origin: Implications for the etiology of tennis elbow. J Orthop Res 17:554–559, 1999.
11. Meyer, NJ, Pennington, W, Haines, B, and Daley, R: The effect of the forearm support band on forces at the origin of the extensor carpi radialis brevis: A cadaveric study and review of literature. J Hand Ther 15:179–185, 2002.
12. National Collegiate Athletic Association, http://www.ncaa.org/library/sports_sciences/sports_med_handbook/2003-04/2003-04_sports_med_handbook.pdf, Sports medicine handbook, 2003–2004.
13. National Federation of State High School Associations. 2004–05 Field Hockey Rules Book. Indianapolis, IN: National Federation of State High School Associations, 2004.
14. Nirschl, RP: Tennis elbow. Orthop Clin North Am 4:787–800, 1973.
15. Nirschl, RP: The etiology and treatment of tennis elbow. J Sports Med 2:308–328, 1974.
16. Nirschl, RP: Prevention and treatment of elbow and shoulder injuries in the tennis player. Clin Sports Med 7:289–308, 1988.
17. Nirschl, RP, and Kraushaar, BS, http://www.physsportsmed.com/issues/1996/05_96/nirschl.htm, Assessment and treatment guidelines for elbow injuries, 1996.
18. Priest, JD: Tennis elbow: The syndrome and a study of average players. Minn Med 59:367–371, 1976.
19. Snyder-Mackler, L, and Epler, M: Effect of standard and Aircast tennis elbow bands on integrated electromyography of forearm extensor musculature proximal to the bands. Am J Sports Med 17:278–281, 1989.
20. Vicenzino, B, Brooksbank, J, Minto, J, Offord, S, and Paungmali, A: Initial effects of elbow taping on pain-free grip strength and pressure pain threshold. J Orthop Sports Phys Ther 33:400–407, 2003.
21. Wadsworth, CT, Nielson, DH, Burns, LT, Krull, JD, and Thompson, CG: Effect of the counterforce armband on wrist extension and grip strength and pain in subjects with tennis elbow. J Orthop Sports Phys Ther 11:192–197, 1989.
22. Wuori, JL, Overend, TJ, Kramer, JF, and MacDermid, J: Strength and pain measures associated with lateral epicondylitis bracing. Arch Phys Med Rehabil 79:832–837, 1998.

Wrist

1. Discuss common injuries and conditions that occur to the wrist.
2. Demonstrate the ability to apply taping, wrapping, bracing, and padding techniques for the wrist when preventing, treating, and rehabilitating injuries.
3. Explain and demonstrate appropriate taping, wrapping, bracing, and padding techniques for the wrist within a therapeutic exercise program.

INJURIES AND CONDITIONS

Acute and chronic injuries and conditions to the wrist may result from compressive forces, excessive range of motion, and repetitive stresses. Normal range of motion and stability of the wrist are required for participation in most athletic, work, and casual activities. Loss of range of motion, as a result of contusions, sprains, fractures, dislocations, and overuse injuries and conditions, can be caused by compressive forces, a fall on the outstretched arm, excessive range of motion, and/or repetitive stresses. Sprains, fractures, and dislocations can occur due to excessive range of motion and shearing forces, and can result in loss of wrist stability. Common injuries to the wrist include:

• Contusions
• Sprains
• Triangular fibrocartilage complex
• Fractures
• Dislocations
• Ganglion cysts
• Overuse injuries and conditions

Contusions

While uncommon, contusions to the wrist do occur; they may be caused by compressive forces. Athletes participating in sports that utilize a stick can be injured as a result of being struck on the wrist by an opponent. Although mandatory gloves normally protect the wrist, an ice hockey forward, for example, can be struck with a stick during a shot on goal.

Sprains

Sprains to the wrist are common in athletic and work activities, and are caused by several mechanisms. A fall on the outstretched arm, rotary forces, and abnormal ranges of motion can result in injury to the ligamentous and capsular tissues of the distal **radioulnar** and **radiocarpal joints** (Illustration 10–1). For example, a wrestler may sprain his wrist during a takedown, when he lands on the outstretched arm and hyperextends his wrist.

Triangular Fibrocartilage Complex (TFCC)

Injury to the **TFCC** can be caused by a fall on the outstretched arm, rotary stress, and excessive range of motion. Athletic participation with the upper extremity in a closed kinetic chain position increases the risk of injury.[20] Excessive forces and abnormal ranges of motion placed on the wrist during gymnastic floor exercises, for instance, can contribute to a TFCC injury.

Fractures

Fractures to the distal radius can be the result of a fall on the outstretched arm. A fall on the outstretched arm and shearing forces can cause fractures of the scaphoid and hamate.

Dislocations

Dislocations of the wrist can occur at the distal radioulnar joint and may be associated with a fracture and soft tissue injury. The causes include excessive extension, pronation, and supination.

Ganglion Cysts

Ganglion cysts may form on the dorsal or **palmar** wrist following a sprain or repetitive hyperextension. A dorsal cyst is more commonly seen. For example, a cyst can develop in a competitive weightlifter as a result of daily training, which can cause repetitive hyperextension and overload.

Overuse

Overuse injuries and conditions are caused by excessive, repetitive stress to the wrist. Repetitive pressure on the palmar aspect of the wrist and palms during athletic and work activities may cause flexor digitorum tendonitis (Illustration 10–2). Flexor carpi radialis and flexor carpi ulnaris tendinitis may be the result of excessive flexion often seen in sports involving a racquet. Excessive gripping and radial and ulnar deviation can cause **de Quervain's tenosynovitis.** Excessive use of a hammer, which requires constant gripping and repetitive wrist motion, can result in tenosynovitis. Nerve

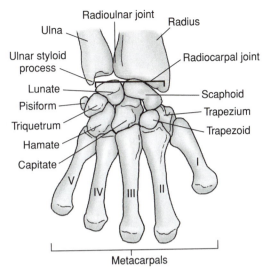

Illustration 10-1 Dorsal view of the bones and joints of the wrist.

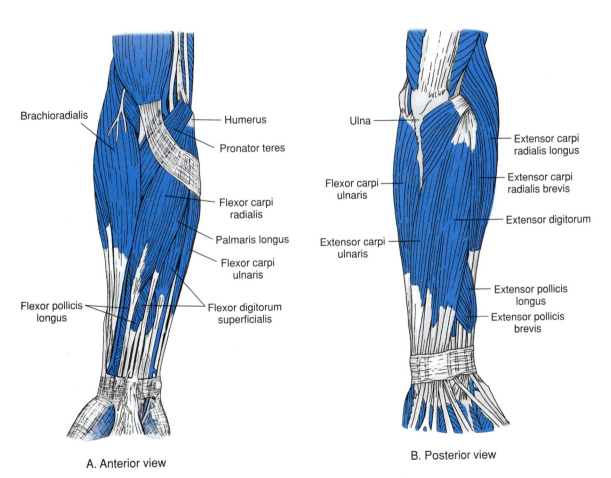

A. Anterior view

B. Posterior view

Illustration 10-2 Superficial muscles of the forearm and wrist.

entrapment and compression syndromes are caused by repetitive wrist flexion and extension, direct forces, structural abnormalities, and repetitive compression and can affect the median, ulnar, and/or radial nerves.

Compression of the median nerve is referred to as **carpal tunnel syndrome.**[22] The excessive wrist flexion and extension experienced in rowing, for example, can lead to carpal tunnel syndrome.

Taping Techniques

Several taping techniques provide support, limit range of motion, and anchor protective padding to the wrist. Many techniques are used to prevent and treat sprains, TFCC injury, fractures, and dislocations and to provide support and lessen excessive range of motion. With proper application, these techniques provide varying amounts of support; the application of the same technique on two individuals may produce different outcomes. Consider the purpose of the technique, the injury, the individual, and the activity when deciding which technique to use. Other taping techniques are used to immobilize the wrist or anchor protective padding. Note that many of these techniques may be used for hand and thumb injuries and conditions as indicated.

CIRCULAR WRIST Figures 10–1, 10–2

▶ **Purpose:** Use the circular wrist technique to provide mild support, limit range of motion, and anchor protective padding to the wrist. Use this technique when preventing and treating contusions, sprains, fractures, and dislocations. Protective padding techniques are illustrated in the Padding section. Two methods are illustrated in the application of the circular wrist technique to accommodate individual preferences and available supplies.

Circular Wrist Technique One

▶ **Materials:**
  • 1½ inch or 2 inch non-elastic tape

  Option:
  • Pre-tape material or self-adherent wrap

▶ **Position of the individual:** Sitting on a taping table or bench with the wrist in a neutral position and the fingers in abduction .

> **Helpful Hint:** Maintain a neutral position of the wrist by having the individual place his or her extended, abducted fingers into your abdomen area. This position also lessens movement of the individual's arm during application.

▶ **Preparation:** Apply circular wrist technique one directly to the skin.

  Option: *Apply pre-tape material or self-adherent wrap around the wrist to lessen irritation* ◀▶.

▶ **Application:**
  STEP 1: Anchor 1½ inch or 2 inch non-elastic tape over the **ulnar styloid process** (Fig. 10–1A).

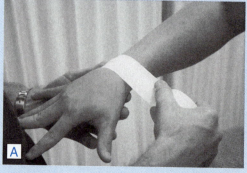

A

Figure 10-1

STEP 2: Continue to apply the tape using a moderate amount of roll tension in a circular, lateral-to-medial direction around the wrist, and return to the anchor (Fig. 10–1B).

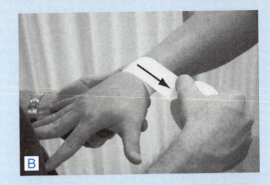

STEP 3: Apply four to five additional circular strips around the wrist, either directly over the last strip or overlapping by ½ of the width of the tape (Fig. 10–1C). Apply the strips in an individual or continuous pattern with moderate roll tension.

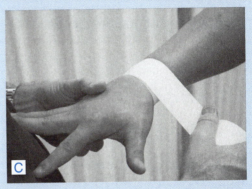

STEP 4: Finish the circular pattern over the dorsum of the wrist to prevent unraveling from contact with equipment during activity (Fig. 10–1D).

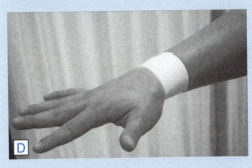

Figure 10-1 *continued*

Circular Wrist Technique Two

▶ **Materials:**
  • 2 inch or 3 inch elastic tape, taping scissors

  Options:
  • Pre-tape material or self-adherent wrap
  • 1½ inch or 2 inch non-elastic tape

▶ **Position of the individual:** Sitting on a taping table or bench with the wrist in a neutral position and the fingers in abduction.

▶ **Preparation:** Apply this circular wrist technique directly to the skin.

  Option: *Apply pre-tape material or self-adherent wrap around the wrist to lessen irritation* ◀▶ .

▶ **Application:**
  STEP 1: Anchor 2 inch or 3 inch elastic tape over the ulnar styloid process and encircle the wrist in a lateral-to-medial circular pattern using moderate roll tension (Fig. 10–2A).

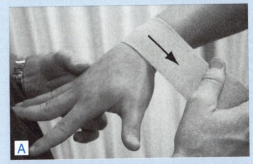

Figure 10-2

STEP 2: Continue with four to five additional circular patterns over the previous strip, or overlap by ½ of the tape width (Fig. 10–2B). Again, apply the strips in an individual or continuous pattern with moderate roll tension.

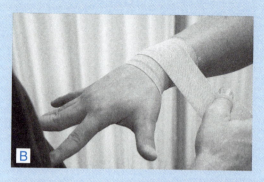

STEP 3: Circular strips may be applied around the proximal hand and palm to provide additional support or anchor protective padding (Fig. 10–2C). These strips should not cause constriction of the thumb and hand.

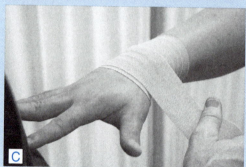

STEP 4: Anchor over the dorsum of the wrist (Fig. 10–2D).

Option: *Apply two to three 1½ inch or 2 inch non-elastic tape circular strips in a lateral-to-medial direction around the wrist with moderate roll tension for additional support.*

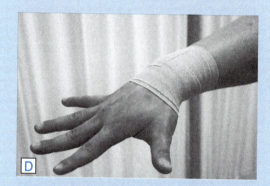

Figure 10-2 *continued*

FIGURE-OF-EIGHT TAPE Figure 10–3

▸ **Purpose:** The figure-of-eight wrist technique provides mild to moderate support, limits range of motion, and anchors custom-made braces and off-the-shelf and custom-made padding when preventing and treating contusions, sprains, TFCC injury, fractures, and dislocations (Fig. 10–3).

▸ **Materials:**
  • 1½ inch or 2 inch non-elastic tape
  Options:
  • Pre-tape material
  • 2 inch elastic tape or self-adherent wrap, taping scissors

▸ **Position of the individual:** Sitting on a taping table or bench with the wrist and hand in a neutral position and the fingers in abduction.

▸ **Preparation:** Apply the figure-of-eight technique directly to the skin.

  Option: *Apply pre-tape material around the hand and wrist to lessen irritation* 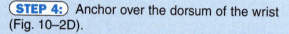 .

▶ **Application:**

STEP 1: Anchor 1½ inch non-elastic tape over the ulnar styloid process and encircle the wrist in a lateral-to-medial direction with moderate roll tension.

Option: *Two inch elastic tape or self-adherent wrap may be used to prevent constriction of the hand.*

STEP 2: At the ulnar styloid process, proceed in a medial direction over the dorsum of the hand (Fig. 10–3A), continue over the **thenar web space,** then across the distal palm (Fig. 10–3B). The tape may need to be partially creased when covering the thenar web space to prevent constriction. Apply the tape with moderate roll tension and remain proximal to the **metacarpophalangeal (MCP) joints** of the hand.

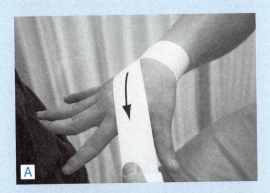

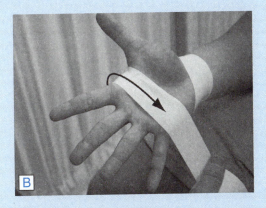

STEP 3: Next, continue from the fifth metacarpal over the dorsum of the hand to the distal radius (Fig. 10–3C), around the wrist, and return to the ulnar styloid process with moderate roll tension (Fig. 10–3D).

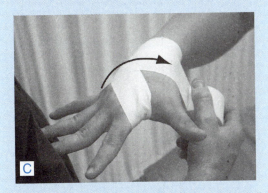

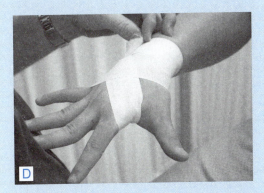

STEP 4: Repeat the figure-of-eight pattern, overlapping by ⅓ of the tape width, and anchor on the dorsal wrist (Fig. 10–3E). The pattern should not cause constriction of the hand and thumb.

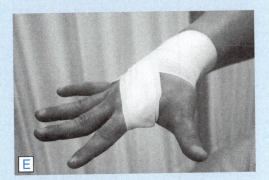

Figure 10-3

FAN TAPE Figure 10–4

- ▶ **Purpose:** Use the fan technique to provide moderate support and limit excessive flexion and extension when preventing and treating sprains, TFCC injury, fractures, and dislocations (Fig. 10–4).

- ▶ **Materials:**
  - 1½ inch or 2 inch non-elastic tape, 2 inch elastic tape, taping scissors

  Options:
  - Pre-tape material or self-adherent wrap, adherent tape spray

- ▶ **Position of the individual:** Sitting on a taping table or bench with the wrist in a neutral position and the fingers in abduction. Determine painful range(s) of motion by placing the forearm on a table. Position the elbow in 90° of flexion and the wrist over the edge of the table with the dorsal hand facing the floor. To determine painful flexion, stabilize the forearm, place a hand on the dorsal fingers, and slowly move the hand and wrist into flexion until pain occurs. Place a hand on the palmar fingers and slowly move the hand and wrist into extension to determine painful extension. Once painful range(s) of motion is (are) determined, place the wrist in a pain-free range and maintain this position during application.

- ▶ **Preparation:** Apply the fan technique directly to the skin.

  Option: *Apply adherent tape spray and pre-tape material or self-adherent wrap around the hand and wrist to provide additional adherence and lessen irritation* ◀━━▶.

- ▶ **Application:**
  STEP 1: Apply an anchor of 1½ inch or 2 inch non-elastic tape around the distal hand, just proximal to the MCP joints, and an anchor around the distal forearm with mild roll tension ◀━━▶ (Fig. 10–4A).

  Option: *Two inch elastic tape may be used for the hand and forearm anchors to prevent constriction.*

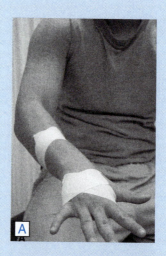

STEP 2: To limit wrist flexion, anchor 1½ inch or 2 inch non-elastic tape on the dorsal lateral hand, proceed in a proximal direction across the hand and wrist, and anchor on the distal forearm (Fig. 10–4B). Monitor the pain-free position of the wrist and apply the tape with moderate roll tension.

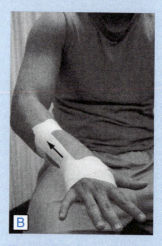

Figure 10-4

STEP 3: Start the next strip on the dorsal hand by overlapping the first by ⅓ of the tape width. Continue across the hand and wrist, and anchor on the distal forearm (Fig. 10–4C).

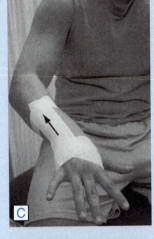

STEP 4: Continue to apply four to five additional strips in this overlapping pattern with moderate roll tension (Fig. 10–4D). Apply enough strips to cover the dorsal hand. The fan should not constrict the thumb. The length from the distal hand to the distal forearm can be measured and a one-piece fan made 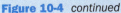.

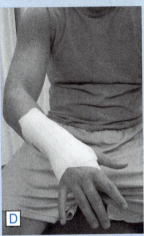

STEP 5: To limit wrist extension, anchor a strip of 1½ inch or 2 inch non-elastic tape on the palmar lateral hand; continue across the hand and wrist with moderate roll tension, and anchor on the distal forearm (Fig. 10–4E). Repeat the overlapping strips in a distal-to-proximal fashion (Fig. 10–4F). Monitor the pain-free position of the wrist.

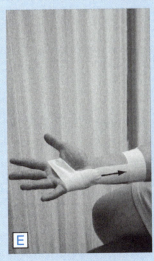

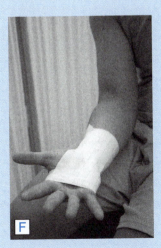

Figure 10-4 *continued*

STEP 6: At the distal hand and forearm, apply two to four closure strips with 1½ inch or 2 inch non-elastic or 2 inch elastic tape with moderate roll tension ◄► (Fig. 10–4G). The closure strips should not cause constriction of the thumb. Partially crease the tape over the thenar web space if necessary.

STEP 7: Use a dorsal and palmar fan to limit multidirectional motion. The circular wrist or figure-of-eight technique may be applied to anchor the strips and provide additional support.

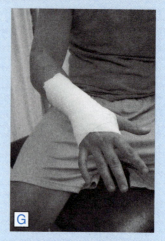

Figure 10-4 *continued*

Helpful Hint: On a taping table or bench, apply a strip of 1½ inch or 2 inch non-elastic tape of a length measured from the distal hand to the distal forearm. Continue to apply strips, overlapping by ⅓ of the tape width, until a 3 inch to 4 inch width fan is constructed. Smooth and adhere the strips together with the hands. Begin to remove the fan by pulling the first strip off the table or bench.

Make two fans by applying strips twice the length measured from the hand to the forearm. Continue to apply the overlapping strips and remove the fan from the table or bench. Bring the non-adherent ends together and cut the fan in half. Use one strip on the dorsal hand and the other on the palmar hand.

STRIP TAPE Figures 10–5, 10–6

▸ **Purpose:** The strip tape technique provides moderate support and limits excessive flexion and extension when preventing and treating sprains, TFCC injury, fractures, and dislocations. Two interchangeable methods are illustrated in the application of the technique. Choose according to individual preferences and available supplies.

Strip Tape Technique One

▸ **Materials:**
- 1½ inch or 2 inch non-elastic tape, 2 inch elastic tape, 4 inch width heavy resistance exercise band, taping scissors

Option:
- Pre-tape material or self-adherent wrap, adherent tape spray

▸ **Position of the individual:** Sitting on a taping table or bench with the wrist in a neutral position and the fingers in abduction. Determine painful range(s) of motion. Once the range is determined, place the wrist in a pain-free range and maintain this position during application.

▸ **Preparation:** Apply strip tape technique one directly to the skin.

Option: *Apply adherent tape spray and pre-tape material or self-adherent wrap around the hand and wrist to provide additional adherence and lessen irritation* ◄► .

Application:

(**STEP 1:**) Apply anchors as illustrated in Figure 10–4A.

(**STEP 2:**) To limit wrist flexion, anchor a piece of 4 inch width heavy resistance exercise band over the dorsal hand with 2 inch elastic tape with mild roll tension 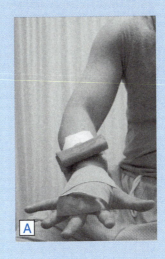. Leave approximately 2–3 inches of the band extending distally beyond the anchor (Fig. 10–5A).

(**STEP 3:**) Pull the band proximally with moderate tension across the hand and wrist, and anchor with mild roll tension on the distal forearm with 2 inch elastic tape 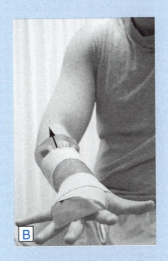 (Fig. 10–5B). Monitor the pain-free position of the wrist and cut the band approximately 2–3 inches beyond the anchor. A second piece of elastic exercise band may be applied directly over the first for additional support.

(**STEP 4:**) To limit wrist extension, anchor the 4 inch heavy resistance exercise band with 2 inch elastic tape on the palmar hand with mild roll tension, leaving approximately 2–3 inches of the band extending distally 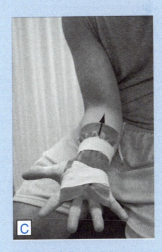. Pull the band across the hand and wrist with moderate tension and anchor on the distal forearm (Fig. 10–5C). Cut the band approximately 2–3 inches beyond the anchor. Monitor the pain-free position of the wrist. Apply a second piece of elastic exercise band if necessary.

Figure 10-5

STEP 5: Fold the excess band over the distal hand and forearm anchors and apply two to three circular closure strips in an individual or continuous pattern with 1½ inch or 2 inch non-elastic or 2 inch elastic tape ◄——► (Fig. 10–5D). Apply the tape with moderate roll tension.

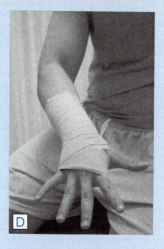

STEP 6: Use the circular wrist or figure-of-eight technique to anchor the exercise band and provide additional support (Fig. 10–5E). Monitor the thumb and thenar web space to prevent constriction. To limit multidirectional motion, apply a dorsal and palmar elastic exercise band.

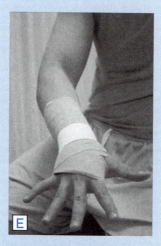

Figure 10-5 *continued*

Strip Tape Technique Two

▶ **Materials:**
   • 1½ inch or 2 inch non-elastic tape, 2 inch elastic tape, 2 inch or 3 inch width heavyweight moleskin, taping scissors

   Option:
   • Pre-tape material or self-adherent wrap, adherent tape spray

▶ **Position of the individual:** Sitting on a taping table or bench with the wrist in a neutral position and the fingers in abduction. Determine painful range(s) of motion. Once the range is determined, place the wrist in a pain-free range and maintain this position during application.

▶ **Preparation:** Apply this strip tape technique directly to the skin.

   Option: *Apply adherent tape spray and pre-tape material or self-adherent wrap around the hand and wrist to provide additional adherence and lessen irritation* ◄——► .

▶ **Application:**

STEP 1: Apply anchors as illustrated in Fig. 10–4A.

STEP 2: Measure and cut a strip of 2 inch or 3 inch heavyweight moleskin from the distal hand to the distal forearm anchors.

STEP 3: To limit wrist flexion, apply the moleskin strip on the dorsal hand, pull the strip across the hand and wrist with moderate tension, and attach on the distal forearm (Fig. 10–6A). Monitor the pain-free position of the wrist.

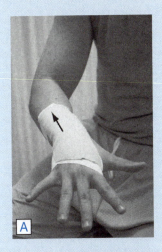

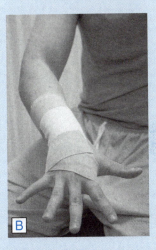

STEP 4: Anchor the moleskin with mild tension on the distal hand and forearm, with 2 inch elastic tape ◀▶ (Fig. 10–6B).

STEP 5: To limit wrist extension, apply a moleskin strip on the palmar hand, continue over the hand and wrist with moderate tension, and anchor on the distal forearm (Fig. 10–6C). Anchor on the distal hand and forearm with 2 inch elastic tape with mild roll tension ◀▶ (Fig. 10–6D). Monitor the pain-free position of the wrist.

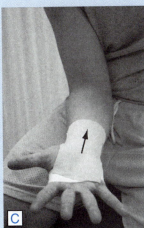

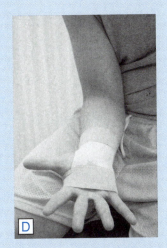

Figure 10-6

STEP 6: Apply two to three individual or continuous circular closure strips with moderate roll tension around the hand and forearm with 1½ inch or 2 inch non-elastic or 2 inch elastic tape ◄━ (Fig. 10–6E).

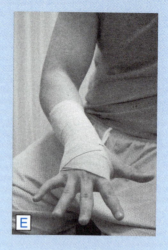

STEP 7: Anchor the moleskin and provide additional support with the application of the circular wrist or figure-of-eight technique (Fig. 10–6F). Monitor the thumb and thenar web space to prevent constriction. Use both moleskin strips to limit multidirectional motion.

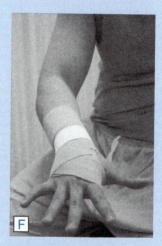

Figure 10-6 *continued*

"X" TAPE Figure 10–7

▸ **Purpose:** The "X" technique provides moderate support and limits excessive flexion and extension when preventing and treating sprains, TFCC injury, fractures, and dislocations (Fig. 10–7).

▸ **Materials:**
   • 1½ inch or 2 inch non-elastic tape, 2 inch elastic tape, taping scissors
   Option:
   • Pre-tape material or self-adherent wrap, adherent tape spray

▸ **Position of the individual:** Sitting on a taping table or bench with the wrist in a neutral position and the fingers in abduction. Determine painful range(s) of motion. Once the range is determined, place the wrist in a pain-free range and maintain this position during application.

▸ **Preparation:** Apply the "X" technique directly to the skin.

   Option: *Apply adherent tape spray and pre-tape material or self-adherent wrap around the hand and wrist to provide additional adherence and lessen irritation* ◄━ .

▶ **Application:**

STEP 1: Apply anchors as illustrated in Figure 10–4A.

STEP 2: To limit wrist flexion, anchor 1½ inch or 2 inch non-elastic tape at an angle on the dorsal hand proximal to the second MCP joint. Continue across the hand and wrist with moderate roll tension, and anchor on the lateral distal forearm (Fig. 10–7A). Monitor the pain-free position of the wrist.

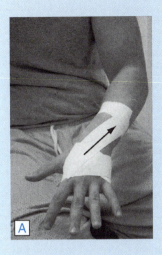

STEP 3: Apply the next strip on the dorsal hand proximal to the fifth MCP joint; proceed across the hand and wrist, and finish on the medial distal forearm (Fig. 10–7B).

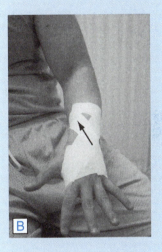

STEP 4: Overlap the tape by ⅓ of the width and apply two to four additional strips in the "X" pattern with moderate roll tension 🔧 (Fig. 10–7C). Monitor the pain-free position of the wrist.

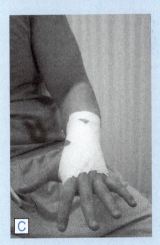

Figure 10-7

STEP 5: To limit wrist extension, place 1½ inch or 2 inch non-elastic tape proximal to the second MCP joint at an angle on the palmar hand. Continue across the hand and wrist, and anchor on the medial distal forearm with moderate roll tension (Fig. 10–7D).

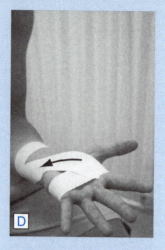

STEP 6: Apply a strip on the palmar hand proximal to the fifth MCP joint, across the hand and wrist, and anchor on the lateral distal forearm (Fig. 10–7E).

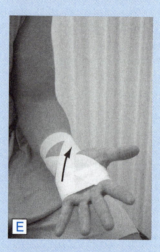

STEP 7: Apply two to four additional strips, overlapping by ⅓ of the tape width, in the "X" pattern with moderate roll tension (Fig. 10–7F). Monitor the pain-free position of the wrist.

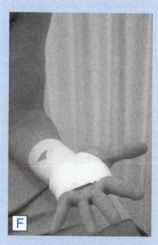

Figure 10-7 *continued*

STEP 8: Place two to three closure strips with moderate roll tension in a circular pattern around the hand and forearm, using 1½ inch or 2 inch non-elastic or 2 inch elastic tape ◄■► (Fig. 10–7G).

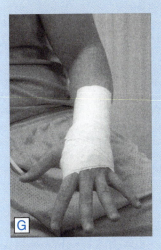

G

STEP 9: Apply the circular wrist or figure-of-eight technique to anchor the strips and provide additional support (Fig. 10–7H). Monitor the thumb and thenar web space to prevent constriction. Use the dorsal and palmar "X" strips to limit multidirectional motion.

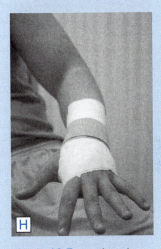

H

Figure 10-7 *continued*

Helpful Hint: Premake the "X" strip on a taping table or bench after determining the length from the distal hand to the distal forearm. Smooth and adhere the tape on the countertop, then place on the individual. Trim any excess tape with taping scissors.

Critical Thinking Question 1

About midway through the Australian Rules Football season, a half forward suffers a right wrist sprain caused by a fall during a match. Following a period of rehabilitation, he is allowed to return to activity with an off-the-shelf functional brace that has been approved for use. During the first match, the half forward falls on his right outstretched arm, but continues to play.

▶ **Question: What taping techniques can you apply at halftime to provide additional stability?**

...IF/THEN...

IF an athlete asks for the wrists to be taped and she or he has no history of injury, **THEN** consider applying the non-elastic tape circular wrist technique; it provides mild support, is quick to apply, and requires less expensive non-elastic tape.

BRACE ANCHOR   Figure 10–8

▸ **Purpose:** Use the brace anchor technique to attach custom-made braces and to provide moderate support and immobilization of the hand and wrist when treating sprains, dislocations, and overuse injuries and conditions (Fig. 10–8).

▸ **Materials:**
- 2 inch or 3 inch elastic tape, pre-tape material, taping scissors

Option:
- Self-adherent wrap

▸ **Position of the individual:** Sitting on a taping table or bench with the hand and wrist in a neutral position. Place the wrist in the desired range of flexion or extension, as indicated by a physician. Maintain this position during application.

▸ **Preparation:** Apply pre-tape material around the distal hand and distal forearm ◀▶.

▸ **Application:**

STEP 1: Position the custom-made brace on the dorsal or palmar hand, wrist, and forearm.

STEP 2: Anchor 2 inch or 3 inch elastic tape directly on the proximal brace and apply three to four circular patterns around the forearm with mild to moderate roll tension without overlapping ◀▶ (Fig. 10–8A). Finish the circular pattern on the dorsal forearm to prevent irritation and unraveling.

Option: *Self-adherent wrap may be used, without pre-tape material, for the circular patterns if elastic tape is not available.*

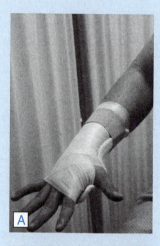

STEP 3: Next, anchor on the top of the distal brace with 2 inch or 3 inch elastic tape and apply three to four circular patterns around the distal hand with mild to moderate roll tension ◀▶ (Fig. 10–8B). Anchor the pattern on the dorsal hand.

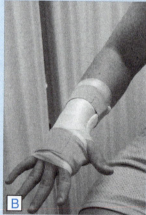

Figure 10-8

WRIST SEMIRIGID CAST   Figure 10–9

▸ **Purpose:** The semirigid cast technique provides maximum support and limits wrist range of motion when treating sprains, TFCC injury, fractures, and dislocations (Fig. 10–9). The cast should be applied by qualified health-care professionals. The cast may be used during athletic and work activities, removed, and then used again.

▸ **Materials:**
- 2 inch or 3 inch semirigid cast tape, gloves, water, self-adherent wrap, ⅛ inch foam or felt, 2 inch elastic tape, taping scissors

Option:
• Thermoplastic material, a heating source

▶ **Position of the individual:** Sitting on a taping table or bench with the hand and wrist in the position to be immobilized, as indicated by a physician, and the fingers in abduction.

▶ **Preparation:** Apply ⅛ inch foam or felt over bony prominences and palmar surface of the thumb to lessen the occurrence of irritation.

▶ **Application:**

(STEP 1:) Apply two to three layers of self-adherent wrap to the hand, wrist, and distal forearm with mild to moderate roll tension ◀ (Fig. 10–9A). The wrap may be applied in a figure-of-eight pattern.

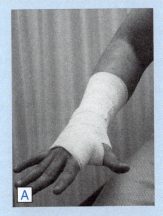

(STEP 2:) With 2 inch or 3 inch semirigid cast tape, anchor on the distal lateral forearm and apply circular, lateral-to-medial patterns with moderate roll tension in a proximal-to-distal direction, overlapping the tape by ½ of its width (Fig. 10–9B).

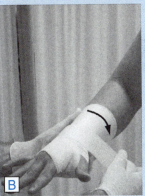

(STEP 3:) At the wrist, continue to apply the tape in a figure-of-eight pattern with moderate roll tension involving the hand and wrist (Fig. 10–9C). Apply the tape proximal to the MCP joints of fingers two through five. Depending on the individual's size, the cast tape may need to be creased or partially cut when covering the thenar web space to prevent constriction.

Option: *Mold and incorporate thermoplastic material over the dorsal and/or palmar hand and wrist to provide additional support (Fig. 10–9D).*

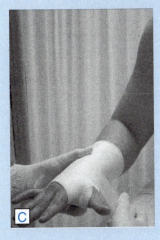
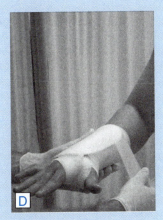

Figure 10-9

STEP 4: Continue to alternate figures-of-eight with circular patterns around the hand, wrist, and distal forearm, overlapping the tape by ⅓ to ½ of its width (Fig. 10–9E).

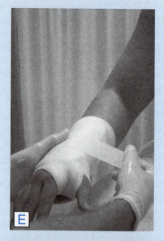

STEP 5: Finish the tape pattern on the dorsal wrist/distal forearm and smooth and mold the cast with the hands (Fig. 10–9F).

STEP 6: Cover the semirigid cast with high-density, closed-cell foam of at least ½ inch thickness for all athletic practices and competitions (see Fig. 10–19A–B).

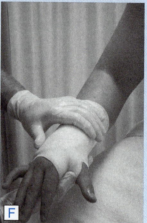

STEP 7: Remove the cast by cutting with taping scissors along the ulnar or radial aspect of the cast (Fig. 10–9G). Choose the side that is opposite from the injured area.

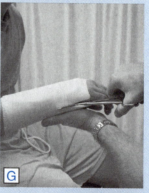

STEP 8: To reuse, apply two to three layers of self-adherent wrap to the hand, wrist, and distal forearm ◀▶ . Place the cast on the hand, wrist, and forearm, and anchor with 2 inch elastic tape or self-adherent wrap with moderate roll tension in a circular pattern ◀▶ (Fig. 10–9H).

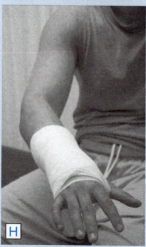

Figure 10-9 *continued*

POSTERIOR SPLINT Figure 10–10

▶ **Purpose:** The posterior splint technique is used to immobilize the wrist and hand when treating sprains, TFCC injury, fractures, dislocations, and overuse injuries and conditions (Fig. 10–10). Use the splint as temporary immobilization prior to further evaluation by a physician. This technique is applied with the same materials listed in Chapter 9 (see Fig. 9–11). Two interchangeable methods are illustrated in the application of the technique to accommodate available supplies.

> ◯ **DETAILS**
>
> Periods of immobilization are normally determined by a physician following evaluation of the individual. Cast technicians and physicians can provide complete immobilization with rigid cast tape applied over stockinet.

▶ **Design:**
  • Purchase off-the-shelf rigid splints in pre-cut and padded designs. The splints are manufactured of several layers of rigid fiberglass material, covered with fabric and foam padding in 2, 3, 4, and 5 inch widths by 10, 12, 15, 30, 35, and 45 inch lengths.

Posterior Splint Technique One

▶ **Materials:**
  • Off-the-shelf rigid, padded splint, water, towel, two 4 inch width by 5 yard length elastic wraps, metal clips, 1½ inch non-elastic tape

▶ **Position of the individual:** Sitting on a taping table or bench with the hand and wrist in a neutral position. Place the wrist in the desired range of flexion or extension as indicated by a physician. Maintain this position during application.

▶ **Preparation:** Mold and apply the padded splint directly to the skin.

▶ **Application:**
  (STEP 1:) Remove the splint from the package and immerse in water of 70° to 75° F. Remove the splint from the water and place lengthwise on a towel. Quickly roll the splint and towel together to remove excess water (Fig. 10–10A).

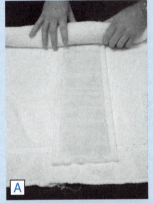
A

  (STEP 2:) Apply the splint from just proximal to the MCP joints of fingers two through five to the mid to proximal forearm (Fig. 10–10B). The splint is most commonly used on the palmar aspect of the hand, wrist, and forearm.

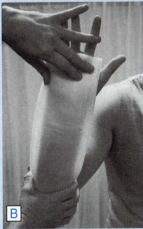
B

Figure 10-10

STEP 3: Apply a 4 inch width by 5 yard length elastic wrap in a spiral pattern with moderate roll tension to mold the splint to the contours of the hand, wrist, and forearm ←→ (Fig. 10–10C). Mold and shape the splint with the hands. Monitor the position of wrist flexion or extension. After 10–15 minutes, the fiberglass should be cured; remove the elastic wrap.

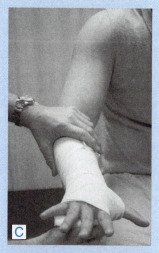

STEP 4: Attach the splint to the hand, wrist, and forearm with another 4 inch width by 5 yard length elastic wrap with moderate roll tension using a distal-to-proximal spiral pattern ←→ (Fig. 10–10D). Anchor the wrap with metal clips or loosely applied 1½ inch non-elastic tape. A sling may be required for daily activities.

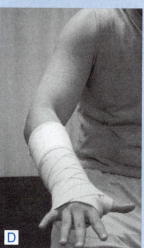

Posterior Splint Technique Two

▶ **Materials:**
- 3 inch, 4 inch, or 5 inch width rigid cast tape, stockinet, gloves, 4 inch width by 5 yard length elastic wrap, metal clips, 1½ inch non-elastic tape, taping scissors

▶ **Position of the individual:** Sitting on a taping table or bench with the hand and wrist in a neutral position. Place the wrist in the desired range of flexion or extension as indicated by a physician. Maintain this position during application.

▶ **Preparation:** Apply one layer of stockinet from the distal fingers to the elbow.

▶ **Application:**
STEP 1: Remove the cast tape from the pouch and immerse in water of 70° to 75° F. Anchor on the palmar aspect of the hand, just proximal to the MCP joints of fingers two through five. Continue to apply the tape in a proximal direction over the hand and wrist, and finish at the mid to proximal forearm (Fig. 10–10E).

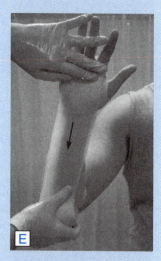

Figure 10-10 *continued*

STEP 2: At the mid to proximal forearm, reverse the tape and continue over the previous strip toward the distal hand (Fig. 10–10F). Repeat this sequence until four to five layers of tape have been applied. Use additional rolls of cast tape if needed and mold the tape with gloved hands. Monitor the position of wrist flexion or extension. Curing should be complete in 10–15 minutes.

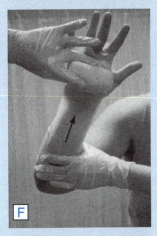

STEP 3: With taping scissors, cut the stockinet lengthwise down the dorsal aspect of the hand, wrist, and forearm. Fold the stockinet over the splint to protect against skin irritation (Fig. 10–10G).

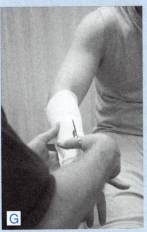

STEP 4: Attach the splint with a 4 inch width by 5 yard length elastic wrap in a spiral, distal-to-proximal pattern with moderate roll tension (Fig. 10–10H). Anchor the wrap with metal clips or loosely applied 1½ inch non-elastic tape. A sling may be required for daily activities.

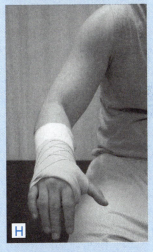

Figure 10-10 *continued*

Wrapping Techniques

Use wrapping techniques to provide compression to assist in controlling swelling following soft tissue injuries and conditions. Use elastic and self-adherent wraps also to anchor protective padding and braces when preventing and treating contusions, sprains, fractures, dislocations, and overuse injuries and conditions. These techniques can also be used for hand injuries and conditions as indicated.

COMPRESSION WRAP Figure 10–11

▶ **Purpose:** The compression wrap technique provides pressure and lessens mild, moderate, or severe swelling and inflammation when treating contusions, sprains, dislocations, and ganglion cysts (Fig. 10–11).

▶ **Materials:**
- 2 inch, 3 inch, or 4 inch width by 5 yard length elastic wrap, metal clips, 1½ inch non-elastic or 2 inch elastic tape, ⅛ inch or ¼ inch foam or felt, taping scissors

  Options:
- Self-adherent wrap
- ¼ inch or ½ inch open-cell foam

▶ **Position of the individual:** Sitting on a taping table or bench with the wrist and hand in a pain-free position and the fingers in abduction.

▶ **Preparation:** Because of the irregular shape of the hand and wrist, place ⅛ inch or ¼ inch foam or felt over the inflamed area directly to the skin to assist in venous return. The pad is particularly useful for providing compression following aspiration of a ganglion cyst.

▶ **Application:**

STEP 1: Anchor the extended end of the elastic wrap on the dorsal surface of the hand just distal to the MCP joints of fingers two through five and encircle the hand ◄▶ (Fig. 10–11A).

Option: *Self-adherent wrap may be used if an elastic wrap is not available.*

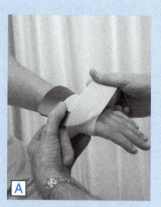

A

STEP 2: Continue around the hand over the thenar web space, overlapping the wrap by ⅓ to ½ of its width (Fig. 10–11B).

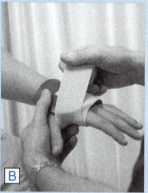

B

STEP 3: Next, proceed across the dorsal hand, encircle the wrist, then across the dorsal hand, and encircle the hand in a figure-of-eight pattern (Fig. 10–11C).

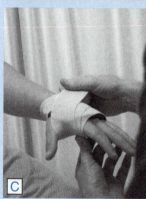

C

Figure 10-11

STEP 4: Repeat the figure-of-eight pattern, overlapping by ⅓ to ½ of the wrap width (Fig. 10–11D). Cover all exposed areas. Roll tension is greatest distally and lessens proximally.

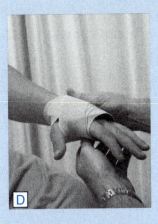

STEP 5: At the wrist, continue the wrap in a distal-to-proximal direction over the distal forearm in a spiral pattern. Anchor over the dorsum of the distal forearm with Velcro, metal clips, or loosely applied 1½ inch non-elastic or 2 inch elastic tape ◄——► (Fig. 10–11E). In order to lessen migration, apply a figure-of-eight pattern loosely through the hand with 2 inch elastic tape or self-adherent wrap ◄——► (Fig. 10–11F).

Option: A ¼ inch or ½ inch open-cell foam pad may be placed over the dorsal hand, extending from the MCP joints to the wrist, for additional compression (see Fig. 11–22). Apply the pad directly on the skin and cover with the compression wrap.

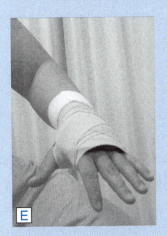 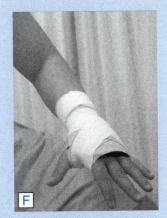

Figure 10-11 *continued*

FIGURE-OF-EIGHT WRAP **Figure 10–12**

▶ **Purpose:** Use the figure-of-eight wrist technique to provide compression and mild support and to anchor custom-made braces and protective padding when preventing and treating contusions, sprains, TFCC injury, fractures, dislocations, and overuse injuries and conditions (Fig. 10–12).

▶ **Materials:**
  • 2 inch, 3 inch, or 4 inch width by 5 yard length elastic wrap, metal clips, 1½ inch non-elastic or 2 inch elastic tape, taping scissors

  Option:
  • Self-adherent wrap

▶ **Position of the individual:** Sitting on a taping table or bench with the wrist and hand in a neutral position and the fingers in abduction.

▶ **Preparation:** To lessen migration, apply adherent tape spray, tape strips, or anchors directly to the skin (see Fig. 1–7).

▶ **Application:**

(STEP 1:) Place the brace or pad over the injured area.

(STEP 2:) Anchor the elastic wrap directly to the skin over the ulnar styloid process and apply the figure-of-eight taping technique with moderate roll tension (Fig. 10–12A).

Option: *Self-adherent wrap may be used if an elastic wrap is not available.*

(STEP 3:) Finish the wrap and anchor over the wrist or distal forearm with Velcro, metal clips, or loosely applied 1½ inch non-elastic or 2 inch elastic tape ◀━▶ (Fig. 10–12B). A figure-of-eight pattern may be applied loosely through the hand with 2 inch elastic tape or self-adherent wrap for additional support.

...IF/THEN...

IF using an elastic or self-adherent wrap to control swelling over the dorsal hand and wrist following a contusion, **THEN** consider applying the compression wrap technique; this technique, along with a foam or felt pad, provides compression over a greater area than the figure-of-eight wrap.

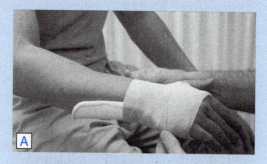

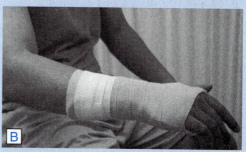

Figure 10-12

Bracing Techniques

Off-the-shelf and custom-made braces are available for the wrist in a variety of designs. The braces can be classified into three categories: prophylactic, rehabilitative, and functional. Use these bracing techniques to prevent and treat acute and chronic injuries and conditions. Note that several of these braces are also used for hand and thumb injuries and conditions.

PROPHYLACTIC Figure 10–13

▶ **Purpose:** Prophylactic braces are designed to prevent or reduce the severity of wrist injuries (Fig. 10–13). These braces, referred to as wrist guards, provide moderate support and are primarily used to protect the wrist from sprains, TFCC injury, fractures, and dislocations.

DETAILS

Prophylactic braces are commonly used to provide wrist stability for individuals in sports such as biking, in-line skating, skiing, and snowboarding, but can also be useful with work and casual activities. Most braces can be used either under or over athletic and work gloves. Prophylactic braces may be used in combination with the circular wrist (Figs. 10–1 and 10–2), figure-of-eight (Fig. 10–3), fan (Fig. 10–4), strip (Figs. 10–5 and 10–6), and "X" (Fig. 10–7) taping techniques to provide additional stability.

▶ **Design:**
- Off-the-shelf prophylactic braces are available in universal fit and right or left styles in predetermined sizes corresponding to wrist circumference measurements or width from the second to the fifth MCP joint.
- The braces are constructed in circumferential and open designs in different lengths based on the amount of protection desired.
- Most designs are manufactured of a nylon mesh material outer shell with an EVA foam or gel pad and moisture-resistant lining.
- Some braces have a high-density plastic or aluminum palmar and/or dorsal bar(s) incorporated into the outer shell to limit wrist flexion and/or extension.
- Other designs are constructed with a plastic, leather, or Kevlar palmar pad that covers the entire or proximal palm.
- Most prophylactic braces are attached to the hand, wrist, and forearm through nylon straps with Velcro closures.
- Some designs allow for unrestricted finger and thumb range of motion, while other designs are available in a glove design.

▶ **Position of the individual:** Sitting on a taping table or bench with the wrist and hand in a neutral position.

▶ **Preparation:** Apply the brace directly to the skin or over a glove.
Follow the manufacturer's instructions, which are included with the braces when purchased, during the application of prophylactic designs. The following guidelines apply to most prophylactic designs.

▶ **Application:**
STEP 1: Begin application by loosening the straps and unfolding the brace.

STEP 2: Place the brace onto the involved hand, wrist, and forearm. Align the bar(s) on the dorsal and/or palmar aspect of the hand, wrist, and forearm (Fig. 10–13A). Reposition the brace if necessary.

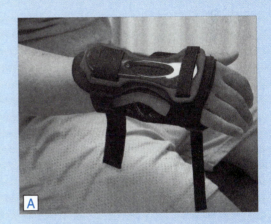

STEP 3: Wrap the outer shell around the hand, wrist, and forearm. Continue with most designs by pulling the straps tight and anchoring with Velcro (Fig. 10–13B).

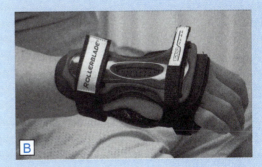

Figure 10-13

RESEARCH BRIEF

Numerous studies have described the high incidence of wrist injury among snowboarders[1,3,23] and in-line skaters.[4,11,19] Off-the-shelf wrist guards are used by many in attempts to protect against or lessen the severity of injury. Although the effects of prophylactic knee and ankle bracing techniques are well documented, few investigations in the literature have examined the effectiveness of wrist guards.

The researchers who have examined the protective value of off-the-shelf wrist guards have produced positive findings. Cadaveric studies have revealed differences in injury patterns with the use of guards. Using a fast, gravity-driven load, guards provided protection against capsular disruption, carpal fractures, and ligamentous injury compared to nonbraced specimens.[13] A significant reduction in wrist dorsiflexion was found with guard use during the application of a compressive load, compared to a control group.[6] During a simulated fall on a snowy surface, specimens fitted with guards required a significantly greater force to produce fracture than specimens without guards.[7] Other investigations revealed no significant differences in the force required to produce fracture using a quasistatic load among braced and nonbraced specimens.[5]

In a prospective, randomized, clinical trial among snowboarders, researchers demonstrated a significant difference in the number of injuries, with braced subjects reporting eight injuries and nonbraced subjects 29 injuries.[17] A 10-snowboarding-season survey among medical facilities in the western United States showed that the wrist was the most commonly injured joint; subjects wearing guards were approximately half as likely to sustain an injury as subjects without wrist protection.[9]

The prophylactic effects of a wrist guard are determined by many factors, one being the amount of energy absorbed by the materials of the guard. A guard too rigid may produce high stress loads at the distal and/or proximal end(s) of the brace. Researchers have reported forearm fractures associated with the use of rigid guards with in-line skaters.[2] The optimal wrist guard should absorb the maximum amount of energy without the production of these high stress points.[17]

Overall, most[7,8,13,17] researchers agree that using prophylactic wrist guards in snowboarding and in-line skating activities can lower the incidence and severity of injuries. However, further research is needed to understand fully the mechanism of wrist injury and the functional role of wrist guards and to provide a framework for future guard design.[7,13]

...IF/THEN...

IF a prophylactic brace is needed to lessen wrist flexion, extension, and ulnar and radial deviation, **THEN** consider a circumferential design, which will provide greater support than an open design.

REHABILITATIVE   Figure 10–14

▶ **Purpose:** Rehabilitative braces are designed to provide compression, immobilization, and mild to moderate support. The braces also limit range of motion and correct structural abnormalities when treating sprains, TFCC injury, fractures, dislocations, tendinitis, tenosynovitis, nerve entrapment and compression syndromes, and postoperative procedures (Fig. 10–14). The braces can replace rigid casting and be removed to accommodate treatment and rehabilitation. Rehabilitative brace designs may be used with the compression wrap technique.

▶ **Design:**
- These off-the-shelf universal fit and right or left style braces are available in predetermined sizes based on wrist circumference measurements or width from the second to the fifth MCP joint.
- The circumferential and open designs are available in various lengths depending on the technique objective.
- Some braces are non-elastic in design while others are elastic.
- Most non-elastic designs are constructed with a polyester/cotton or foam laminate, nylon/fiber, canvas, soft leather, or perforated suede material outer shell lined with nylon, cotton or suede stockinet, or polypropylene felt material.

- Non-elastic braces have dorsal and/or palmar aluminum or plastic bar(s) incorporated into the outer shell to lessen wrist extension and/or flexion. Many of these are **malleable** as well as removable.
- The non-elastic braces are anchored to the hand, wrist, and forearm with adjustable D-ring closures, pull-tab laces, and Velcro straps.
- Elastic designs consist of a cotton, nylon, polyester, or neoprene material outer shell with a polypropylene felt, cotton, or Lycra material lining.
- Most of these designs are available with adjustable dorsal and/or palmar aluminum or plastic bar(s) attached to the outer shell.
- D-ring closures, laces, and Velcro straps attach the braces to the hand, wrist, and forearm.
- Some non-elastic and elastic designs allow unrestricted motion of the fingers and thumb while other designs are available with an attached thumb spica to place the thumb in a neutral position.

> **DETAILS**
>
> The non-elastic braces are commonly used to immobilize the wrist in a neutral or **cock-up position;** most designs allow for adjustments in fit depending on the injury or condition. Although most elastic designs also immobilize the wrist in a neutral or cock-up position, limited range of motion is allowed.

▶ **Position of the individual:** Sitting on a taping table or bench with the involved hand and wrist in a pain-free range of motion.

▶ **Preparation:** Apply the brace directly to the skin.
　　Instructions for the application of rehabilitative braces are included with each brace when purchased. The following guidelines pertain to most designs.

▶ **Application:**
　STEP 1: Loosen the straps and unfold the brace.

　STEP 2: Apply the brace onto the involved hand, wrist, and forearm. Align the bar(s) on the dorsal and/or palmar aspect of the hand, wrist, and forearm (Fig. 10–14A). Remold and reposition the bars if necessary.

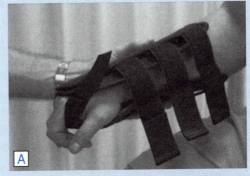

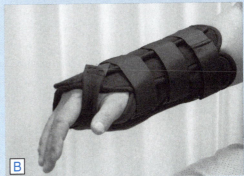

　STEP 3: Wrap the outer shell around the hand, wrist, and forearm. The application of straps will depend on the specific brace design. Begin application of most designs by pulling the strap through the hand and anchoring. Next, pull the most distal wrist strap and anchor. Continue in a proximal direction and anchor the remaining straps (Fig. 10–14B). When using other designs, pull the tab lacing closure(s) tight and anchor. The individual may require a sling for daily activities.

Figure 10-14

Critical Thinking Question 2

A retired circus clown is seen in a local outpatient orthopedic clinic for treatment of de Quervain's tenosynovitis of the left wrist. He was placed in an off-the-shelf thumb, hand, and wrist brace by a physician 1 week ago and restricted from his daily fly-fishing activities. The retired clown complains of itching underneath the brace; upon removal, mild redness and swelling are present on the dorsal left wrist. The physician originally ordered the brace to be worn for 3 weeks.

▶ **Question: How can you manage this situation?**

FUNCTIONAL Figure 10–15

▶ **Purpose:** Functional braces provide compression and moderate stability to the wrist when preventing and treating sprains, TFCC injury, fractures, dislocations, tendinitis, tenosynovitis, nerve entrapment and compression syndromes, and postoperative procedures (Fig. 10–15). These designs are commonly used following injury during a return to work and athletic activities.

DETAILS

Functional braces are commonly used to provide wrist stability for athletes in sports such as baseball, basketball, diving, fencing, field hockey, football, gymnastics, ice hockey, lacrosse, soccer, skiing, softball, volleyball, and wrestling, but can also be useful with work and casual activities. Functional braces may be used in combination with the circular wrist, figure-of-eight, fan, strip, and "X" taping techniques to provide additional stability.

▶ **Design:**
- Off-the-shelf functional braces are available in universal and right or left styles, corresponding to wrist circumference measurements or width from the second to the fifth MCP joint.
- These braces are available in circumferential and open designs of various lengths and are commonly lower profile in construction and lighter in weight than rehabilitative braces.
- Some designs are constructed of neoprene with adjustable, interchangeable dorsal and/or palmar foam insert(s) or aluminum bar(s) to restrict excessive range of motion.
- Other braces are manufactured of a cotton/elastic, nylon, or polyester material outer shell with a Lycra, cotton stockinet, or polypropylene felt lining. Adjustable dorsal and/or palmar aluminum or plastic bars, metal springs, or rubber tubing are used to limit excessive range of motion.
- Several designs contain a viscoelastic polymer pad incorporated into the palmar aspect of the brace to lessen compressive forces.
- Velcro straps and D-ring closures anchor the braces to the hand, wrist, and forearm, and provide for adjustments in fit. Some designs use one strap to anchor the brace around the hand, wrist, and forearm.
- Most of the functional braces allow for unrestricted motion of the fingers and thumb.

▶ **Position of the individual:** Sitting on a taping table or bench with the wrist and hand in a neutral position.

▶ **Preparation:** Apply the brace directly to the skin. Loosen all straps.
   Application of functional designs should follow manufacturer's instructions, which are included with the braces when purchased. The following guidelines pertain to most braces.

▶ **Application:**

STEP 1: Apply most of the designs by placing the brace onto the involved hand, wrist, and forearm. Align the dorsal and/or palmar bar(s), wrap the outer shell around the hand, wrist, and forearm, and anchor the strap(s) (Fig. 10–15A). Reposition the bars if necessary.

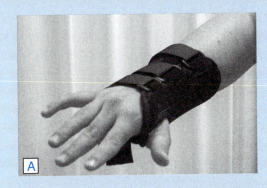

STEP 2: When using other designs, place the neoprene material outer shell over the fingers and pull in a proximal direction until positioned over the wrist (Fig. 10–15B). Anchor the straps.

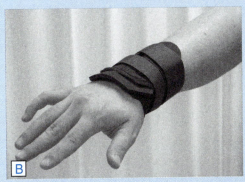

Figure 10-15

Critical Thinking Question 3

A nuclear lab technician has been suffering from numbness and tingling in the fingertips of the right thumb, index, and middle fingers for the past month. Two weeks ago, she was seen by a physician and diagnosed with carpal tunnel syndrome. She was fitted with an off-the-shelf brace to immobilize the right wrist in a position of neutral-to-slight extension. She wore the brace at night only. Ergonomic changes to her office and lab have been made, and, in only 2 weeks, she responded well to the treatment. Nonetheless, her symptoms have now returned despite the ergonomic changes and continued night splinting. The lab technician awakens with pain in the right wrist and wonders if any damage occurred to the brace in her luggage during a recent airline trip to a national meeting.

▶ **Question: What can be done in this situation?**

CUSTOM-MADE Figure 10–16

▶ **Purpose:** Construct custom-made braces from thermoplastic material to provide moderate support and to immobilize, limit range of motion, and correct structural abnormalities for a variety of wrist injuries and conditions (Fig. 10–16). Use these braces when preventing and treating sprains, TFCC injury, fractures, dislocations, tendinitis, tenosynovitis, nerve entrapment and compression syndromes, and postoperative procedures. This technique is effective when off-the-shelf brace designs are not available. Custom-made braces can be used during rehabilitative, work, and casual activities. Custom-made braces may be used with the compression wrap technique.

▶ **Materials:**
- Paper, felt tip pen, thermoplastic material, ⅛ inch or ¼ inch foam or felt or 2 inch or 3 inch moleskin, a heating source, an elastic wrap, taping scissors

▶ **Position of the individual:** Sitting on a taping table or bench with the wrist and hand in a neutral position.

▶ **Preparation:** Design the brace with a paper pattern (see Fig. 1–14) on the dorsal aspect from the MCP joints, across the wrist, and finish at the distal forearm. For the palmar aspect, begin at the MCP joints, continue across the wrist, and finish at the distal forearm. The pattern should cover the entire dorsal or palmar surface of the hand, wrist, and forearm and not cause constriction of finger and thumb motion. Mold and shape the material over the area in the desired range of wrist motion as indicated by a physician.

▶ **Application:**

STEP 1: Attach ⅛ inch or ¼ inch foam or felt or 2 inch or 3 inch moleskin to the inside surface of the material (Fig. 10–16) to prevent irritation.

STEP 2: Place the brace on the dorsal or palmar hand, wrist, and forearm directly to the skin. Anchor the brace with the brace anchor taping technique or the figure-of-eight taping or wrapping technique.

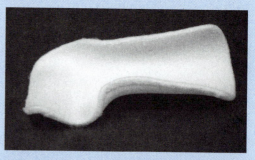

Figure 10-16 Custom-made thermoplastic palmar wrist splint with moleskin lining.

RESEARCH BRIEF

To lessen compression on the medial nerve, most physicians recommend splinting the wrist in a neutral position when treating carpal tunnel syndrome.[16,21,24] Splinting the wrist during sleep—night splinting—is commonly attempted first in the conservative treatment of the condition.[16,18,21,24] Full-time splinting may be indicated initially or with unsuccessful night splinting. Some physicians suggest splinting is most effective when used within 3 months of the onset of symptoms.[10]

Several studies have examined the effectiveness of splinting in the treatment of carpal tunnel syndrome. Using a unique brace design, a 4-week period of night splinting was shown to be more effective in lessening symptoms compared to no treatment.[12] The construction of the brace applied pressure over the metacarpal heads of fingers two through five and positioned the third and fourth fingers in extension. Other studies have demonstrated a greater reduction in symptoms with full-time brace use than night splinting alone.[25] However, the researchers cautioned that compliance issues with full-time brace use are greater than with night splinting.

Bracing techniques play a large role in the overall conservative treatment of carpal tunnel syndrome. Selection and use of bracing techniques should be based on the individual's symptoms and compliance with the treatment protocol.

...IF/THEN...

IF off-the-shelf functional braces excessively restrict sport- or work-specific movements, **THEN** consider designing a custom-made brace; mold the brace with the wrist in a functional position while maintaining the necessary support and/or limits in range of motion.

SLINGS

▶ **Purpose:** Slings provide support and immobilization when treating wrist injuries and conditions.
  • Use sling technique one (see Fig. 8–11) when treating sprains, TFCC injury, fractures, dislocations, overuse injuries and conditions, and postoperative procedures.

Padding Techniques

Use viscoelastic polymers, foam, felt, and thermoplastic materials to absorb shock, lessen compressive and repetitive stresses, and provide protection to the wrist. The techniques are used when preventing and treating contusions, ganglion cysts, fractures, dislocations, carpal tunnel syndrome, and postoperative procedures.

VISCOELASTIC POLYMERS Figure 10–17

▶ **Purpose:** Viscoelastic polymers absorb shock and lessen compressive stress when preventing and treating ganglion cysts and carpal tunnel syndrome (Fig. 10–17). The sleeves may be cleaned and reused multiple times.

▶ **Materials:**
- Off-the-shelf wrist and hand sleeves lined with padding and pads (see Fig. 10–17A).

▶ **Position of the individual:** Sitting on a taping table or bench with the wrist and hand in a neutral position.

▶ **Preparation:** Apply the viscoelastic polymer sleeves and pads directly to the skin.

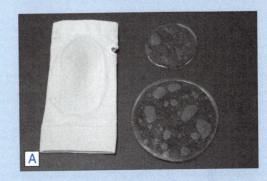

▶ **Application:**
STEP 1: Place the sleeve over the fingers and pull onto the hand and wrist in a proximal direction (Fig. 10–17B). No additional anchors are required.

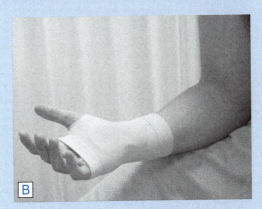

STEP 2: Place the pads directly onto the skin and anchor with the figure-of-eight taping or wrapping technique or adhesive gauze material (see Figs. 3–13 and 10–17C).

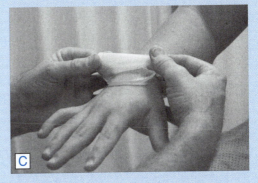

Figure 10-17 A Viscoelastic polymers. (Left) Hand and wrist sleeve. (Right) Pads.

DONUT PADS

▶ **Purpose:** When treating fractures and ganglion cysts, use a donut pad to lessen the amount of compression over an area by dispersing the stress outward (see Fig. 3–27).

- Construct the pads from ⅛ inch or ¼ inch foam or felt or purchase them pre-cut with adhesive backing.
- Pre-cut viscoelastic donuts may also be purchased in a variety of sizes.
- Attach the pad directly to the skin over the hook of the hamate with adhesive gauze material (see Fig. 3–13) or with the figure-of-eight taping or wrapping technique.

CUSTOM-MADE Figure 10–18

▶ **Purpose:** Custom-made pads constructed of thermoplastic material absorb shock and provide protection when preventing and treating wrist contusions (Fig. 10–18).

▶ **Materials:**
- Paper, felt tip pen, thermoplastic material, ⅛ inch or ¼ inch foam or felt, a heating source, 2 inch or 3 inch elastic tape, an elastic wrap, soft, low-density foam, rubber cement, taping scissors

▶ **Position of the individual:** Sitting on a taping table or bench or standing with the hand, wrist, and forearm placed in a functional position.

▶ **Preparation:** Design the pad with a paper pattern (see Fig. 1–14). Cut, mold, and shape the thermoplastic material on the hand, wrist, and/or forearm over the injured area. Attach soft, low-density foam to the inside surface of the material (see Fig. 1–15).

▶ **Application:**

STEP 1: Apply the pad over the injured area and attach with the circular wrist or figure-of-eight taping, or figure-of-eight wrapping technique (Fig. 10–18). Prior to all practices and competitions, pad all nonpliable materials to meet NCAA[14] and NFHS[15] rules.

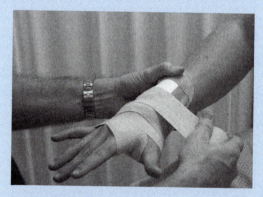

Figure 10-18

CAST PADDING Figure 10–19

▶ **Purpose:** With approval from a physician, an athlete can return early to activity following a fracture, dislocation, or surgery by placing the hand and wrist in a rigid or semirigid cast. NCAA and NFHS rules require padding casts to protect the injured athlete and her or his competitors from injury (Fig. 10–19).

▶ **Materials:**
- Paper, felt tip pen, high-density, closed-cell foam or similar material of at least ½ inch thickness, 2 inch or 3 inch width by 5 yard length elastic wrap, 2 inch or 3 inch elastic tape and pre-tape material, or self-adherent wrap, taping scissors

- **Position of the individual:** Sitting on a taping table or bench with the hand and wrist in the casted position.

- **Preparation:** Construct a paper pattern of the cast area to be padded. Trace this pattern onto high-density, closed-cell foam or similar material and cut out the pad with taping scissors.

- **Application:**

  STEP 1: Place the foam over the cast (Fig. 10–19A). Anchor the padding with a 2 inch or 3 inch elastic wrap, 2 inch or 3 inch elastic tape, or self-adherent wrap with moderate roll tension ◀▶ (Fig. 10–19B). When using elastic tape, first apply pre-tape material over the padding to protect the foam from the tape adhesive. The foam may be reused multiple times.

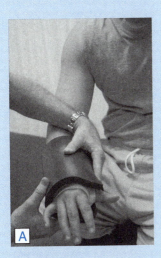
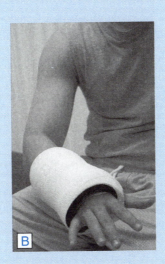

Figure 10-19

Critical Thinking Question 4

The offensive center on the football team comes in after practice complaining of pain in the dorsal right wrist. An evaluation reveals a small palpable lump over the area. He sustained a second degree right wrist sprain last season, but has returned to full activities, including his hobby of weightlifting. The team physician examines the athlete and believes a ganglion cyst has formed. At this time, the physician recommends symptomatic treatment and prevention of any known causative factors.

▶ **Question: What techniques are appropriate in this situation?**

...IF/THEN...

IF padding is required to cover a rigid or semi-rigid cast, **THEN** consider using thermomold-able foam; after heating and molding, the foam retains the shape of the cast, allowing for easy reapplication.

CASE STUDY

Tracey Haney agrees to go in-line skating with her office co-workers on Saturday morning. Tracey has never been in-line skating before, but believes her background in soccer will provide for a quick learning curve. She visits an in-line skating store and purchases skates and elbow and knee pads, but does not feel comfortable wearing wrist guards and decides not to purchase them.

On Saturday morning, Tracey arrives at the park and receives instructions and tips from her co-workers. She immediately begins to skate on the asphalt path. Lacking skate control and the ability to stop, Tracey soon loses control when the front wheel of the right skate strikes a small rock on the path. She falls on her right outstretched arm, forcing her wrist into excessive extension upon contact with the path. Her co-workers help Tracey to her feet and advise her to see a physician. Tracey is able to drive to the local hospital and is seen in the Emergency Department. The attending physician evaluates Tracey and finds tenderness over the ulnar aspect of the wrist and pain with active extension, flexion, and radial and ulnar deviation. Radiographs are obtained and demonstrate no bony pathology. The physician believes she has sustained a second degree right wrist sprain. He immobilizes the right wrist and refers her to Lozman Orthopedic Clinic, located next to the hospital. Which taping, wrapping, and bracing techniques can you use to provide compression, support, and immobilization at this time?

Three days later, Tracey is seen in the clinic by JoAnn Ochoa, a PT/AT who worked with Tracey last year for a soccer-related injury. JoAnn and an orthopedic physician are conducting the weekly in-house clinic for the local high school athletes and examine Tracey when they finish. The physician agrees with the earlier diagnosis and decides to immobilize Tracey's right wrist for 2 weeks. Tracey is to avoid in-line skating and soccer activities during this time. What taping, wrapping, and bracing techniques would provide compression, support, immobilization, and limit range of motion of the wrist during this period?

Tracey returns to the clinic after 2 weeks of immobilization for her follow-up evaluation. The physician finds a decrease in pain with the available active range of motion and no fractures on follow-up radiographs. The physician allows Tracey to begin a therapeutic exercise program with JoAnn, including two additional weeks of night splinting. What wrapping and bracing techniques are appropriate to use during the therapeutic exercise program to provide support and immobilization?

The therapeutic exercise program is moving ahead well, and the physician allows Tracey to progress back into her athletic activities if adequate support is provided to her wrist. Which taping and bracing techniques could you apply to provide support during in-line skating and soccer activities?

WRAP UP

- Compressive, shear, rotary, and repetitive forces, abnormal ranges of motion, and structural abnormalities can result in acute and chronic injuries and conditions to the wrist.
- The circular wrist and figure-of-eight taping techniques provide support, limit range of motion, and anchor protective padding.
- The fan, strip, "X," and semirigid cast taping techniques support and limit range of motion of the wrist.
- The brace anchor taping technique is used to attach braces to the wrist.
- Posterior splints and slings provide immobilization following injury and/or surgery.

- Elastic and self-adherent wraps provide compression and anchor braces and pads.
- Prophylactic, rehabilitative, functional, and custom-made bracing techniques provide compression, protection, stability, and immobilization; limit range of motion; and correct structural abnormalities.
- Viscoelastic, donut, and custom-made padding techniques absorb shock, lessen stress, and provide protection.
- Cast padding techniques are used to protect the injured athlete and his or her opponents during practices and competitions, and are required by NCAA and NFHS rules.

■ WEB REFERENCES

American Physical Therapy Association
http://www.apta.org//AM/Template.cfm?Section=Home
· This Web site allows you access to information about the prevention, treatment, and rehabilitation of a variety of wrist injuries and conditions.

emedicine
http://www.emedicine.com/
· This site provides access to online manuscripts of acute and chronic wrist injuries and conditions.

MDAdvice
http://www.mdadvice.com/
· This Web site provides information on various wrist injuries and conditions.

MDchoice
http://mdchoice.com
· This site allows you to search for information about wrist injuries and conditions, including photo links.

REFERENCES

1. Abu-Laban, RB: Snowboarding injuries: An analysis and comparison with alpine skiing injuries. CMAJ 145:1097–1103, 1991.

2. Cheng, SL, Rajaratnam, K, Raskin, KB, Hu, RW, and Axelrod, TS: Splint-top fracture of the forearm: A description of an in-line skating injury associated with the use of protective wrist splints. J Trauma 39:1194–1197, 1995.

3. Chow, TK, Corbett, SW, and Farstad, DJ: Spectrum of injuries from snowboarding. J Trauma 41:321–325, 1996.

4. Ellis, JA, Kierulf, JC, and Klassen, TP: Injuries associated with in-line skating from the Canadian hospitals injury reporting and prevention program database. Can J Public Health 86:133–136, 1995.

5. Giacobetti, FB, Sharkey, PF, Bos-Giacobetti, MA, Hume, EL, and Taras, JS: Biomechanical analysis of the effectiveness of in-line skating guards for preventing wrist fractures. Am J Sports Med 25:223–225, 1997.

6. Grant-Ford, M, Sitler, MR, Kozin, SH, Barbe, MF, and Barr, AE: Effect of a prophylactic brace on wrist and ulnocarpal joint biomechanics in a cadaveric model. Am J Sports Med 31:736–743, 2003.

7. Greenwald, RM, Janes, PC, Swanson, SC, and McDonald, TR: Dynamic impact response of human cadaveric forearms using a wrist brace. Am J Sports Med 26:825–830, 1998.

8. Heitkamp, H-C, Horstmann, T, and Schalinski, H: In-line skating: Injuries and prevention. J Sports Med Phys Fitness 40:247–253, 2000.

9. Idzikowski, JR, Janes, PC, and Abbott, PJ: Upper extremity snowboarding injuries: Ten-year results from the Colorado snowboard injury survey. Am J Sports Med 28:825–832, 2000.

10. Kruger, VL, Kraft, GH, Deitz, JC, Ameis, A, and Polissar, L: Carpal tunnel syndrome: Objective measures and splint use. Arch Phys Med Rehabil 72:517–520, 1991.

11. Malanga, GA, and Stuart, MJ: In-line skating injuries. Mayo Clin Proc 70:752–754, 1995.

12. Manente, G, Torrieri, F, Di Blasio, F, Staniscia, T, Romano, F, and Uncini, A: An innovative hand brace for carpal tunnel syndrome: A randomized controlled trial. Muscle Nerve 24:1020–1025, 2001.

13. Moore, MS, Popovic, NA, Daniel, JN, Boyea, SR, and Polly, DW: The effect of a wrist brace on injury patterns in experimentally produced distal radial fractures in a cadaveric model. Am J Sports Med 25:394–401, 1997.

14. National Collegiate Athletic Association, http://www.ncaa.org/library/sports_sciences/sports_med_handbook/2003-04/2003-04_sports_med_handbook.pdf, Sports medicine handbook, 2003–2004.

15. National Federation of State High School Associations. 2004 Football Rules Book. Indianapolis, IN: National Federation of State High School Associations, 2004.

16. Prentice, WE: Rehabilitation Techniques for Sports Medicine and Athletic Training, ed 4. McGraw-Hill, Boston, 2004.

17. Rønning, R, Rønning, I, Gerner, T, and Engebretsen, L: The efficacy of wrist protectors in preventing snowboarding injuries. Am J Sports Med 29:581–585, 2001.

18. Sailer, SM: The role of splinting and rehabilitation in the treatment of carpal and cubital tunnel syndrome. Hand Clin 12:223–241, 1996.

19. Schieber, RA, Branche-Dorsey, CM, Ryan, GW, Rutherford, GW, Stevens, JA, and O'Neil, BS. Risk factors for injuries from in-line skating and the effectiveness of safety gear. N Engl J Med 335:1630–1635, 1996.

20. Starkey, C, and Ryan, JL: Evaluation of Orthopedic and Athletic Injuries, ed 2. FA Davis, Philadelphia, 2002.

21. Steele, M, http://www.emedicine.com/emerg/topic83.htm, Carpal tunnel syndrome, 2004.

22. Sternbach, G: The carpal tunnel syndrome. J Emerg Med 17:519–523, 1999.

23. Sutherland, AG, Holmes, JD, and Myers, S: Differing injury patterns in snowboarding and alpine skiing. Injury 27:423–425, 1996.

24. Viera, AJ: Management of carpal tunnel syndrome. Am Fam Physician 68:265–272, 279–280, 2003.

25. Walker, WC, Metzler, M, Cifu, DX, and Swartz, Z: Neutral wrist splinting in carpal tunnel syndrome: A comparison of night-only versus full-time wear instructions. Arch Phys Med Rehabil 81:424–429, 2000.

Hand, Fingers, and Thumb

LEARNING OBJECTIVES

1. Identify common injuries and conditions that occur to the hand, fingers, and thumb.

2. Demonstrate taping, wrapping, bracing, and padding techniques to the hand, fingers, and thumb when preventing, treating, and rehabilitating injuries.

3. Explain and demonstrate the ability to apply taping, wrapping, bracing, and padding techniques to the hand, fingers, and thumb within a therapeutic exercise program.

INJURIES AND CONDITIONS

The hand, fingers, and thumb are essential to athletic, work, and casual activities such as catching a basketball, typing, and gardening. Because of the significant role the hand, fingers, and thumb play in daily activities, injuries occur frequently. Although gloves do offer protection, shearing forces, compressive forces, and excessive range of motion often result in bony and soft tissue injury. Common injuries to the hand, fingers, and thumb include:

• Contusions
• Sprains
• Dislocations
• Fractures
• Tendon ruptures
• Blisters

Contusions

Contusions to the hand, fingers, and thumb are frequent in sports because of the minimal protection for the bony structures.[8] Contusions are also common with work activities. Accumulation of edema is more frequently seen in the dorsal rather than the palmar hand because of the differences in the loose and elastic properties of the dorsal skin compared to the inelastic properties of the palmar skin.[4] Mechanisms of injury include shear and compression forces. A contusion can result, for instance, when a diver strikes the diving board with her hand, fingers, and/or thumb while twisting in the air, sustaining a compressive force to the structures.

Sprains

Sprains typically occur to the fingers and thumb as a result of hyperextension and varus or valgus forces.[1] Finger and thumb sprains involve injury to the collateral ligaments and often to the capsular and tendinous tissues (Illustration 11–1). Sprains may occur at the metacar-

pophalangeal (MCP), **proximal interphalangeal (PIP), or distal interphalangeal (DIP) joints.** A sprain of the ulnar collateral ligament (**gamekeeper's thumb**) results from forceful abduction and hyperextension of the proximal phalanx.[5] For example, a sprain to the ulnar collateral ligament can happen as a softball player slides headfirst into third base, making initial contact with the thumb, causing abduction and hyperextension.

> ### DETAILS
> The name gamekeeper's thumb originates from actual gamekeepers who were subjected to the abduction/hyperextension mechanism during their job-related tasks, which included snapping the necks of fowl with their hands.

Dislocations

Dislocations can occur at the MCP, PIP, and DIP joints of the fingers and thumb. The causes are extreme flexion, or extension, rotation, or compressive loads to the tip of the fingers or thumb.[2] Only qualified health-care professionals should attempt reductions. All individuals with dislocations should be referred to a physician for radiographic examination. A dislocation at the PIP joint can result, for instance, when a bare-handed fan at a baseball game catches a line drive foul ball over the first base dugout, causing a compressive load to the distal finger and hyperextension at the PIP joint.

Fractures

Fractures are seen in the carpals, metacarpals, or phalanges and are caused by compressive or rotational forces (Illustration 11–2).[8] Compressive forces that may cause a fracture include, for example, dropping a dumbbell on the hand or having an opponent fall on a player's fingers while tackling in football.

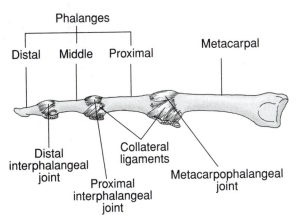

Illustration 11-1 Bones and collateral ligaments of the metacarpophalangeal, proximal interphalangeal, and distal interphalangeal joints of the fingers.

Tendon Ruptures

A rupture of the extensor digitorum tendon at its distal attachment (**mallet finger**) often causes an accompanying avulsion fracture of the distal phalanx. The distal phalanx is forced into flexion, while being held in extension, from a direct blow to the tip of the finger.[10] For example, an extensor digitorum rupture can occur as a basketball player extends the fingers and thumb to receive a pass from a teammate and the ball strikes the tip of the second finger, causing violent flexion of the distal phalanx.

Blisters

Blisters are commonly seen in athletic and work activities that involve the use of the hands on equipment. Shearing forces on the palmar aspect of the fingers and thumb in sports such as baseball, softball, rowing, and weight training can result in the development of blisters.

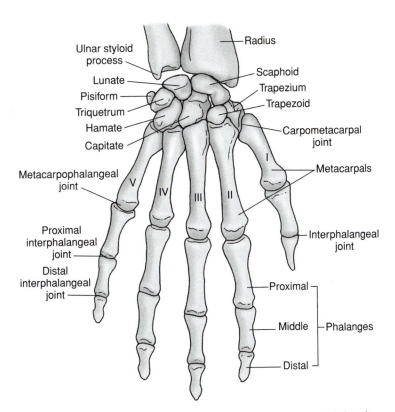

Illustration 11-2 Bones and joints of the hand, fingers, and thumb.

Hand, Fingers, and Thumb

Taping Techniques

Taping techniques for the hand, fingers, and thumb can be used for a variety of injuries and conditions. Most techniques are used to provide support and lessen excessive range of motion when preventing and treating sprains and postdislocation and postfracture injuries. Other techniques are used to prevent and treat injuries to the skin.

BUDDY TAPE Figure 11–1

▶ **Purpose:** Use the buddy tape technique to provide mild to moderate support to the collateral ligaments of the fingers following sprains and postdislocation and postfracture injuries. As the name implies, the injured finger is taped together with its buddy, the largest adjacent finger, to provide support (Fig. 11–1).

▶ **Materials:**
  • ½ inch non-elastic tape, ⅛ inch foam or felt, adherent tape spray, taping scissors
  Option:
  • 1 inch non-elastic or elastic tape

▶ **Position of the individual:** Sitting on a taping table or bench with the hand and fingers in a neutral position.

▶ **Preparation:** Apply adherent tape spray to the fingers. Cut the ⅛ inch foam or felt to the length of the shortest finger to be taped. The buddy tape technique may be applied directly to the skin or over sports-specific gloves.

▶ **Application:**

STEP 1: Apply a strip of ½ inch non-elastic tape around the foam or felt at the proximal end, then place the foam or felt between the fingers to retain anatomical alignment ◀▬▶ (Fig. 11–1A).

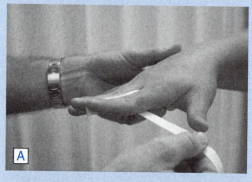

A

STEP 2: Encircle the fingers between the MCP and PIP joints with the ½ inch non-elastic tape strip with moderate roll tension ◀▬▶ (Fig. 11–1B). This *lock-in* strip will prevent the foam or felt from dislodging and loosening during activity as perspiration and moisture begin to affect the tape adhesive.

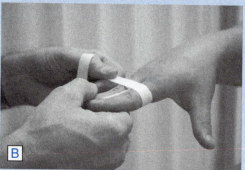

B

STEP 3: Maintaining alignment of the fingers, tape the fingers together with ½ inch non-elastic tape between the MCP and PIP joints, between the PIP and DIP joints, and around the distal phalanx, if necessary, with three to five circular strips with moderate roll tension ◀▬▶ (Fig. 11–1C). End the tape strips on the dorsal aspect of the fingers to prevent unraveling due to contact with equipment during activity. Do not place tape directly over the joints.

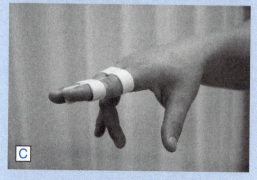

C

Figure 11-1

Option: *1 inch non-elastic or elastic tape may be used for the circular strips on large fingers to provide adequate support or prevent constriction. Note, the use of elastic tape may allow for less support and greater range of motion.*

STEP 4: Apply an additional lock-in strip following completion of these circular strips

 Helpful Hint: Begin the additional lock-in technique by anchoring a strip of tape under the proximal circular strip on the dorsal aspect of the finger (Fig. 11–1D). Continue distally over the distal end of the foam or felt with moderate roll tension and finish by anchoring under the proximal circular strip on the palmar aspect of the finger (Fig. 11–1E). Apply an additional proximal circular strip with moderate roll tension to serve as an anchor (Fig. 11–1F).

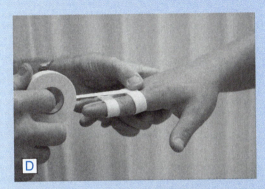

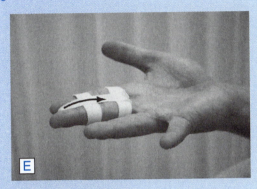

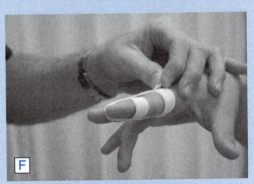

Figure 11-1 *continued*

"X" TAPE Figure 11–2

▶ **Purpose:** The "X" technique also provides mild to moderate support to the collateral ligaments of the PIP joint of the finger following sprains and postdislocation and postfracture injuries. Use this technique with individuals who require support, but also desire independent motion of all fingers (Fig. 11–2).

▶ **Materials:**
  • ½ inch non-elastic tape, adherent tape spray, taping scissors

▶ **Position of the individual:** Sitting on a taping table or bench with the hand and fingers in a neutral position.

▶ **Preparation:** Apply adherent tape spray to the involved finger.

Application:

STEP 1: Using ½ inch non-elastic tape, alternate the application of angled strips directly to the skin over the lateral (Fig. 11–2A) and medial (Fig. 11–2B) joint lines of the PIP joint with moderate roll tension, forming an "X." Each strip should reach proximal and distal to the PIP joint, but not over the DIP or MCP joints.

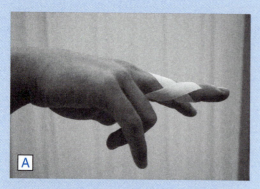

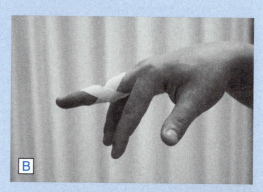

STEP 2: After applying an "X" on each side of the PIP joint, repeat the procedure, overlapping the tape ⅛–¼ inch (Fig. 11–2C).

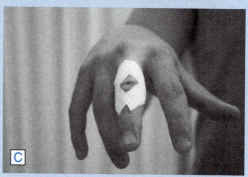

STEP 3: Place circular anchors at the proximal and distal ends of the "X" strips with moderate roll tension, leaving the ends of the anchors on the dorsal aspect of the finger ◀▬▶ (Fig. 11–2D).

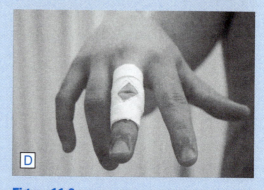

Figure 11-2

 Helpful Hint: Use a cotton-tipped applicator to apply adherent tape spray to the finger. This method will concentrate adherent on the specific areas and prevent spreading to adjacent fingers. The use of adherent is recommended, especially in warm environments.

Critical Thinking Question 1

While diving for a loose ball during practice, a guard on the women's basketball team dislocates the PIP joint of her left fourth finger. Following a reduction and evaluation by a physician, she is cleared to return to practice. You apply the buddy tape technique to support the injured finger. Shortly, she approaches and reports that the technique is uncomfortable.

▶ **Question: What actions can you take in this situation?**

ELASTIC MATERIAL Figures 11–3, 11–4, 11–5

▶ **Purpose:** Several methods are available to cover wound dressings and attach pads to the hand, fingers, and thumb when treating wounds, contusions, and blisters. The material should possess elastic properties and great adhesive strength and not impede hand, finger, and thumb motion. Three methods are illustrated in the application of the technique; they differ based on the site of the wound or contusion.

Elastic Material Technique One

▶ **Materials:**
• Adhesive gauze material, taping scissors

▶ **Position of the individual**: Sitting on a taping table or bench with the hand and fingers in a neutral position.

▶ **Preparation:** Apply adhesive gauze material directly to the skin and use without adherent tape spray.

▶ **Application:**

(**STEP 1:**) Cut the piece of material to overlap a sterile wound dressing or pad from ½ inch to 1 inch to provide an effective anchor base to the skin .

(**STEP 2:**) After application of sterile materials, donut pad, or friction-reducing lubricant, place the piece of the adhesive gauze material directly on the skin (Fig. 11–3).

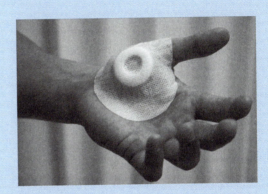

Figure 11-3

Helpful Hint: It is best to round all corners of the material to prevent the edges from being removed by contact with clothing or equipment.

Elastic Material Technique Two

▶ **Materials:**
• Adhesive gauze material, 1 inch or 1½ inch non-elastic tape, taping scissors
Option:
• 2 inch or 3 inch lightweight or heavyweight elastic tape

▶ **Position of the individual**: Sitting on a taping table or bench with the hand and fingers in a neutral position.

▶ **Preparation:** Apply sterile materials, donut pad, or friction-reducing lubricant to the palmar hand. Apply technique two directly to the skin.

▶ **Application:**

(**STEP 1:**) Cut adhesive gauze material into a 12–16 inch strip.

Option: *If adhesive gauze material is not available, use 2 inch or 3 inch lightweight or heavyweight elastic tape.*

STEP 2: Fold the strip and cut a hole in the middle slightly smaller than the finger (Fig. 11–4A).

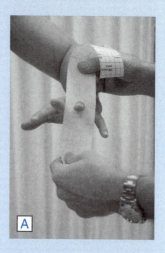

A

STEP 3: Place the hole in the strip over the fingertip. Pull the strip firmly in a proximal direction to the web space between the fingers (Fig. 11–4B). If necessary, trim the strip to prevent irritation of the web space of adjacent fingers.

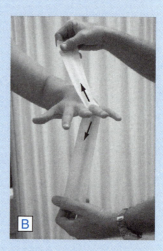

B

STEP 4: Smooth the adhesive gauze material to the palmar and dorsal hand (Fig. 11–4C).

STEP 5: Finish the strip at the wrist, cutting any excess with taping scissors.

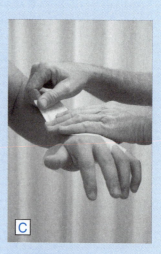

C

Figure 11-4

STEP 6: Anchor the strip in a circular pattern with 1 inch or 1½ inch non-elastic tape around the wrist with moderate roll tension ◀━▶ (Fig. 11–4D).

Elastic Material Technique Three

> ○ **DETAILS**
> Use adhesive gauze material or lightweight elastic tape also to manage finger, thumb, and fingertip wounds and blisters. Fingertip bandages often are too large, resulting in excess bandage material affecting use and sensation of the finger.

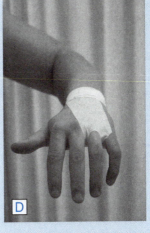

Figure 11-4 *continued*

▸ **Materials:**
- Adhesive gauze material, taping scissors

Options:
- 2 inch or 3 inch lightweight elastic tape
- ½ inch non-elastic tape

▸ **Position of the individual**: Sitting on a taping table or bench with the hand, fingers, and thumb in a neutral position.

▸ **Preparation:** Apply sterile materials, donut pad, or friction-reducing lubricant to the finger or thumb. Apply technique three directly to the skin.

▸ **Application:**
STEP 1: Cut a piece of the adhesive gauze material to cover an area from the fingertip to just proximal to the DIP or PIP joint.

Option: 2 inch or 3 inch lightweight elastic tape may be used if adhesive gauze is not available.

STEP 2: Place the fingertip in the center of the adhesive gauze material (Fig. 11–5A).

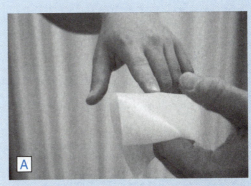

STEP 3: Fold the sides over the finger, avoiding wrinkles (Fig. 11–5B).

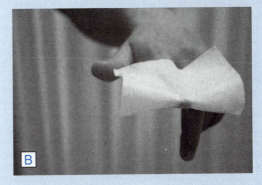

Figure 11-5

STEP 4: Press the sides of the material firmly together against the finger (Fig. 11–5C).

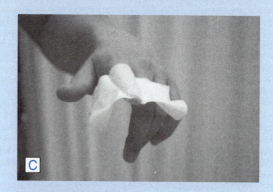

STEP 5: Cut the excess material away from the sides, leaving enough of the material to maintain adherence (Fig. 11–5D).

Option: *Place circular strips of ½ inch non-elastic tape around the distal, middle, and/or proximal phalanx with moderate roll tension to anchor the material or tape* ◀▶ *(Fig. 11–5E). End the tape strips on the dorsal finger to prevent unraveling.*

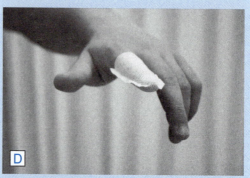

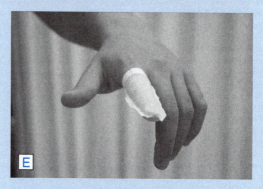

Figure 11-5 *continued*

THUMB SPICA Figures 11–6, 11–7, 11–8, 11–9, 11–10, 11–11

The thumb spica technique is simply a figure-of-eight pattern encircling the wrist and thumb. This technique provides mild to moderate support and limits excessive abduction and extension at the MCP joint. Use the technique when preventing and treating thumb sprains and postdislocation and postfracture injuries. The spica may be applied with varying amounts of support and in combination with sports-specific gloves. This section first illustrates the basic spica and then explores several variations and discusses the addition of other materials for maximum support.

Basic Thumb Spica

▶ **Purpose:** The basic thumb spica provides mild to moderate support and lessens excessive range of motion of the MCP joint when preventing and treating thumb sprains and postdislocation and postfracture injuries (Fig. 11–6).

▶ **Materials:**
  • ½ inch or 1 inch non-elastic tape or 1 inch elastic tape, 1½ inch non-elastic tape
  Option:
  • Pre-tape material or self-adherent wrap

▶ **Position of the individual**: Sitting on a taping table or bench with the hand and thumb in a neutral position.

▶ **Preparation:** Apply the basic thumb spica directly to the skin.

Option: *Apply one to three layers of pre-tape material around the wrist and continue around the thumb, returning to the wrist to lessen irritation* ◀▶ *. Self-adherent wrap may be applied in place of pre-tape material. Apply the self-adherent wrap as illustrated in Step 1 below (Fig. 11–6A).*

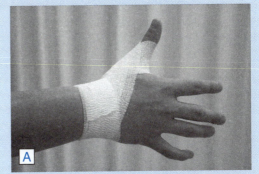

▶ **Application:**
STEP 1: Anchor a strip of ½ inch or 1 inch non-elastic or 1 inch elastic tape to the medial dorsal surface of the wrist and continue in a medial-to-lateral direction around the wrist to the MCP joint of the thumb with moderate roll tension (Fig. 11–6B).

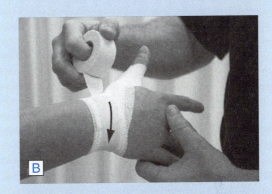

STEP 2: Next, cross the MCP joint, encircle the thumb, and anchor on the dorsal surface of the wrist with moderate roll tension (Fig. 11–6C). Slightly adduct and flex the thumb while applying the anchor dorsally.

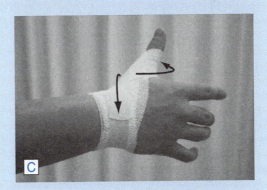

STEP 3: Apply two to three strips of ½ inch or 1 inch non-elastic or 1 inch elastic tape in the medial-to-lateral pattern with moderate roll tension, overlapping each by ¼ to ½ of the tape width in a proximal direction on the thumb (Fig. 11–6D). The tape strips should remain proximal to the **interphalangeal joint (IP)** of the thumb. The strips may be applied in an individual or continuous figure-of-eight pattern around the thumb and wrist.

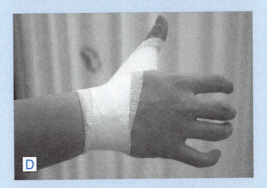

Figure 11-6

STEP 4: Anchor the strips with moderate roll tension around the wrist with 1 inch or 1½ inch non-elastic tape in a circular pattern ◀▶ (Fig. 11–6E).

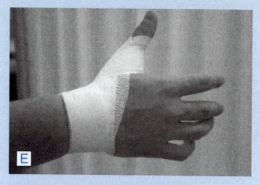

Figure 11-6 *continued*

Variation One

▸ **Purpose:** This variation to the basic thumb spica technique provides mild to moderate support and limits range of motion of the MCP joint without restricting wrist motion (Fig. 11–7).

▸ **Materials:**
  • 1 inch non-elastic or elastic tape

▸ **Position of the individual**: Sitting on a taping table or bench with the hand and thumb in a neutral position.

▸ **Preparation:** Apply variation one directly to the skin or over pre-tape material or self-adherent wrap.

▸ **Application:**
  STEP 1: Using 1 inch non-elastic or elastic tape, anchor on the medial dorsal aspect of the hand and continue in a medial-to-lateral pattern around the hand with moderate roll tension, remaining distal to the ulnar styloid process (Fig. 11–7A).

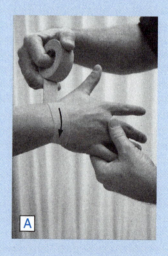

STEP 2: At the MCP joint, encircle the thumb, and finish on the dorsal hand with moderate roll tension (Fig. 11–7B).

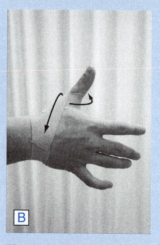

Figure 11-7

STEP 3: Apply two to three additional spica strips with 1 inch non-elastic or elastic tape in an individual or continuous medial-to-lateral pattern, overlapping by ¼ to ½ of the tape width in a proximal direction on the thumb, and anchor on the dorsal hand (Fig. 11–7C). The tape should remain distal to the ulnar styloid process and proximal to the IP joint of the thumb. Do not apply anchor strips around the wrist.

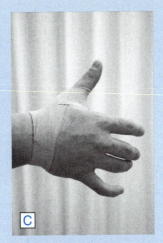

> **...IF/THEN...**
>
> **IF** a thumb spica technique is required for a basketball player to support the MCP joint following a sprain, **THEN** consider using variation one, which will provide support and allow for full range of motion at the wrist with minimal effect on wrist flexion and extension during shooting.

Figure 11-7 *continued*

Variation Two

▶ **Purpose:** Another variation to provide mild to moderate support and limit range of motion of the MCP joint involves applying individual strips in a loop fashion around the joint (Fig. 11–8).

▶ **Materials:**
  • 1 inch non-elastic or elastic tape, 1½ inch non-elastic tape

▶ **Position of the individual**: Sitting on a taping table or bench with the hand and thumb in a neutral position.

▶ **Preparation:** Apply variation two directly to the skin or over pre-tape material or self-adherent wrap.

▶ **Application:**

STEP 1: Using 1 inch non-elastic or elastic tape, anchor a strip on the medial palmar aspect of the wrist, proceed over the MCP joint in a lateral direction, encircle the thumb, and finish the strip just proximal to the first carpometacarpal joint with moderate roll tension 𝄢 (Fig. 11–8A).

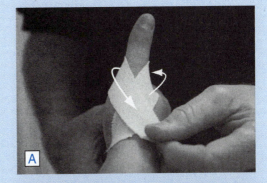

STEP 2: Next, apply a strip from the medial dorsal aspect of the wrist, continue over the MCP joint in a medial direction, encircle the thumb, and finish just proximal to the first carpometacarpal joint with moderate roll tension (Fig. 11–8B).

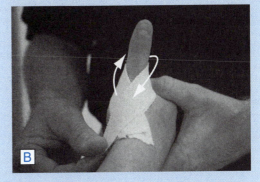

Figure 11-8

STEP 3: Repeat the two strips two to three times in a proximal overlapping pattern on the thumb (Figs. 11–8C and 11–8D). The tape should remain proximal to the IP joint of the thumb.

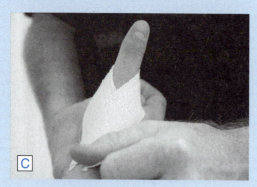

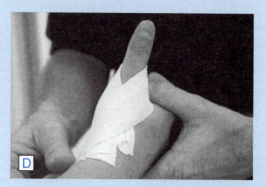

STEP 4: Anchor the strips with 1 inch or 1½ inch non-elastic tape around the wrist in a circular pattern with moderate roll tension 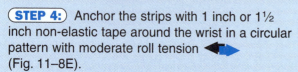 (Fig. 11–8E).

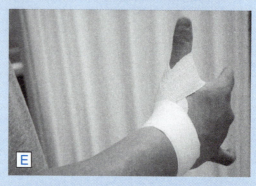

Figure 11-8 *continued*

Helpful Hint: As the strip encircles the thumb, crease or pinch the tape, if needed, to allow for smooth contact on the palmar surface of the thumb.

Variation Three

▶ **Purpose:** When an injury requires greater support and reduction in range of motion of the MCP joint, use circular wrist taping technique one (see Fig. 10–1) or two (see Fig. 10–2), or the following additional materials with the thumb spica taping (Fig. 11–9).

▶ **Materials:**
- 1 inch non-elastic and elastic tape, 1½ inch non-elastic tape, pre-tape material or self-adherent wrap, discarded tape core from 2 inch or 3 inch tape, taping scissors

▶ **Position of the individual:** Sitting on a taping table or bench with the hand and thumb in a neutral position.

▶ **Preparation:** Apply two to three layers of pre-tape material or self-adherent wrap as shown with the basic spica technique. Cut a discarded tape core to form a teardrop shape slightly larger than the MCP joint (Fig. 11–9A). Round the corners to prevent sharp edges and irritation to the skin.

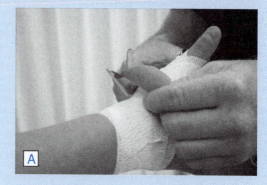

Figure 11-9

▶ **Application:**

STEP 1: Apply two to three basic spica strips with 1 inch elastic tape in an individual or continuous pattern with moderate roll tension (Fig. 11–9B).

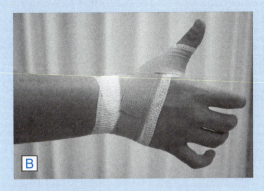

B

STEP 2: Place the tape core over the MCP joint (Fig. 11–9C) and apply three to five additional 1 inch elastic tape basic spica strips with moderate roll tension in an overlapping fashion (Fig. 11–9D). The tape should remain proximal to the IP joint of the thumb.

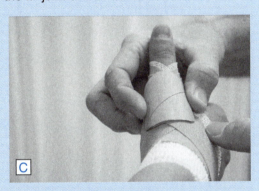

C

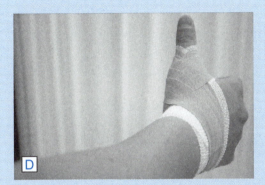

D

STEP 3: Apply one to two 1 inch non-elastic tape basic spica strips with moderate roll tension and anchor at the wrist (Fig. 11–9E).

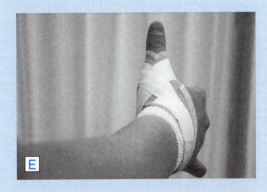

E

STEP 4: Anchor the strips with 1 inch or 1½ inch non-elastic tape around the wrist in a circular pattern with moderate roll tension ◀▬▶ (Fig. 11–9F).

STEP 5: Apply circular wrist taping technique one or two for additional support.

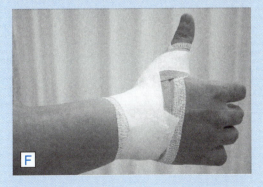

F

Figure 11-9 *continued*

Variation Four

▶ **Purpose:** Mold and apply thermoplastic material to provide additional support to the MCP joint. The size and shape of the material depend on the amount of support needed. Use a small teardrop shape to cover the MCP joint and provide moderate support, or use a custom-made brace to encase the entire thumb for moderate support and immobilization (Fig. 11–10).

▶ **Materials:**
• Paper, felt tip pen, thermoplastic material, a heating source, 1 inch non-elastic and elastic tape, 1½ inch non-elastic tape, pre-tape material or self-adherent wrap, 2 inch width moleskin, taping scissors

▶ **Position of the individual**: Sitting on a taping table or bench with the hand and thumb in a neutral position.

▶ **Preparation:** Apply two to three layers of pre-tape material or self-adherent wrap as shown with the basic spica technique. Design the teardrop shape with a paper pattern (see Fig. 1–14). Cut, mold, and shape the thermoplastic material on the MCP joint (Fig. 11–10A). Apply 2 inch moleskin to the inside surface of the material to prevent irritation.

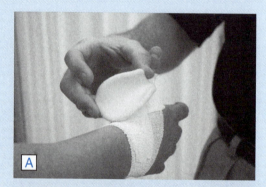

A

▶ **Application:**
STEP 1: Apply two to three 1 inch elastic tape basic spica strips with moderate roll tension (Fig. 11–10B). Apply the strips in an individual or continuous pattern.

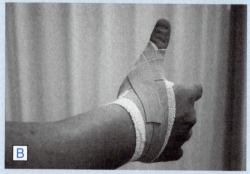

B

STEP 2: Next, place the thermoplastic material over the MCP joint and secure with three to four overlapping 1 inch elastic tape basic spica strips with moderate roll tension (Fig. 11–10C). The tape should remain proximal to the IP joint of the thumb. One to two 1 inch non-elastic tape basic spica strips may be applied to provide additional support.

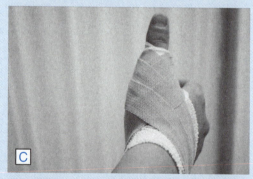

C

STEP 3: Anchor at the wrist in a circular pattern with 1 inch or 1½ inch non-elastic tape with moderate roll tension (Fig. 11–10D).

STEP 4: Circular wrist taping technique one or two may be applied for additional support.

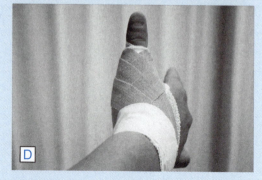

D

Figure 11-10

Anchor Technique to the Basic Spica and Spica Variations

- **Purpose:** Place horizontal strips over the MCP joint following application of the basic spica or spica variations to aid in limiting joint motion (Fig. 11–11). Consider using these strips to provide additional support to the MCP joint when preventing and treating sprains and postdislocation and postfracture injuries.

- **Materials:**
  - ½ inch or 1 inch non-elastic tape

- **Position of the individual:** Sitting on a taping table or bench with the hand and thumb in a neutral position.

- **Preparation:** Apply the basic thumb spica or one of the spica variations.

- **Application:**
  STEP 1: Begin proximal to the MCP joint and apply individual ½ inch or 1 inch non-elastic tape strips with equal tension inward toward the joint. Anchor each strip on the medial and lateral aspect of the thumb. Continue the strips in a distal direction, overlapping by ½ of the tape width, and finish just distal to the MCP joint (Figs. 11–11A and 11–11B).

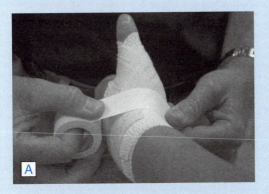

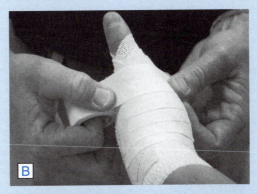

STEP 2: Anchor the horizontal strips by placing a ½ inch non-elastic tape strip with mild to moderate roll tension from the wrist, under and around the thumb, and finish on the wrist (Fig. 11–11C).

STEP 3: Apply a 1 inch non-elastic tape circular anchor around the wrist with moderate roll tension ◀▶.

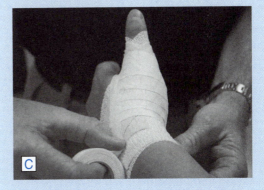

Figure 11-11

...IF/THEN...

IF applying a thumb spica taping technique for football linemen to prevent and treat MCP injuries, **THEN** consider using variation three, four, and/or the anchor technique; these techniques provide additional support and can be applied under or over gloves.

THUMB SPICA SEMIRIGID CAST Figure 11–12

▶ **Purpose:** A semirigid cast provides maximum support and limits MCP joint and wrist range of motion (Fig. 11–12). This cast should be applied only by qualified health-care professionals. Use the thumb spica cast when treating sprains and postdislocation and postfracture injuries upon a return to activity. The cast may be applied and reused, if removed carefully following athletic or work activities.

▶ **Materials:**
- 2 inch or 3 inch semirigid cast tape, gloves, water, self-adherent wrap, ⅛ inch foam or felt, 2 inch elastic tape, taping scissors

Option:
- Thermoplastic material, a heating source

▶ **Position of the individual:** Sitting on a taping table or bench with the hand, thumb, and wrist in the position to be immobilized (as indicated by a physician) and the fingers in abduction.

▶ **Preparation:** Pad bony prominences with ⅛ inch foam or felt to lessen the occurrence of irritation.

▶ **Application:**

STEP 1: Apply two to three layers of self-adherent wrap to the hand, thumb, and wrist with mild to moderate roll tension with the basic thumb spica and figure-of-eight patterns (see Figs. 10–3 and 11–12A).

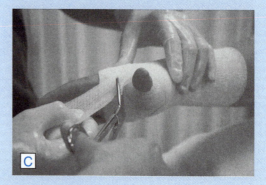

STEP 2: Using 2 inch or 3 inch semirigid cast tape, anchor on the medial dorsal surface of the wrist and proceed around the wrist and thumb with the basic thumb spica pattern with moderate roll tension (Fig. 11–12B).

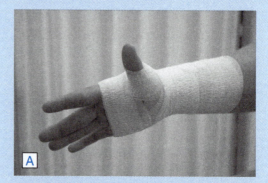

STEP 3: Depending on the individual's size, the cast tape may need to be cut partially when encircling the thumb (Fig. 11–12C).

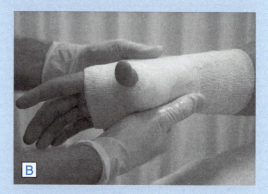

Figure 11-12

STEP 4: Alternate the basic thumb spica pattern with figures-of-eight involving the hand and wrist with moderate roll tension, overlapping the tape by ⅓ to ½ of its width (Fig. 11–12D). The cast tape should remain proximal to the MCP joints of fingers two through five, and proximal to the IP joint of the thumb.

Option: *Incorporate thermoplastic material over the MCP joint for additional support (Figs. 11–12E and 11–21F).*

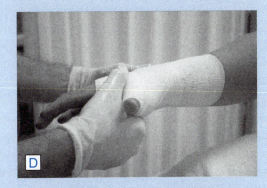

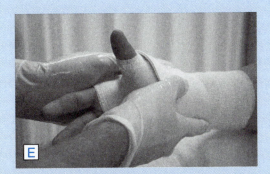

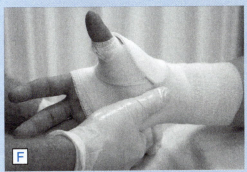

STEP 5: Finish the tape on the dorsal wrist and smooth and mold the cast with the hands (see Fig. 11–12G).

STEP 6: Prior to athletic practices and competitions, cover the semirigid cast with high-density, closed-cell foam of at least ½ inch thickness (Figs. 11–21A and 11–21B).

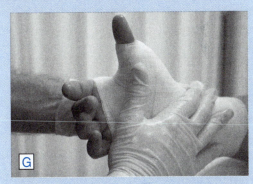

STEP 7: Following athletic or work activities, remove the cast with taping scissors along the ulnar aspect of the cast (Fig. 11–12H). Allow the inside of the cast to dry overnight by removing the self-adherent wrap and placing the cast in a well-ventilated area.

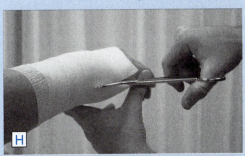

STEP 8: When reusing, apply two to three layers of self-adherent wrap to the hand, thumb, and wrist with the basic thumb spica and figure-of-eight patterns with moderate roll tension. Replace the cast on the hand, thumb, and wrist, and anchor with 2 inch elastic tape or self-adherent wrap in a circular pattern with moderate roll tension (Fig. 11–12I).

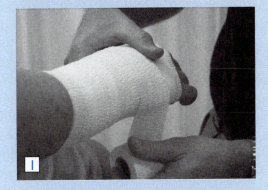

Figure 11-12 *continued*

Helpful Hint: Place a tongue depressor inside the cast to spread the edges apart to ensure drying.

FIGURE-OF-EIGHT TAPE

▸ **Purpose:** The figure-of-eight tape technique is used to anchor padding when preventing and treating hand injuries and conditions.
  • Use the figure-of-eight tape technique (see Fig. 10–3) to attach protective padding when preventing and treating contusions.

Critical Thinking Question 2

During the middle of the season, an offensive tackle on the football team sustains a third degree right thumb ulnar collateral ligament sprain during practice. After surgery, he is immobilized in a rigid thumb spica cast for 3 weeks. Rehabilitation begins, after which he and the surgeon begin to discuss his return to activity. The surgeon allows a return to activity based on the following guidelines:

  Postop weeks 3 to 6: Return to practice and competition at postop week 4 with maximum support, splinting of the right thumb during nonathletic activities.

  Postop weeks 6 to 8: Continue athletic participation with moderate support, discontinue nonathletic activity splinting.

▸ **Question: What techniques can be used in this situation?**

Wrapping Techniques

Wrapping techniques provide compression and support when treating hand, finger, and thumb injuries and conditions. Elastic wraps, tapes, and sleeves, self-adherent wrap, and conforming gauze are used to control swelling following injury. Wraps may be used to anchor protective padding following soft tissue and bone injuries.

COMPRESSION WRAP Figure 11–13

▸ **Purpose:** Compression wraps for the hand, fingers, and thumb reduce mild, moderate, or severe swelling and inflammation by applying mechanical pressure[9] when treating contusions, sprains, dislocations, and tendon ruptures (Fig. 11–13).

▸ **Materials:**
  • 2 inch, 3 inch, or 4 inch width by 5 yard length elastic wrap, metal clips, 1½ inch non-elastic or 2 inch elastic tape, ⅛ inch or ¼ inch foam or felt, taping scissors
  • 1 inch elastic tape or self-adherent wrap for the fingers or thumb

  Options:
  • Self-adherent wrap
  • ¼ inch or ½ inch open-cell foam

▸ **Position of the individual:** Sitting on a taping table or bench with the wrist and hand in a pain-free position and the fingers in abduction.

▸ **Preparation:** Place ⅛ inch or ¼ inch foam or felt over the inflamed area directly on the skin.

▶ **Application:**

STEP 1: For the hand, anchor the elastic wrap on the dorsal hand in a circular pattern just distal to the MCP joints of fingers two through five and apply the hand compression wrap technique (see Figs. 10–11 and 11–13A).

Options: *Self-adherent wrap may be used if an elastic wrap is not available. Place a ¼ inch or ½ inch open-cell foam pad over the dorsal hand for additional compression to assist in venous return (see Fig. 11–22A). Apply the pad directly on the skin and cover with the hand compression wrap.*

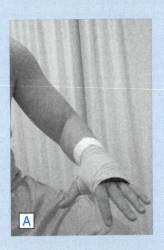

STEP 2: For the fingers or thumb, apply 1 inch elastic tape or self-adherent wrap in a distal-to-proximal circular pattern over the finger or thumb (Fig. 11–13B). Apply pressure greatest at the distal end and less toward the proximal end. The tip of the finger or thumb should remain exposed to monitor circulation. No additional anchor is required.

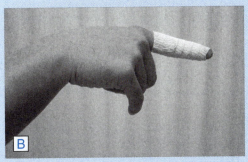

Figure 11-13

FINGER SLEEVES Figure 11–14

▶ **Purpose:** Use finger sleeves to provide mild to moderate support and compression to the PIP joint to reduce mild, moderate, or severe swelling when treating sprains (Fig. 11–14). The benefit of this technique is that the individual can apply the sleeve without assistance following application instruction.

▶ **Design:**
  • The sleeves are available off-the-shelf in predetermined sizes based on finger width measurements.
  • Most sleeves are constructed of nylon and elastic materials in a single or double finger design.
  • The design of the sleeve allows for normal range of motion at the DIP joint.

▶ **Materials:**
  • Off-the-shelf single or double finger sleeve

▶ **Position of the individual:** Sitting on a taping table or bench with the hand, fingers, and thumb in a pain-free position.

▶ **Preparation:** Apply the finger sleeve directly to the skin.

▶ **Application:**

STEP 1: To apply, pull the sleeve onto the finger(s) in a proximal direction (Fig. 11–14A). No anchors are necessary; the sleeves are washable and reusable.

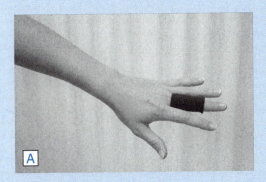

Figure 11-14

BOXER'S WRAP Figure 11–15

▶ **Purpose:** The boxer's wrap is similar to the technique used under boxing gloves to pad the hands, but this technique can also be used as a compression wrap for the hand to lessen mild, moderate, or severe swelling following contusions (Fig. 11–15). The boxer's wrap padding technique is discussed later in the chapter.

▶ **Materials:**
• 1½ inch, 2 inch, or 3 inch conforming gauze or self-adherent wrap, 1½ inch non-elastic tape, ⅛ inch or ¼ inch foam or felt, taping scissors

Option:
• ¼ inch or ½ inch open-cell foam

▶ **Position of the individual:** Sitting on a taping table or bench with the hand, fingers, and thumb in a pain-free position and the fingers in abduction.

▶ **Preparation:** Apply the boxer's wrap directly to the skin. Eighth of an inch or ¼ inch foam or felt may be placed over the inflamed area to assist in venous return.

▶ **Application:**

STEP 1: Anchor 1½ inch, 2 inch, or 3 inch conforming gauze or self-adherent wrap to the medial dorsal surface of the wrist and continue in a medial-to-lateral direction around the wrist with moderate roll tension (Fig. 11–15A).

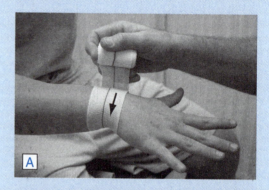

STEP 2: From the wrist, continue to apply the conforming gauze or wrap across the dorsal aspect of the hand, encircle the second finger at the MCP joint with mild to moderate roll tension, then return and anchor around the wrist in a medial-to-lateral direction (Fig. 11–15B).

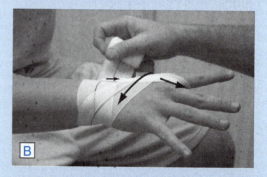

STEP 3: Continue with this pattern, encircling the third, fourth, and fifth fingers at the MCP joint (Fig. 11–15C). Instruct the individual to flex the fingers actively and make a fist when making each pass around the MCP joint ⚖.

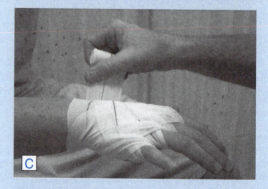

Figure 11-15

STEP 4: Next, apply two to three basic thumb spicas with moderate roll tension with the gauze or wrap (Fig. 11–15D).

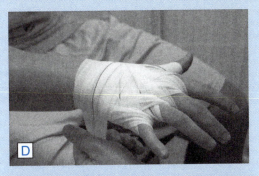

STEP 5: Cover the remainder of the hand with overlapping figures-of-eight (see Fig. 10–3) with moderate roll tension and anchor loosely around the wrist (Fig. 11–15E).

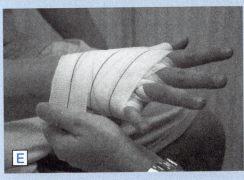

STEP 6: Apply a loose anchor of 1½ inch non-elastic tape around the wrist 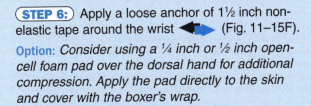 (Fig. 11–15F).

Option: *Consider using a ¼ inch or ½ inch open-cell foam pad over the dorsal hand for additional compression. Apply the pad directly to the skin and cover with the boxer's wrap.*

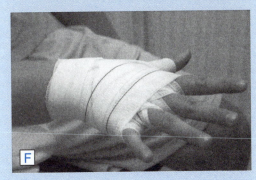

Figure 11-15 *continued*

Helpful Hint: Allowing active flexion of the fingers during the technique will prevent the conforming gauze or self-adherent wrap from constricting and abrading the finger web space.

FIGURE-OF-EIGHT WRAP

▶ **Purpose:** The figure-of-eight wrap technique anchors protective padding when preventing and treating hand injuries and conditions.
• Use the technique illustrated in Chapter 10 (see Fig. 10–12) to attach pads when preventing and treating contusions.

...IF/THEN...

IF using a finger or thumb brace and swelling and inflammation are present, **THEN** apply a compression wrap technique underneath the brace to control swelling and inflammation; note, a larger size brace may be needed to ensure proper fit, support, and immobilization of the finger and/or thumb.

Bracing Techniques

Bracing techniques are used to prevent and treat acute and chronic finger and thumb injuries and conditions. The off-the-shelf and custom-made designs provide compression, support, and immobilization and lessen range of motion. Several other braces used for hand and thumb injuries and conditions were discussed in Chapter 10.

FINGER BRACES Figure 11–16

▶ **Purpose:** Use off-the-shelf and custom-made finger braces to provide support and immobilization and to limit range of motion when treating sprains, fractures, and tendon ruptures (Fig. 11–16). Three methods are illustrated in the application of the technique. Choose a technique according to individual preferences and available supplies.

Off-the-Shelf

▶ **Purpose:** Several off-the-shelf bracing techniques may be used to treat an extensor digitorum tendon rupture and/or distal phalanx fracture. Use these braces to provide moderate support and complete immobilization of the DIP joint. Regardless of which design is used, rotate the brace from the dorsal to the palmar aspect of the finger frequently to prevent maceration of the skin. While the brace is being changed, maintain extension in the DIP joint.

○ DETAILS

Depending on the finger and hand involvement in activities, these braces are commonly used to provide support for athletes in sports such as baseball, basketball, fencing, field hockey, football, gymnastics, ice hockey, lacrosse, soccer, skiing, softball, track and field, volleyball, and wrestling, but can also be useful with work and casual activities.

▶ **Design:**
- Off-the-shelf braces are available in predetermined sizes in universal fit designs based on finger length or width measurements.
- Some designs are constructed of plastic materials and are purchased in kits that include several types of braces in pre-molded sizes.
- These braces allow for minimal adjustments in fit and are attached to the finger with non-elastic or elastic tape.
- Other braces are constructed of malleable aluminum with an open-cell foam pad lining.
- These designs allow for adjustments in fit depending on the injury and condition.
- Attach these braces to the finger with non-elastic or elastic tape.

▶ **Materials:**
- ½ inch non-elastic or 1 inch non-elastic or elastic tape, taping scissors

▶ **Position of the individual:** Sitting on a taping table or bench with the hand, fingers, and thumb in a neutral position. Place the DIP joint of the involved finger or thumb in extension.

▶ **Preparation:** Apply the off-the-shelf braces directly to the skin.

▶ **Application:**

(**STEP 1:**) Apply some designs by placing the brace over the tip of the finger or thumb. Continue to apply the brace in a distal-to-proximal direction until the tip of the finger or thumb contacts the distal end of the brace. The finger or thumb should fit snugly in the brace (Fig. 11–16A).

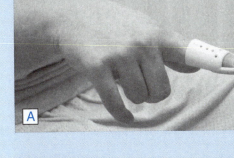

(**STEP 2:**) Anchor with mild to moderate roll tension at the proximal end of the brace with ½ inch non-elastic or 1 inch non-elastic or elastic tape. Apply three to five continuous circular patterns ◀▬▶ (Fig. 11–16B). End the pattern on the dorsal aspect of the finger or thumb to prevent unraveling.

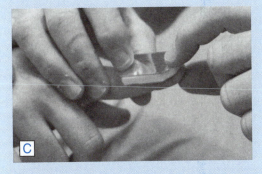

(**STEP 3:**) Other designs require cutting and molding to the finger or thumb. Cut a piece of the aluminum material in a length from proximal to the DIP joint to the distal end of the finger or thumb (Fig. 11–16C).

(**STEP 4:**) Trim any sharp edges of the aluminum to prevent injury and slightly bend the distal end of the brace to maintain full extension in the DIP joint.

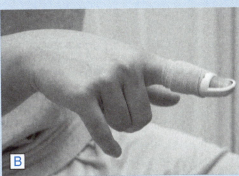

(**STEP 5:**) Apply the brace on the dorsal or palmar aspect of the finger or thumb. Anchor ½ inch or 1 inch non-elastic tape on top of the brace and apply three to five continuous circular patterns around the distal and proximal ends of the brace with moderate roll tension, positioning the DIP joint in full extension ◀▬▶ (Fig. 11–16D). End the pattern on the dorsal aspect of the finger or thumb.

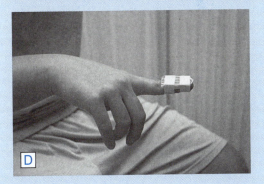

Figure 11-16

Custom-Made

▶ **Purpose:** Use thermoplastic material to custom fit a brace to the finger and thumb when off-the-shelf designs are not available. This technique also provides moderate support and immobilization of the DIP joint when treating an extensor digitorum tendon rupture and/or distal phalanx fracture. Rotate these braces from the dorsal to the palmar aspect of the finger or thumb frequently to prevent maceration of the skin. Maintain extension in the DIP joint while the brace is being changed. Custom-made finger and thumb designs are useful in athletic, work, and casual activities and are reusable.

Hand, Fingers, and Thumb

▶ **Materials:**
- Paper, felt tip pen, thermoplastic material, ⅛ inch foam or 2 inch width moleskin, a heating source, ½ inch or 1 inch non-elastic tape, taping scissors

▶ **Position of the individual:** Sitting on a taping table or bench with the hand, fingers, and thumb in a neutral position. Place the DIP joint of the involved finger or thumb in extension.

▶ **Preparation:** Design the brace with a paper pattern or estimate the width and length from proximal to the DIP joint to the distal end of the finger or thumb. Heat the thermoplastic material. Apply this technique directly to the skin.

▶ **Application:**

STEP 1: Fit and mold the material to the dorsal or palmar aspect of the finger or thumb (Fig. 11–16E). Remember to keep the DIP joint in full extension during fitting. Trim the edges of the material to prevent injury and cover the inside surface with ⅛ inch foam or 2 inch moleskin for comfort.

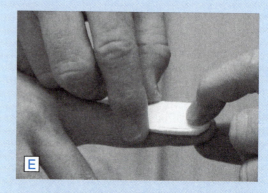

STEP 2: Apply the brace on the dorsal or palmar finger or thumb. Place ½ inch or 1 inch non-elastic tape on top of the brace and anchor with three to five continuous circular patterns around the distal and proximal ends of the brace with moderate roll tension ◀▶ (Fig. 11–16F). Maintain full extension of the DIP joint. End the pattern on the dorsal aspect of the finger or thumb.

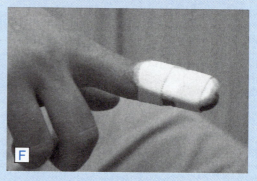

Figure 11-16 *continued*

◯ **DETAILS**─────────────

Whether off-the-shelf or custom-made braces are worn on the dorsal or on the palmar aspect of the fingers and thumb depends on the activities of the individual. Away from sport or work, apply the brace on the palmar aspect. During sport or work activity, **tactile** sensation of the finger and thumb is often required. In these cases, apply the brace to the dorsal aspect of the finger and thumb.

Spencer Splint

▶ **Purpose:** Use the Spencer splint when treating MCP joint sprains to provide mild to moderate support and limit abduction, flexion, and extension at the MCP joint.[3] This brace can be used with individuals who require use of the distal portion of their fingers for gripping or athletic skills, such as shooting a basketball.

▶ **Materials:**
- Paper, felt tip pen, thermoplastic material, a heating source, taping scissors

Option:
- ½ inch non-elastic or 1 inch elastic tape

▶ **Position of the individual:** Sitting on a taping table or bench with the hand, fingers, and thumb in a neutral position.

▶ **Preparation:** Design the brace with a paper pattern.

▶ **Application:**

STEP 1: Using paper, make a pattern from the palmar surface of the second finger, continue around the finger in a medial-to-lateral direction to the dorsal surface of the second finger (Fig. 11–16G), then through the web space to the palmar surface of the third finger (Fig. 11–16H), and around the third finger in a lateral-to-medial direction to the dorsal surface of the finger to form an S-shaped pattern (Fig. 11–16I). The width of the pattern should not limit MCP or PIP joint flexion excessively. A pattern may be made for fingers three and four or four and five.

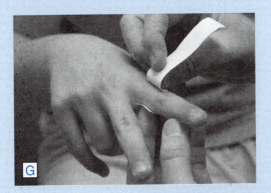

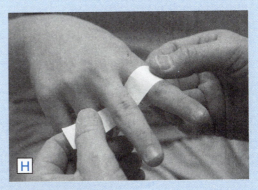

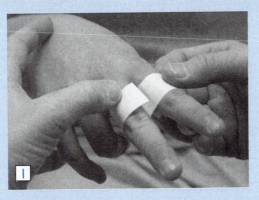

STEP 2: Using the pattern, cut the thermoplastic material, then heat. While molding the material, allow the individual to position the fingers and hand in a pain-free, **functional position** (Fig. 11–16J). Trim the brace if necessary to prevent excessive restriction of range of motion at the MCP and PIP joints.

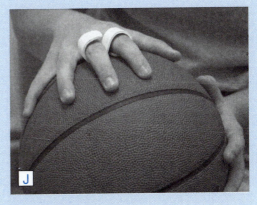

Figure 11-16 *continued*

STEP 3: Place the brace over the fingertips and pull in a proximal direction until the brace is positioned on the proximal fingers (Fig. 11–16K). Reuse the brace; the individual can apply it daily.

Option: *Apply ½ inch non-elastic or 1 inch elastic tape over the brace with mild roll tension to supplement stability* ◀▬▶ *(Fig. 11–16L).*

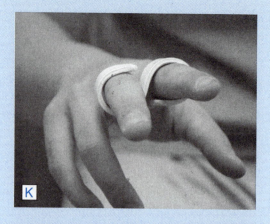

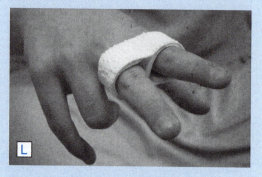

Figure 11-16 *continued*

THUMB BRACES Figure 11–17

▶ **Purpose:** Off-the-shelf and custom-made thumb braces provide compression and support, and limit range of motion during athletic and work activities. These braces also provide compression and immobilization when away from these activities. Use these designs when preventing and treating sprains, dislocations, and postfracture injuries of the thumb (Fig. 11–17). Note that some rehabilitative wrist braces, discussed in Chapter 10, can be used to treat thumb sprains, dislocations, and postfracture injuries. Two methods are illustrated in the application of the thumb bracing technique. Choose according to individual preferences and available supplies.

Off-the-Shelf

▶ **Purpose:** Use off-the-shelf thumb braces to provide compression, moderate support, and immobilization and lessen range of motion when preventing and treating sprains, dislocations, and postfracture injuries.

○ **DETAILS**──────────────

Thumb braces are commonly used to provide support for athletes in sports such as baseball, basketball, fencing, field hockey, football, ice hockey, lacrosse, soccer, skiing, softball, track and field, and wrestling, but can also be useful with work and casual activities.

▶ **Design:**
  • Off-the-shelf universal fit and right or left style designs are available in predetermined sizes corresponding to wrist circumference measurements. Some designs are available in universal sizes.

- Most braces are constructed of a neoprene or nylon material outer shell with a Lycra or cotton material lining.
- Some designs have a dorsal thermoplastic bar incorporated into the outer shell to prevent excessive abduction and extension at the MCP joint.
- Other braces have a viscoelastic polymer pad incorporated into the lining to absorb shock and lessen stress.
- The braces are attached to the thumb and wrist with polyethylene or neoprene straps with Velcro or D-ring closures and allow for adjustments in fit.
- Most of the designs cover the wrist, but allow for unrestricted motion of the hand and fingers two through five.

▸ **Position of the individual:** Sitting on a taping table or bench with the hand and thumb in a neutral position.

▸ **Preparation:** Apply the brace directly to the skin or over sports-specific gloves.

Follow the manufacturer's application instructions during the application of the braces. The following guidelines apply to most designs.

▸ **Application:**

STEP 1: Loosen the straps and unfold the brace.

STEP 2: Place the brace onto the involved thumb (Fig. 11–17A). Wrap the outer shell around the thumb and/or wrist. If a bar is included, align the bar on the dorsal thumb.

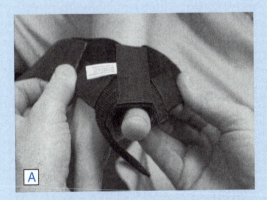

STEP 3: The application of straps will depend on the specific brace design. Apply most by pulling the strap(s) at the wrist tight and anchoring with Velcro (Fig. 11–17B). When using other designs, wrap the strap around the thumb and/or wrist and anchor.

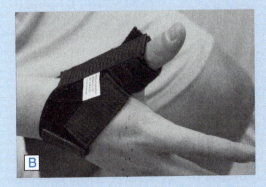

Figure 11-17

Custom-Made

▸ **Purpose:** Construct custom-made designs from thermoplastic material to provide moderate support and immobilization and to limit range of motion to prevent and treat sprains, dislocations, and postfracture injuries. These braces are commonly used when off-the-shelf designs are not available and when away from athletic and work activities, but can be useful in athletic, work, and casual activities as well.

▸ **Materials:**
- Paper, felt tip pen, thermoplastic material, ⅛ inch foam or 2 inch width moleskin, a heating source, an elastic wrap, taping scissors

▶ **Position of the individual**: Sitting on a taping table or bench with the hand and thumb in a neutral position.

▶ **Preparation:** Design the brace with a paper pattern from just distal to the IP joint, over the MCP joint, and partially incorporate the wrist. Mold and shape the material to the thumb and wrist. Apply ⅛ inch foam or 2 inch moleskin to the inside surface of the brace to prevent irritation.

　　Apply the brace directly to the skin or over pre-tape material or self-adherent wrap (see Fig. 11–6A). These braces may also be applied over sports-specific gloves.

▶ **Application:**
　STEP 1: Position the brace on the thumb (Fig. 11–17C).

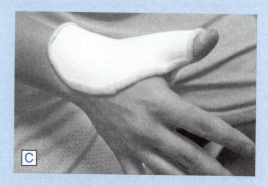

　STEP 2: Anchor the brace with the basic thumb spica pattern with a 2 inch or 3 inch width by 5 yard length elastic wrap, self-adherent wrap, or pre-tape material and 1 inch elastic tape with mild to moderate roll tension (Fig. 11–17D).

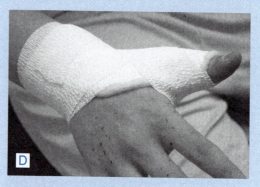

Figure 11-17 *continued*

Critical Thinking Question 3

The center fielder on the baseball team suffers a first degree left thumb ulnar collateral ligament sprain while sliding into second base. Following an evaluation, your team physician allows the center fielder to return to play if protected from further injury. The athlete bats and throws right handed and is the leading base stealer on the team.

▶ **Question: What techniques are appropriate for practices and competitions?**

...IF/THEN...

IF a finger brace is required for support in individuals participating in athletic and/or work activities, **THEN** consider constructing a custom-made design; these designs are lower-profile, and dorsal application will allow for tactile sensation.

Padding Techniques

A variety of materials provide shock absorption, protection, and compression and lessen stress for hand, finger, and thumb injuries and conditions. Felt, foam, and viscoelastic polymers may prevent and treat contusions, sprains, and blisters. Use thermoplastic material and foam to cover rigid and semirigid casts when returning to activity postoperatively or while treating sprains, dislocations, and fractures.

BOXER'S WRAP Figure 11–18

▶ **Purpose:** As previously discussed, padding is the traditional use of the boxer's wrap. The wrap is effective in absorbing shock and preventing contusions and in treating injuries to the hand that require padding (Fig. 11–18). The wrap is useful for athletes in baseball, field hockey, football, gymnastics, ice hockey, lacrosse, softball, and boxing activities and can also be used in combination with sports-specific gloves.

▶ **Materials:**
- 1½ inch, 2 inch, or 3 inch conforming gauze or self-adherent wrap, 1½ inch non-elastic tape, 2 inch elastic tape, 1 inch non-elastic or elastic tape, ⅛ inch or ¼ inch foam or felt, taping scissors

▶ **Position of the individual:** Sitting on a taping table or bench with the hand, fingers, and thumb in a neutral position and the fingers in abduction.

▶ **Preparation:** Cut a piece of ⅛ inch or ¼ inch foam or felt to cover the dorsal area of the hand. The pad may be extended to cover the MCP joints of the fingers. Apply the boxer's wrap directly to the skin or over a sports-specific glove.

▶ **Application:**

STEP 1: Place the pad on the dorsal hand directly on the skin (Fig. 11–18A). Anchor 1½ inch, 2 inch, or 3 inch conforming gauze or self-adherent wrap to the medial dorsal surface of the wrist and apply the boxer's wrap with moderate roll tension as illustrated in Figure 11–15.

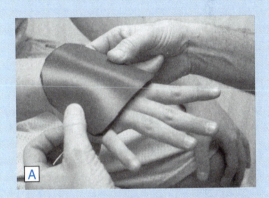

STEP 2: Using 2 inch elastic tape or self-adherent wrap, cover the boxer's wrap with two to four additional figure-of-eight (see Fig. 10–3) patterns with moderate roll tension (Fig. 11–18B).

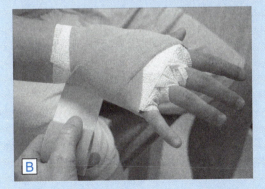

Figure 11-18

STEP 3: Apply two to three basic thumb spicas with 1 inch non-elastic or elastic tape with moderate roll tension for additional support (Fig. 11–18C).

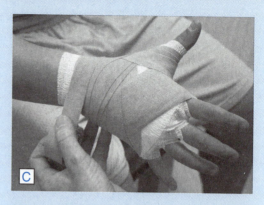

STEP 4: Finish the figure-of-eight and/or basic thumb spica on the dorsal wrist and anchor with 1½ inch non-elastic tape in a circular pattern with moderate roll tension ◀▬▶ (Fig. 11–18D). Note that circular wrist taping technique one (see Fig. 10–1) or two (see Fig. 10–2) may also be applied for additional support.

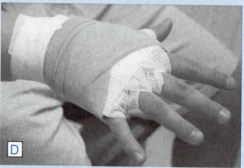

Figure 11-18 *continued*

VISCOELASTIC POLYMERS Figure 11–19

▶ **Purpose:** Use viscoelastic polymers to absorb shock and lessen friction and pressure when preventing and treating hand, finger, and thumb contusions and blisters (Fig. 11–19).

▶ **Materials:**
  • Off-the-shelf elastic finger and thumb sleeves fully lined with padding, elastic finger and thumb caps lined with padding, elastic hand sleeves lined with padding, pads (Fig. 11–19A), adhesive gauze material

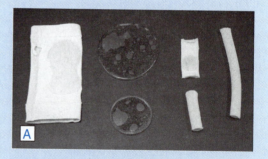

Figure 11-19A Viscoelastic polymers. (Left) Hand and wrist sleeve. (Middle) Pads. (Right) Finger sleeves and cap.

▶ **Position of the individual:** Sitting on a taping table or bench with the hand, fingers, and thumb in a neutral position.

▶ **Preparation:** Cut and fit the appropriate size of the material to overlap the injured area on the hand, fingers, and thumb.

▶ **Application:**
  STEP 1: Pull the sleeve and cap designs onto the hand, finger, and thumb, in a distal-to-proximal direction, directly to the skin (Fig. 11–19B). No adherent tape spray or anchor strips are required.

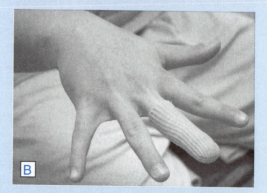

Figure 11-19

STEP 2: Place the pads directly onto the skin and anchor with elastic material or the figure-of-eight taping or wrapping (see Fig. 10–12) technique (Fig. 11–19C). Clean and reuse the sleeves, caps, and pads.

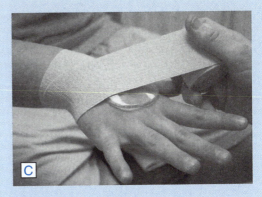

Figure 11-19 *continued*

FOAM PADS Figure 11–20

▶ **Purpose:** Several padding designs constructed of foam absorb shock and lessen friction and pressure when preventing and treating finger and thumb contusions and blisters (Fig. 11–20).

▶ **Materials:**
- Off-the-shelf finger and thumb sleeves in predetermined sizes based on finger width measurements
- Off-the-shelf foam donuts or ¼ inch or ½ inch closed-cell foam, taping scissors

▶ **Position of the individual:** Sitting on a taping table or bench with the hand, fingers, and thumb in a neutral position.

▶ **Preparation:** Cut and fit the appropriate size of the sleeve to overlap the injured area on the fingers and thumb. Quarter inch or ½ inch closed-cell foam may be cut to the appropriate size donut. If the area of the finger or thumb allows, cut the pad to extend in all directions ½ inch to 1 inch beyond the painful area. Mark the painful area on the piece of foam and cut out the area with taping scissors, creating a hole (Fig. 11–20A). This hole protects the painful area from stress and/or impact.

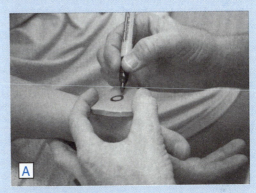

▶ **Application:**
STEP 1: Pull the sleeve onto the finger and thumb directly on the skin, in a distal-to-proximal pattern (Fig. 11–20B). No adherent tape spray or anchor strips are required. Clean and reuse the sleeves.

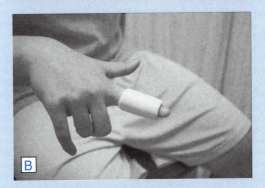

Figure 11-20

STEP 2: Prevent and treat contusions of the thumb and palm associated with athletic bat usage by using an off-the-shelf or custom-made closed-cell foam donut. Place the donut over the thumb directly on the skin under a sports-specific glove or use over a glove (Fig. 11–20C). The donut does not require anchors and is reusable.

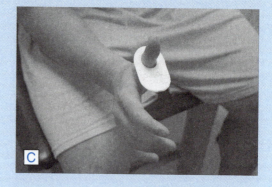

STEP 3: The off-the-shelf or custom-made pad may be attached to the thumb using the basic thumb spica technique with 1 inch elastic tape or self-adherent wrap with moderate roll tension (Fig. 11–20D).

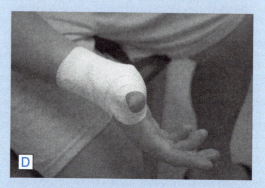

Figure 11-20 *continued*

CAST PADDING Figure 11–21

- **Purpose:** The cast padding technique protects the injured athlete and her or his competitors from injury, and meets NCAA[6] and NFHS[7] rules (Fig. 11–21). Use the technique to cover rigid or semirigid casts when an athlete returns to activity following a fracture, dislocation, or surgery.

- **Materials:**
  - Paper, felt tip pen, high-density, closed-cell foam or similar material of at least ½ inch thickness, 2 inch or 3 inch width by 5 yard length elastic wrap, 2 inch or 3 inch elastic tape and pre-tape material, or self-adherent wrap, taping scissors

  Option:
  - Thermoplastic material, a heating source

- **Position of the individual:** Sitting on a taping table or bench with the hand, fingers, and thumb in the casted position.

- **Preparation:** Begin by making a paper pattern of the cast area to be padded. Trace the pattern onto high-density, closed-cell foam or similar material, then cut the pad with taping scissors.

- **Application:**
  STEP 1: Apply the foam over the cast and anchor with a 2 inch or 3 inch elastic wrap, 2 inch or 3 inch elastic tape, or self-adherent wrap with moderate roll tension ◀▶ (Fig. 11–21A). If using elastic tape, first cover the padding with pre-tape material to protect the foam from the tape adhesive ◀▶. The foam may be reused.

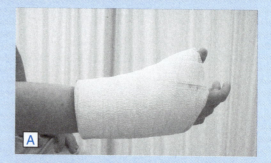

Figure 11-21

Option: *A decision to cover the fingers and/or thumb for additional protection depends on the activity and sport-position of the individual. For example, a semirigid, padded hood of thermoplastic material may be constructed for a football lineman to protect the fingers and thumb from injury (Fig. 11–21B). Because a linebacker or defensive back requires use of his fingers and thumb, a hood may not be necessary. Pad the hood with appropriate material to meet NCAA[6] and NFHS[7] rules.*

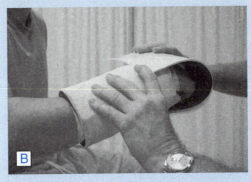

Figure 11-21 *continued*

COMPRESSION WRAP PAD Figure 11–22

- **Purpose:** The compression wrap pad assists in reducing mild, moderate, or severe swelling when treating hand contusions and sprains (Fig. 11–22).

- **Materials:**
  - ¼ inch or ½ inch open-cell foam, taping scissors

- **Position of the individual:** Sitting on a taping table or bench with the wrist and hand in a pain-free position and the fingers in abduction.

- **Preparation:** Apply the pad directly to the skin.

- **Application:**
  STEP 1: Extend the pad across the dorsal hand, from the first MCP joint to the fifth MCP joint, and from the MCP joints to the wrist (Fig. 11–22A).

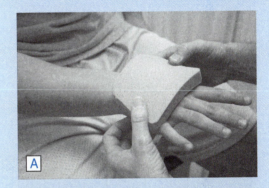

  STEP 2: Place the pad over the dorsal hand and apply the compression (see Fig. 10–11) or boxer's wrap technique (see Fig. 11–15) (Fig. 11–22B).

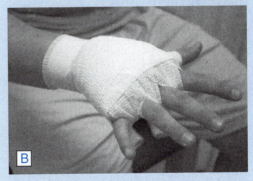

Figure 11-22

Critical Thinking Question 4

At the company picnic, the data entry department won the horseshoe tossing contest, but several members sustained blisters to the palmar aspect of the fingertips. On Monday, the members could not use their keyboards because of pain and pressure associated with the blisters.

- **Question: How can you manage this situation?**

MANDATORY PADDING

Protective equipment for the hand, fingers, and thumb is required in several high school and intercollegiate sports. The NCAA[6] and the NFHS[7] require that athletes participating in fencing, field hockey, ice hockey, and lacrosse wear protective padding during all practices and competitions. The majority of these pads are purchased off-the-shelf; the designs are constructed for specific sports and positions. Chapter 13 will provide a more in-depth discussion of these padding techniques.

> **...IF/THEN...**
>
> **IF** padding of the dorsal hand and support of the first MCP joint are needed for a field hockey or lacrosse athlete following injury, **THEN** consider applying the boxer's wrap with foam or felt over the dorsal hand and a tape core or thermoplastic material over the first MCP joint for additional padding or support, respectively.

CASE STUDY

After the first few days of football practice in August, Dennis Maccini, a freshman defensive lineman at Buckley University, enters the Athletic Training Room with complaints of pain and swelling in his hands and fingers. While taking his history, Scott Garro, ATC, discovers several interesting facts. The practice drills and equipment used with the drills are different from what Dennis used in high school. One particular drill requires each lineman to strike and move around a sled, mimicking a pass rush technique. Dennis estimates that he goes through 15 repetitions of the drill each practice. The sled has appropriate padding, but Dennis does not wear gloves or any other type of protection on his hands and fingers during practice. He continued to participate because he did not want to miss any repetitions or practices. After a complete evaluation, Scott determines Dennis has sustained contusions on the dorsal aspect of his hands and over the PIP joints of fingers two, three, and four, as a result of striking the sled. He has moderate dorsal swelling, no crepitus or deformity, no ligamentous laxity, no neurological symptoms, bilateral strength and range of motion, but moderate pain with finger flexion and extension. That evening, the team physician stops by the Athletic Training Room and evaluates Dennis. The physician agrees with Scott that Dennis has sustained contusions to the dorsal aspect of his hands and PIP joints of the fingers and clears him to return to practice pending a reduction of the swelling. The team physician and Scott discuss an appropriate therapeutic plan that includes padding of the area.

In managing the case, Dennis has been receiving cryotherapy and electrical muscle stimulation for anti-inflammatory effects. What compression wrap technique could you use to help reduce swelling in his hands and fingers? Dennis will wear the wraps in a continuous fashion except during treatments. Which preventive padding techniques for his hands and fingers can be worn upon his return to practice? Dennis wants to continue to be able to have full functional use of his hands and fingers without restrictions in range of motion. Dennis also does not want to wear padded gloves, because he feels they will restrict him in tackling.

WRAP UP

- Shear, compression, and rotational forces and extreme ranges of motion can cause injury to the hand, fingers, and thumb.
- The buddy and "X" taping techniques support the collateral ligaments of the fingers.
- Elastic material and tape provide protection when treating hand, finger, and thumb wounds.
- The thumb spica taping technique and its variations and the thumb spica semirigid cast technique provide support to the MCP joint when

preventing and treating sprains and postdislocation and postfracture injuries.

- The figure-of-eight taping and wrapping techniques are used to attach protective padding to the hand.
- The hand, finger sleeves, and boxer's wrap compression techniques reduce swelling and inflammation following injury.
- Off-the-shelf and custom-made brace designs support, limit range of motion, and immobilize the fingers and thumb following sprains, dislocations, fractures, and tendon ruptures.
- The boxer's wrap, viscoelastic polymers, foam, and compression wrap padding techniques provide shock absorption, protection, and compression.
- Cast padding techniques provide protection for both injured athletes and opponents, and are required by NCAA and NFHS rules.
- The NCAA and NFHS require that protective equipment be used for the hand, fingers, and thumb in several sports.

■ WEB REFERENCES

American Society for Surgery of the Hand
http://www.assh.org/
· This site allows you to search for information on hand injuries and conditions.

HandUniversity
http://www.handuniversity.com/index.html
· This Web site allows access to information regarding the prevention, treatment, and rehabilitation of hand, fingers, and thumb injuries and conditions.

Medline plus Health Information
http://www.nlm.nih.gov/medlineplus/handinjuriesanddisorders.html
· This site provides general hand, finger, and thumb information on a variety of injuries and treatments.

■ REFERENCES

1. Anderson, MK, Hall, SJ, and Martin, M: Sports Injury Management, ed 2. Lippincott Williams & Wilkins, Philadelphia, 2000.
2. Cahalan, TD, and Cooney, WP: Biomechanics. In Jobe, FW, Pink, MM, Glousman, RE, Kvitne, RS, and Zemel, NP (eds): Operative Techniques in Upper Extremity Sports Injuries. Mosby, St. Louis, 1996.
3. Conway, DP, and Decker, AS: "Spencer splint" for metacarpophalangeal joint sprains. J Athl Train 28:268–269, 1993.
4. Houglum, PA: Therapeutic Exercise for Athletic Injuries. Human Kinetics, Champaign, 2001.
5. Laimore, JR, and Enger, WD: Serious, often subtle finger injuries. Phys Sportsmed 26:57, 1997.
6. National Collegiate Athletic Association, http://www.ncaa.org/library/sports_sciences/sports_med_ handbook/2003-04/2003-04_sports_med_ handbook.pdf, Sports medicine handbook, 2003–2004.
7. National Federation of State High School Associations. 2004 Field Hockey Rules Book. Indianapolis, IN: National Federation of State High School Associations, 2004.
8. Prentice, WE: Arnheim's Principles of Athletic Training, ed 11. McGraw-Hill, Boston, 2003.
9. Prentice, WE: Rehabilitation Techniques, ed 3. McGraw-Hill, Boston, 1999.
10. Wilson, RL, and Hazen, J: Management of joint injuries and intraarticular fractures of the hand. In Hunter, JM, Mackin, EJ, and Callahan, AD (eds): Rehabilitation of the Hand: Surgery and Therapy, ed 4. Mosby, St. Louis, 1995.

Thorax, Abdomen, and Spine

LEARNING OBJECTIVES

1. Discuss common injuries and conditions that occur to the thorax, abdomen, and spine.
2. Demonstrate the application of taping, wrapping, bracing, and padding techniques for the thorax, abdomen, and spine when preventing, treating, and rehabilitating injuries.
3. Discuss and demonstrate appropriate taping, wrapping, bracing, and padding techniques for the thorax, abdomen, and spine within a therapeutic exercise program.

INJURIES AND CONDITIONS

Injury to the thorax, abdomen, and spine can occur during athletic and work activities as a result of acute and chronic forces, stresses, and movements. Direct and indirect forces can cause a contusion, fracture, and costochondral injury. Sprains can occur from excessive range of motion and strains from violent muscular movements and overload. Participation in collision and contact sports can predispose an athlete to brachial plexus and overuse injuries and conditions of the spine, all of which are caused by excessive range of motion, compression, and repetitive stress. Common injuries to the thorax, abdomen, and spine include:

- Contusions
- Sprains
- Strains
- Fractures
- Costochondral injury
- Brachial plexus injury
- Overuse injuries and conditions

Contusions

Contusions to the thorax, abdomen, and spine are the result of compressive forces and can involve soft tissue and/or bony structures. A direct blow to the thorax can result in a contusion of the ribs, breasts, and intercostal musculature (Illustrations 12–1 and 12–2). Although uncommon in sports, a severe fall on the ground or on rigid sports equipment may cause a **pulmonary contusion.** A pulmonary contusion can result, for example, as a football wide receiver is violently tackled by two defensive backs on the sideline, landing on unattended helmets near the benches. Contusions of the abdominal wall and kidneys are more likely to occur in collision sports and in sport and work activities with high-speed projectiles.[24] Because of external exposure, the male genitalia can be injured by direct forces. These injuries are common in athletic activities as a result of being kicked or struck with equipment. The thoracic and/or lumbar areas are

susceptible to contusions in sports that do not require protective padding over these areas, such as basketball, football, and soccer. A contusion to the right lumbar musculature can occur, for instance, when a right-handed football quarterback releases the ball for a pass downfield and is struck with an opponent's shoulder pads (Illustration 12–3). A fall from a height or a direct blow can lead to a contusion of the coccyx (Illustration 12–4).

Sprains

Sprains to the thorax, cervical, and lumbar areas are caused by excessive range of motion and repetitive stress. Repetitive movement of the female breasts during athletic activities, as a result of inadequate support, can cause injury to the **Cooper's ligament.** Forced neck flexion, extension, or rotation or sudden contractions of the musculature can lead to a cervical facet joint sprain. A cervical sprain can result, for example, when a wrestler's head and neck are held in a headlock by an opponent during a takedown, causing flexion and rotation of the neck. Abnormal positioning of the head and neck over an extended length of time can also result in a sprain or acute torticollis **(wryneck).** Sleeping with a too-small or too-large pillow and sitting hunched over a desk reading without support for the head and neck can lead to a sprain or acute torticollis.

Activities that require maximal trunk flexion and/or extension with rotation can cause injury to the lumbar facet joints. Injury can occur acutely or through repetitive stress. Improper lifting and/or spotting techniques during the performance of a power clean or dead lift strengthening exercise can cause a lumbar sprain. Sacroiliac joint sprains are the result of acute and chronic stresses associated with trunk bending, twisting, and lifting activities. Repetitive downhill running and unilateral sport movements such as punting, hurdling, and swinging a golf club may also contribute to a sacroiliac joint sprain.

Strains

Overload and sudden, violent movements can cause strains to the musculature of the thorax, abdomen, and

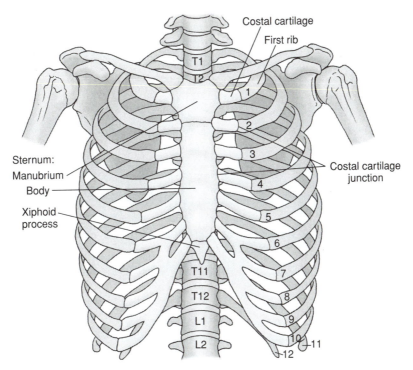

Costal cartilage
First rib
T1
T2
1
2
3
Costal cartilage junction
4
Sternum:
Manubrium
5
Body
6
Xiphoid process
T11
7
T12
8
L1
9
L2
10 — 11
— 12

Illustration 12-1   Bones of the anterior thorax.

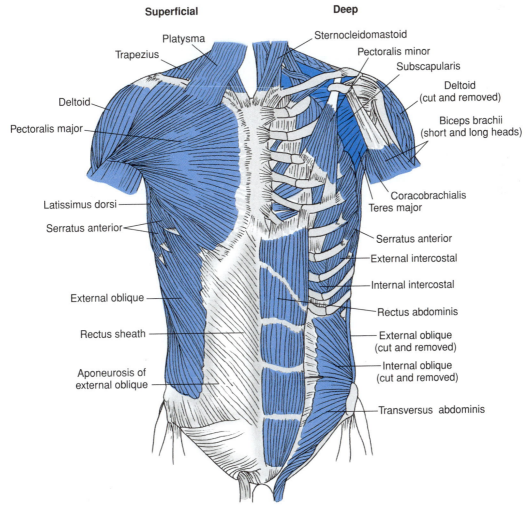

Superficial	Deep

Platysma
Trapezius
Sternocleidomastoid
Pectoralis minor
Subscapularis
Deltoid
Deltoid (cut and removed)
Pectoralis major
Biceps brachii (short and long heads)
Latissimus dorsi
Coracobrachialis
Teres major
Serratus anterior
Serratus anterior
External intercostal
Internal intercostal
External oblique
Rectus abdominis
Rectus sheath
External oblique (cut and removed)
Internal oblique (cut and removed)
Aponeurosis of external oblique
Transversus abdominis

Illustration 12-2   Superficial and deep muscles of the anterior thorax and abdomen.

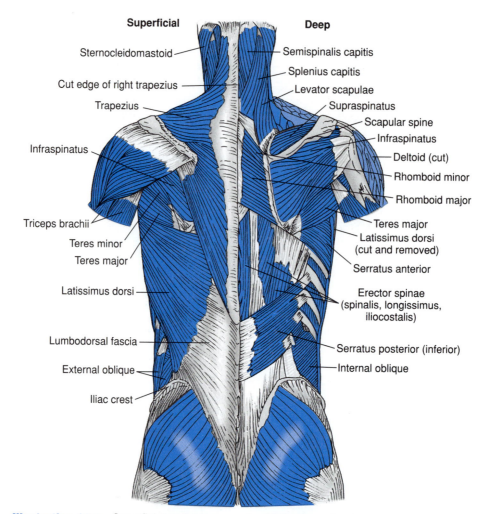

Superficial

- Sternocleidomastoid
- Cut edge of right trapezius
- Trapezius
- Infraspinatus
- Triceps brachii
- Teres minor
- Teres major
- Latissimus dorsi
- Lumbodorsal fascia
- External oblique
- Iliac crest

Deep

- Semispinalis capitis
- Splenius capitis
- Levator scapulae
- Supraspinatus
- Scapular spine
- Infraspinatus
- Deltoid (cut)
- Rhomboid minor
- Rhomboid major
- Teres major
- Latissimus dorsi (cut and removed)
- Serratus anterior
- Erector spinae (spinalis, longissimus, iliocostalis)
- Serratus posterior (inferior)
- Internal oblique

Illustration 12-3   Superficial and deep muscles of the posterior thorax and spine.

spine. Overload during active contractions and violent deceleration movements can result in a pectoralis major strain. A strain can occur as a recreational weight lifter increases the amount of weight on the bar during a maximum repetition bench press, resulting in overload of the musculature. Sudden rotation of the trunk can cause injury to the intercostal musculature. Injury to the rectus abdominis can be the result of sudden, violent trunk movements, such as twisting and extension. For example, a strain can occur as a tennis player serves a ball with an overhand motion during a match, resulting in excessive extension and twisting of the thorax. Cervical strains occur in the same manner as sprains—forced range of motion and sudden muscular contractions; both injuries can occur simultaneously.[1] Trunk extension, in combination with overload stresses and structural abnormalities of the spine, can result in a lumbar strain. Repetitive lifting, **scoliosis,** and **lumbar lordosis** can contribute to a lumbar strain.

Fractures

Fractures to the thorax, abdomen, and spine may involve the ribs, vertebrae, and coccyx. Rib fractures can result

from direct and indirect forces. A direct force to the anterior or posterior thorax severe enough to produce a fracture commonly injures the lateral and anterior portions of the fifth through the ninth ribs.[22,33] A lateral/anterior fracture to the sixth and seventh ribs can occur, for example, as a baseball base runner attempts to score with the catcher blocking home plate, colliding with the catcher's helmet and face guard. Acute and stress fractures can also be the result of indirect forces, such as violent muscular contractions, repetitive stresses, and training errors. Stress fractures have been reported among athletes participating in crew, golf, volleyball, tennis, gymnastics, and baseball.[9,10] Faulty sport movements and excessive training without appropriate recovery, causing abnormal muscular contractions and overload, can also result in a rib fracture. Forced hyperflexion, hyperextension, and axial loading of the head and neck can cause a cervical vertebral fracture. For example, a fracture can occur as a defensive football player, leading with his head and helmet (spearing), tackles a ball carrier, causing hyperflexion or hyperextension and axial loading of the head and neck. A coccygeal fracture can occur through direct forces resulting from a fall from a height. A fracture can

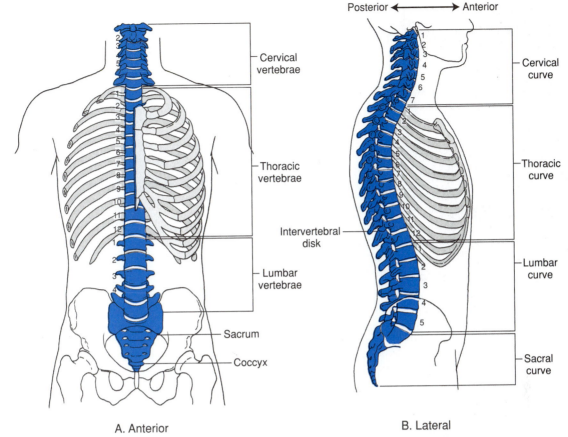

Posterior ◄────► Anterior

- Cervical vertebrae
- Thoracic vertebrae
- Intervertebral disk
- Lumbar vertebrae
- Sacrum
- Coccyx

- Cervical curve
- Thoracic curve
- Lumbar curve
- Sacral curve

A. Anterior   B. Lateral

Illustration 12-4   Vertebral column demonstrating the normal spinal curves.

result as a gymnast dismounts from the uneven bars and loses her balance, landing violently on the mat in a seated position.

Costochondral Injury

Separation of the costal cartilage junction at the sternum and/or ribs is commonly referred to as a dislocation or sprain (see Illustration 12–1). Mechanisms of injury include direct compression, violent trunk rotation, and forced flexion and horizontal abduction of the arm. For example, a dislocation or sprain can occur as a basketball guard dives toward a loose ball and is struck and turned to the left by an opponent, causing trunk rotation and direct compression upon contact with the court.

Brachial Plexus Injury

A stretch/traction or compression brachial plexus injury (**burner** or **stinger**) is most common among athletes participating in football.[15,27,28,31,36] A stretch/traction injury can occur when the shoulder and clavicle are depressed and the neck is forced into lateral flexion in the opposite direction away from the involved brachial plexus. A stretch/traction injury to the left brachial plexus can result as a football fullback is tackled and falls directly onto his left shoulder with his neck forced into lateral flexion to

the right. Violent external rotation, abduction, and extension of the arm can also result in a stretch/traction injury. A compression injury to the brachial plexus can be the result of neck extension and rotation to the same side or with impingement of the brachial plexus between the scapula and football shoulder pads at **Erb's point** on the anterior lateral neck. At this location, the brachial plexus is most superficial. A compression injury of the right brachial plexus can occur, for example, as a football linebacker, using his right shoulder, tackles a tight end, causing impingement of the brachial plexus between the scapula and shoulder pads.

Overuse

Overuse injuries and conditions are caused by excessive, repetitive stress to the spine. Repetitive axial loading and compression, common in collision and contact sports, may result in a herniation of a cervical disk (see Illustration 12–4). Over time, repetitive diving, tackling and blocking in football, and heading the ball in soccer can contribute to degenerative changes of the cervical disk. Congenital weakness and hyperextension of the trunk associated with gymnastics, weightlifting, blocking in football, and spiking in volleyball can cause a defect in the pars interarticularis.[8,16,30] This defect, referred to as spondylolysis, typically leads to a unilateral stress fracture of the pars interarticularis. With continued stress, the defect can progress bilaterally. The resulting condition, spondylolisthesis, allows movement of the superior verte-bra on the vertebra beneath it. Spondylolysis and spondy-lolisthesis can occur at any point along the spine, but are most common at the L4–L5 or L5–S1 levels.[19,23]

Taping Techniques

Taping techniqes are used when preventing and treating wounds, contusions, and fractures of the thorax, abdomen, and spine to anchor wound dressings and off-the-shelf and custom-made protective padding. Padding techniques are illustrated in the Padding section.

ELASTIC MATERIAL Figure 12–1

▶ **Purpose:** Elastic material is used to cover wound dressings and attach off-the-shelf and custom-made pads to the thorax, abdomen, and spine when treating wounds and contusions (Fig. 12–1). The thin profile and great adhesive strength of the material lessen dressing and pad migration and allow for unrestricted range of motion.

▶ **Materials:**
• Adhesive gauze material, taping scissors

▶ **Position of the individual:** Sitting on a taping table or bench or standing with the arms at the side of the body.

▶ **Preparation:** Apply adhesive gauze material directly to the skin; use without adherent tape spray. Apply the sterile wound dressing or pad.

▶ **Application:**

STEP 1: Cut a piece of the adhesive gauze material to extend ½ inch to 1 inch beyond the dressing or pad. Round all corners of the material to prevent the edges from rolling upon contact with clothing.

STEP 2: Apply the gauze material over the dressing or pad and smooth to the skin with the hands (Fig. 12–1).

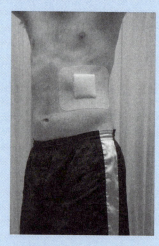

Figure 12-1

CONTUSION/FRACTURE TAPE Figure 12–2

▶ **Purpose:** Use the contusion/fracture technique to absorb shock while anchoring off-the-shelf and custom-made pads to the thorax, abdomen, and spine to prevent and treat contusions and fractures (Fig. 12–2).

▶ **Materials:**
• 2 inch or 3 inch heavyweight elastic tape, adherent tape spray, taping scissors

▶ **Position of the individual:** Sitting on a taping table or bench or standing with the arms at the side of the body.

▶ **Preparation:** Apply the contusion/fracture technique directly to the skin.

▶ **Application:**

STEP 1: Apply adherent tape spray over the pad area and 4–6 inches beyond, over the thorax, abdomen, and/or spine. Allow the spray to dry.

STEP 2: Cut several strips of 2 inch or 3 inch heavyweight elastic tape in lengths that will cover the pad and extend 4–6 inches beyond the pad on the two sides. Place the pad over the injured area.

STEP 3: Next, apply the tape strips with the release-stretch-release sequence illustrated in Chapter 8 (see Fig. 8–2) ◀▶ . Overlap the strips by ½ the width of the tape and apply enough strips to cover the majority of the pad (Fig. 12–2).

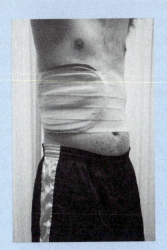

Figure 12-2

Wrapping Techniques

Use wrapping techniques to provide compression, support, and immobilization and to anchor protective padding to the thorax, abdomen, and spine when preventing and treating soft tissue and bony injuries. Elastic wraps and tapes are used following contusions, strains, and fractures to lessen swelling and to provide immobilization following rib fractures. These materials may also be used to anchor protective padding to prevent and treat contusions, strains, fractures, and costochondral injury.

○ **DETAILS**

Exercise care when applying elastic wraps to the thorax, abdomen, and spine. Follow application guidelines and have the individual inhale during application to prevent restriction of chest movement and normal breathing patterns. Should the individual experience shortness of breath, an increase in pain, and/or have a rapid, weak pulse or low blood pressure,[1] suspect a serious thoracic injury/condition and immediately refer the individual to a physician.

COMPRESSION WRAP TECHNIQUE ONE Figure 12–3

▶ **Purpose:** This compression wrap technique is used to control mild to moderate swelling when treating thorax, abdomen, and spine contusions, strains, and fractures (Fig. 12–3).

▶ **Materials:**
• 6 inch width by 5 yard length elastic wrap, metal clips, 2 inch or 3 inch elastic tape, taping scissors

Option:
• ¼ inch or ½ inch foam or felt

▶ **Position of the individual:** Standing on the ground with the arms placed on the lateral hips in a relaxed position.

▸ **Preparation:** To lessen migration, apply adherent tape spray, tape strips, or anchors directly to the skin (see Fig. 1–7).

Option: *Place a ¼ inch or ½ inch foam or felt pad over the inflamed area directly on the skin to provide additional compression and assist in controlling swelling.*

▸ **Application:**

STEP 1: Anchor the end of the wrap directly to the skin just inferior to the injured area and encircle the anchor ◀▬▶ (Fig. 12–3A).

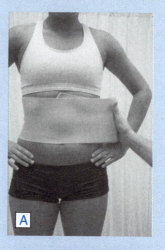

A

STEP 2: Continue to apply the wrap in a spiral pattern in a distal-to-proximal direction, overlapping by ⅓ to ½ of the wrap width (Fig. 12–3B). Apply the greatest amount of roll tension distally and lessen tension as the wrap continues proximally.

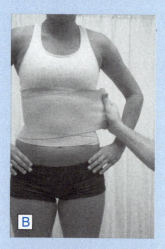

B

STEP 3: Anchor the wrap with Velcro, metal clips, or loosely applied 2 inch or 3 inch elastic tape ◀▬▶ (Fig. 12–3C). Finish and anchor the tape over the circular tape pattern on the anterior thorax or abdomen to ensure adherence and prevent unraveling and irritation.

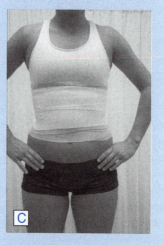

C

Figure 12-3

COMPRESSION WRAP TECHNIQUE TWO Figure 12–4

▶ **Purpose:** Use this compression wrap technique to lessen moderate to severe swelling when treating thorax, abdomen, and spine contusions, strains, and fractures (Fig. 12–4). This technique is particularly useful when treating swelling in large individuals because of the length of the wrap.

▶ **Materials:**
- 4 inch or 6 inch width by 10 yard length elastic wrap, metal clips, 2 inch or 3 inch elastic tape, taping scissors

Option:
- ¼ inch or ½ inch foam or felt

▶ **Position of the individual:** Standing on the ground with the arms placed on the lateral hips in a relaxed position.

▶ **Preparation:** To lessen migration, apply adherent tape spray, tape strips, or anchors directly to the skin.

Option: *Place a ¼ inch or ½ inch foam or felt pad over the inflamed area directly on the skin to assist in venous return.*

▶ **Application:**
STEP 1: Anchor the extended end of the wrap directly to the skin just inferior to the inflamed area and encircle the anchor ◀▶ .

STEP 2: Apply the wrap in a distal-to-proximal direction in a spiral pattern with the greatest roll tension distally and over the inflamed area, lessening as the wrap continues proximally (Fig. 12–4A). Overlap the wrap by ⅓ to ½ of its width.

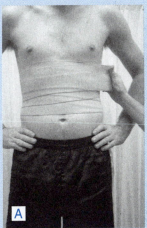

STEP 3: Anchor the wrap with Velcro, metal clips, or loosely applied 2 inch or 3 inch elastic tape ◀▶ (Fig. 12–4B).

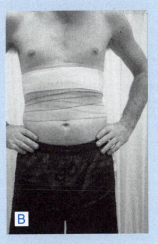

Figure 12-4

CIRCULAR WRAP Figure 12–5

▶ **Purpose:** The circular wrap technique is used to provide compression and mild support and to anchor off-the-shelf and custom-made pads to the thorax, abdomen, and spine when preventing and treating contusions, strains, fractures, and costochondral injury (Fig. 12–5).

▶ **Materials:**
  • 6 inch width by 5 yard length or 4 inch or 6 inch width by 10 yard length elastic wrap, 2 inch or 3 inch elastic tape, taping scissors

▶ **Position of the individual:** Standing on the ground with the arms placed on the lateral hips in a relaxed position.

▶ **Preparation:** To lessen migration, apply adherent tape spray, tape strips, or anchors directly to the skin.

▶ **Application:**
  STEP 1: To provide support, anchor the end of the wrap directly on the skin and encircle the anchor ◀▬▶ (Fig. 12–5A).

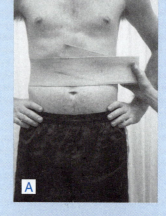

A

STEP 2: Continue to apply the wrap in a circular pattern, overlapping by ⅓ to ½ of its width, with moderate roll tension in a distal-to-proximal or proximal-to-distal direction (Fig. 12–5B).

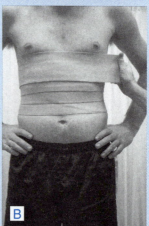

B

STEP 3: To attach a pad, place the pad over the injured area directly on the skin (Fig. 12–5C). Apply the circular wrap technique, leaving a small area in the middle of the pad exposed (Fig. 12–5D).

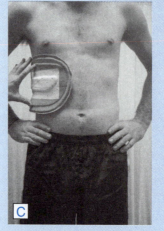

C

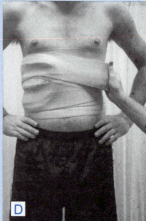

D

Figure 12-5

STEP 4: Anchor the support wrap with Velcro or 2 inch or 3 inch elastic tape with moderate roll tension with two to three continuous circular patterns ◀▬▶. Finish the tape on the circular tape pattern over the anterior thorax or abdomen to prevent unraveling.

STEP 5: When using a pad, anchor 2 inch or 3 inch elastic tape directly on the exposed portion of the pad (Fig. 12–5E) and apply one to two continuous circular patterns over the wrap and pad with moderate roll tension ◀▬▶ (Fig. 12–5F). Anchor the tape over the anterior thorax or abdomen on the circular tape pattern. To prevent migration, a distal circular strip of elastic tape may be applied with distal-to-proximal tension; anchor the loose end on the circular tape pattern. No additional anchors are needed.

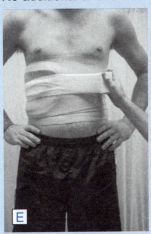 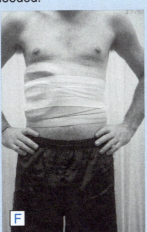

Figure 12-5   *continued*

SWATHE RIB WRAP Figure 12–6

▸ **Purpose:** Use the swathe rib wrap technique in the immediate treatment of rib fractures to provide mild to moderate support and immobilization to the ribs by anchoring the arm to the involved side of the thorax, immobilizing the shoulder (Fig. 12–6).

▸ **Materials:**
   • 4 inch or 6 inch width by 10 yard length elastic wrap, metal clips, 2 inch or 3 inch elastic tape, taping scissors

▸ **Position of the individual:** Sitting or standing with the **ipsilateral** arm (arm on the same side of the injured ribs) across the abdomen with the elbow in 90° of flexion.

▸ **Preparation:** Apply the swathe wrap directly to the skin or over a shirt.

▸ **Application:**
   STEP 1: Anchor the extended end of the wrap over the hand of the ipsilateral arm (Fig. 12–6A).

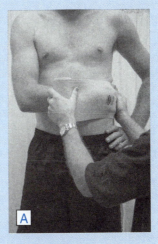

Figure 12-6

Thorax, Abdomen, and Spine

STEP 2: Continue to apply the wrap in a lateral-to-medial direction over the wrist, forearm, and elbow, encircle the trunk, and return to the hand (Fig. 12–6B). Apply the wrap with moderate roll tension.

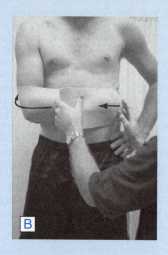

STEP 3: Continue to encircle the arm and trunk with circular patterns, just slightly overlapping the wrap in a proximal direction (Fig. 12–6C). Leave the thumb exposed to monitor circulation.

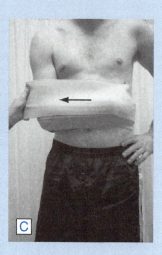

STEP 4: Anchor with Velcro, metal clips, or 2 inch or 3 inch elastic tape in a lateral-to medial circular pattern with moderate roll tension (Fig. 12–6D). Anchor the tape over the ipsilateral hand on the tape pattern.

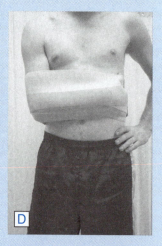

Figure 12-6   *continued*

Bracing Techniques

Bracing techniques for the thorax, abdomen, and spine provide compression and support, lessen range of motion, and correct structural abnormalities. The braces are available in off-the-shelf designs and can be used for a variety of injuries and conditions.

RIB BELTS Figure 12–7

▶ **Purpose:** Rib belts are designed to provide compression and mild to moderate support to the thorax following injury (Fig. 12–7). Use these braces to treat rib contusions and fractures, intercostal strains, and costochondral injury.

○ **DETAILS**

Rib belts are commonly used to provide compression and support for athletes in sports such as baseball, basketball, fencing, field hockey, football, gymnastics, ice hockey, lacrosse, soccer, skiing, softball, track and field, volleyball, and wrestling. The braces can also be used with work and casual activities and are reusable.

▶ **Design:**
 • Off-the-shelf braces are available in universal fit and male and female designs in predetermined sizes based on circumference measurements of the thorax. Some designs are available in universal sizes.
 • Most designs are constructed of elastic materials with a foam/flannel, soft laminated foam, or cotton knit inner lining.
 • The braces measure between 4 and 6 inches in width; most female designs are contoured for comfort and fit.
 • Some designs have elastic or plastic inserts or stays incorporated into the belt to provide additional support.
 • The braces are anchored to the thorax with Velcro closures.

▶ **Position of the individual:** Standing on the ground with the arms placed on the lateral hips in a relaxed position.

▶ **Preparation:** Apply the brace directly to the skin or over a tight-fitting shirt.
  Follow the manufacturer's instructions when applying the braces. The following guidelines pertain to most designs.

▶ **Application:**
 STEP 1: Loosen the closures and place the belt around the thorax. Position the foam inner lining over the injured area (Fig. 12–7A).

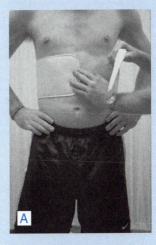

A

Figure 12-7

STEP 2: As the individual inhales, pull the belt with moderate tension and anchor with Velcro closures over the abdomen or back (Fig. 12–7B). Adjust the belt if needed to prevent constriction of chest movement and breathing patterns.

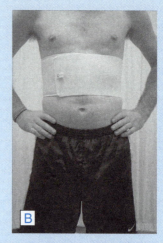

Figure 12-7 *continued*

RESEARCH BRIEF

When treating rib fractures, using compression and support has been questioned. For some individuals, compression and support wraps and/or belts may reduce pain levels significantly.[22,35] For other individuals, compression and support may restrict the already limited ability to inspire.[9] Mechanical restriction may also increase pain levels further[1] and predispose the individual to **hypostatic pneumonia,** which may occur from hypoventilation due to the pain and mechanical restriction.[22,24]

Critical Thinking Question 1

During training for an upcoming triathlon, a preschool teacher sustains a costal cartilage separation while performing medicine ball exercises in the gym. She is seen by a physician and allowed to continue training using an off-the-shelf rib belt after several days of rest. She progresses back into training and is symptom-free until reaching preinjury intensity levels. At this level, she has difficulty with normal breathing patterns and experiences an increase in pain as a result of wearing the belt.

 Question: How can you manage this situation?

...IF/THEN...

IF an athlete requires compression and support to the thorax when being treated for a costochondral injury during a return to activity, **THEN** consider using an off-the-shelf rib belt rather than an elastic wrap; with repetitive trunk flexion and extension and perspiration, the elastic wrap and tape may roll and/or bunch distally and become uncomfortable.

LUMBAR SACRAL BRACE Figure 12–8

▶ **Purpose:** Use lumbar sacral braces when preventing and treating lumbar sprains, rectus abdominis and lumbar strains, spondylolysis, and spondylolisthesis (Fig. 12–8). These braces provide compression and moderate support, lessen range of motion, and correct structural abnormalities.

◯ **D E T A I L S**────────────

Use lumbar sacral braces to provide compression and support, lessen range of motion, and correct structural abnormalities for athletes in sports such as baseball, basketball, fencing, field hockey, football, gymnastics, ice hockey, lacrosse, soccer, skiing, softball, track and field, volleyball, weightlifting, and wrestling. The braces can also be useful with work and casual activities.

▶ **Design:**
- The braces are available off-the-shelf in universal fit designs in predetermined sizes based on waist circumference measurements. Some braces are available in universal sizes.
- These braces are constructed of a cotton/polyester, perforated elastic or vinyl, polyester/nylon, or neoprene material outer shell with a soft foam or neoprene inner lining.
- Most designs have adjustable nylon, elastic, or neoprene strap(s) incorporated in the outer shell to provide additional compression and support. With some braces, these straps may be removed when not in use.
- The braces measure between 4 and 11 inches in width; some female designs are contoured for comfort and fit.
- Many designs use rigid or semirigid neoprene, plastic, thermoplastic, foam, air or gel bladder, silicone, or steel spring stays or inserts over the lumbar, sacral, and/or abdominal areas to provide additional compression and support.
- Most of the stays/inserts can be molded and/or adjusted for individual fit, while others can be removed when not in use.
- Several designs incorporate the brace into nylon/spandex shorts to lessen brace migration during activity.
- Some designs commonly used in weightlifting are manufactured of leather and are available with a foam inner lining.
- Other designs are available with detachable shoulder straps to lessen migration.
- The braces are attached to the trunk through Velcro and/or D-ring closures or buckles and allow for adjustments in fit.

▶ **Position of the individual:** Standing on the ground with the arms placed on the lateral hips in a relaxed position.

▶ **Preparation:** Apply the brace directly to the skin or over a tight-fitting shirt and pant.
    Specific instructions for applying the braces are included with each design. Carefully follow the step-by-step procedures for proper fit and support. The following application guidelines pertain to most braces.

▶ **Application:**
STEP 1: Begin by loosening the straps. Position the brace over the lumbar/sacral area and wrap the ends around the waist (Fig. 12–8A).

STEP 2: When using some braces, position the stays/inserts over the lumbar/sacral and/or abdominal area to achieve the objective of the technique ⨍.

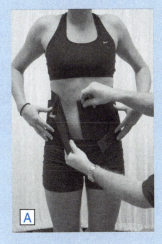

A

Figure 12-8

STEP 3: When using most designs, pull the ends with moderate tension as the individual inhales and anchor over the abdomen with Velcro and/or D-ring closures (Fig. 12–8B).

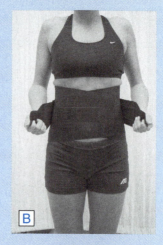

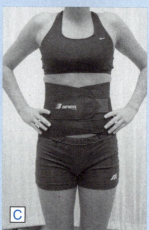

STEP 4: Applying and adjusting straps will depend on the specific brace design. When using many designs, pull the straps incorporated into the outer shell around the waist toward the abdomen and anchor with Velcro closures (Fig. 12–8C). Adjust the brace and/or straps for comfort and fit if necessary.

Figure 12-8 *continued*

 Helpful Hint: If plastic or metal stays/inserts are incorporated into rib belts or lumbar sacral braces, monitor the position of the stays/inserts during use; the stays/inserts can migrate superiorly or inferiorly from the outer shell and injure the soft tissue.

RESEARCH BRIEF

Lumbar sacral braces are used to prevent and treat various injuries and conditions, but the effectiveness of these braces has not been investigated adequately in the literature. Examining the prophylactic benefit of these designs in the work setting, researchers have demonstrated that bracing, along with a back education program, reduced time lost from work.[37] Other researchers have shown that the braces failed to prevent low back injury when used in the workplace.[40] Using these braces appears to have little effect on dynamic lifting capacity or lumbosacral biomechanics, suggesting that a correct lifting technique alone may afford more protection than a brace.[26,34,35] Some researchers believe the brace designs act as a proprioceptive reminder to use proper spine biomechanics during lifting and bending movements.[14]

Most researchers agree that, following injury, bracing may benefit the individual when used within a comprehensive treatment program. However, when and for how long to use the braces remains question. Some researchers have suggested brace use immediately in the treatment program.[3,5,18] Other researchers have recommended brace use with worsening of symptoms during therapy.[17] And still other researchers have recommended using braces when there is continued pain despite removal from aggravating athletic activities.[29] Routine bracing for symptomatic treatment is probably not necessary, as the brace may only serve as a reminder to maintain a correct posture.[17] The effectiveness of lumbar sacral braces in providing athletes with an earlier return to activity has not been addressed in the literature. Health-care professionals should base decisions regarding brace use on an individual basis and the objective of the technique.[32]

SACROILIAC BELTS   Figure 12–9

▶ **Purpose:** Sacroiliac belts are used to provide compression and moderate support when treating sprains (Fig. 12–9). Sacroiliac braces may be used during rehabilitative, athletic, work, and casual activities.

▶ **Design:**
- Off-the-shelf braces are manufactured in universal fit designs in predetermined sizes corresponding to pelvic circumference measurements just inferior to the iliac crest or just superior to the greater trochanter.
- The braces are constructed of a nylon or semi-elastic material outer shell with an inner lining of foam or neoprene.
- Some braces are circular in design, while others are contoured for comfort and fit.
- Several designs use a detachable semirigid foam pad located over the sacral area to provide additional compression.
- Other designs have an adjustable nylon belt incorporated in the outer shell to provide additional compression.
- Most designs are anchored to the sacroiliac area with Velcro and/or D-ring closures and allow for adjustments in fit.

▶ **Position of the individual:** Standing on the ground with the arms placed on the lateral hips in a relaxed position.

▶ **Preparation:** Apply sacroiliac braces over undergarments or other tight-fitting clothing.
   Follow manufacturer's instructions when applying the braces. The following guidelines apply to most designs.

▶ **Application:**
   STEP 1: To apply the brace, loosen the straps and wrap it around the pelvis at the level recommended by the manufacturer (Fig. 12–9A). When using some designs, position the pad over the sacral area.

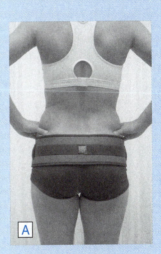

A

   STEP 2: Using moderate tension, pull the straps together and anchor with Velcro and/or D-ring closures (Fig. 12–9B). Reposition the brace if necessary.
   STEP 3: When using other designs, pull the outer shell belt with moderate tension and anchor. Adjust the brace, straps, and/or belt for comfort and fit if necessary.

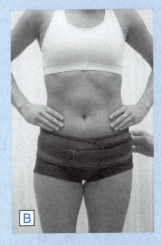

B

Figure 12-9

Thorax, Abdomen, and Spine

CERVICAL COLLAR Figures 12–10, 12–11

▶ **Purpose:** Cervical collars are used to provide support and immobilization and to lessen range of motion when preventing and treating sprains, acute torticollis, strains, stable fractures, disk herniation of the cervical spine, and brachial plexus injury. Two cervical collar designs are illustrated below.

Rehabilitative Technique

▶ **Purpose:** The rehabilitative brace technique is designed to provide moderate to maximal support and complete immobilization of the cervical spine following injury and surgery (Fig. 12–10).

▶ **Design:**
- Rehabilitative braces are available in two basic designs: a rigid and semirigid collar.
- These off-the-shelf braces are available in predetermined sizes based on neck circumference measurements in universal fit designs. Some designs are available in universal sizes.
- The rigid designs consist of an outer shell constructed of polyethylene or thermoplastic materials with a foam inner lining.
- Some of the rigid designs are used for the acute immobilization of the cervical spine following injury (extrication collar) while others are used when complete immobilization is required for extended periods of time.
- Most acute designs allow for adjustments in neck circumference and length measurements during application.
- These braces are typically one piece in design; some can be purchased in various neck lengths.
- The braces are manufactured with openings to allow for pulse checks, airway procedures, and visual inspection.
- Acute braces are attached to the cervical spine through Velcro closures and can be used in most acute injury situations. Most designs are reusable.
- Most rigid, extended wear designs consist of two pieces and are constructed with extra inner padding for comfort. These braces can also be adjusted for comfort and fit and are attached with Velcro closures.
- Semirigid collar designs are manufactured of soft, medium-density foam covered with stockinet.
- The braces are one piece in design, contoured and adjustable for fit, and available in various neck lengths. These braces are anchored with Velcro closures.

⭕ **DETAILS**

Rigid, extended wear braces can be used during rehabilitative and low intensity work and casual activities. Semirigid designs can be used during rehabilitative and low intensity work and casual activities, and are washable and reusable.

 Helpful Hint: To lessen soiling and excessive wear, cover the semirigid brace with stockinet. The stockinet can be changed and washed as needed.

▶ **Position of the individual:** Lying, sitting, or standing on the ground with the neck in a pain-free position.

▶ **Preparation:** Apply rehabilitative braces directly to the skin.
   Instructions for application of the braces are included with each design. For proper application, follow the step-by-step procedure. The following general application guidelines apply to most rigid and semirigid designs.

Application:

STEP 1: When using some rigid acute designs, measure the length from the shoulder to the chin of the individual and adjust the brace to this measurement (Fig. 12–10A). Do not adjust the brace while on the individual.

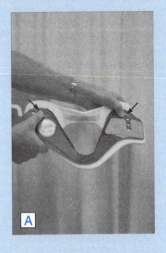

A

STEP 2: Continue application of adjustable and most other acute designs by placing the anterior brace under the chin (Fig. 12–10B).

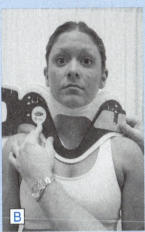

B

STEP 3: Next, position and wrap the brace around the neck (see Fig. 12–10C). Anchor the brace with Velcro closures with moderate tension (Fig. 12–10D).

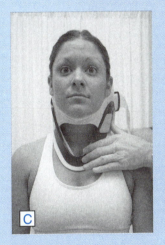 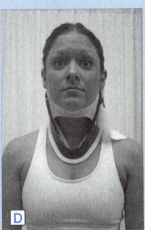

C   D

Figure 12-10

○ **DETAILS**

Note, these are general application guidelines—appropriate care of suspected cervical spine injuries is vital to prevent further trauma. For more complete information, see the Web References.

STEP 4: Begin applying rigid, extended wear designs by placing the anterior piece of the brace under the chin (Fig. 12–10E). When using some designs, wrap the elastic strap around the neck and anchor on the anterior brace.

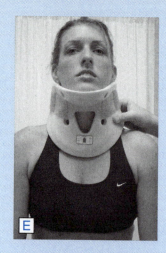

STEP 5: Next, place the posterior piece of the brace around the posterior neck (Fig. 12–10F).

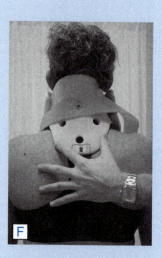

STEP 6: Using moderate tension, anchor the brace with Velcro closures (Fig. 12–10G). Readjust the brace if necessary.

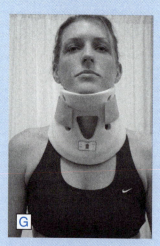

Figure 12-10   *continued*

STEP 7: When using semirigid designs, position the contoured area of the brace under the chin and wrap the ends around the neck with moderate tension (Fig. 12–10H). Anchor with Velcro closures. If necessary, readjust the brace.

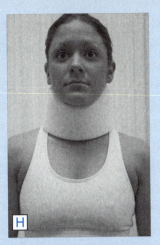

H

Figure 12-10 *continued*

Functional Technique

▶ **Purpose:** Functional braces are designed to provide moderate support, absorb shock, and limit range of motion when preventing and treating cervical sprains, strains, disk herniation, and brachial plexus injury (Fig. 12–11). The designs lessen excessive cervical extension and lateral flexion, but allow for normal flexion. Use these functional braces combined with football shoulder pads.

▶ **Design:**
  • The braces are available off-the-shelf in predetermined sizes corresponding to neck circumference measurements or the weight of the individual in universal fit designs. Some designs can be purchased in universal sizes.
  • Some designs consist of a pre-molded, closed-cell polyethylene foam collar incorporated into a padded foam vest.
  • The collar on some vest designs can be adjusted to lessen specific ranges of motion.
  • One vest design uses an optional plate manufactured from rigid plastic materials that attaches directly to the collar to provide additional support.
  • Vest designs are worn underneath football shoulder pads and are attached either to the pads with laces and/or straps or to the trunk with straps.
  • Another design worn underneath football shoulder pads consists of a molded foam collar incorporated into adjustable nylon straps that anchor the brace to the shoulders and trunk.
  • Other functional braces are manufactured of rigid materials and are bolted directly to football shoulder pads .

Helpful Hint: Because some functional collar designs are anchored directly to shoulder pads, the pads must be properly fitted and correctly worn. With contact, braces that attach to the top of shoulder pads may migrate away from the cervical area, allowing for excessive range of motion and/or compression.[2] Belts and/or buckles that anchor shoulder pads to the shoulder and upper torso should always be applied and worn snugly to lessen migration of the pads and collar.

  • Some functional designs are constructed of both open- and closed-cell foams and are attached to football shoulder pads with laces and/or bolts.
  • These foam braces are available in flat and roll designs in various thicknesses based on the injury and the desired range of motion.

▶ **Position of the individual:** Standing with the arms at the side of the body.

▶ **Preparation:** Attach the functional brace to the shoulder pads, directly to the skin or over a tight-fitting shirt. Apply the shoulder pads directly to the skin or over a shirt.
    Follow the step-by-step application instructions included with each design. The following general application guidelines pertain to most functional designs.

▶ **Application:**

STEP 1: When using vest designs, position the collar through the neck opening of the shoulder pads (Fig. 12–11A). Anchoring of the brace to the pads depends on the design. When using most designs, anchor the vest with laces (Fig. 12–11B).

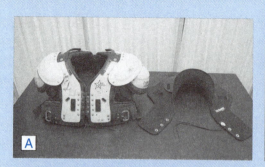

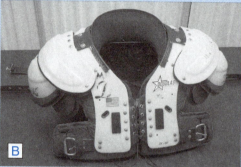

Figure 12-11 A Functional cervical collar. (Left) Football shoulder pads. (Right) Vest design. **B** Vest design attached to football shoulder pads.

STEP 2: If using an adjustable design, position and anchor the collar in the desired range of motion.

STEP 3: When using the strap design, position the collar directly to the skin or over a shirt on the posterior neck and the straps across the anterior thorax. Place the straps under the axillae and anchor across the back with the buckle (Fig. 12–11C).

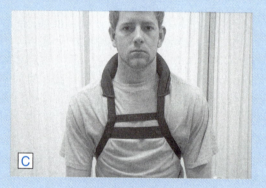

STEP 4: Attach other designs directly to the shoulder pads with bolts and/or laces (Fig. 12–11D).

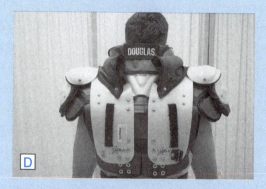

Figure 12-11

┌─────────────────────────────────────┐

...IF/THEN...

IF a functional cervical collar technique is indicated to treat a compression brachial plexus injury, **THEN** consider using a padded foam vest design; this brace will limit range of motion, and the foam vest may lessen compression/impingement over Erb's point.

└─────────────────────────────────────┘

RESEARCH BRIEF

Most discussions of brachial plexus injury include mention of functional cervical collars. A variety of designs are available to reduce cervical hyperextension and lateral flexion in an attempt to prevent brachial plexus injury. While use of cervical collars is common in football, few objective data examining their effectiveness are available.[7]

Two investigations found in the literature provide some support for the use of functional cervical collars. Examining vest, nylon strap, and foam roll designs among football players in a controlled setting, researchers[7] found a significant reduction in active cervical hyperextension when compared with shoulder pads alone. Although the vest brace permitted significantly less hyperextension than the foam roll, all three designs allowed for additional hyperextension when a passive overload was applied. Other investigators have demonstrated a significant limitation of cervical hyperextension among football athletes with vest, foam roll, and custom-made designs compared with shoulder pads alone.[12] Both investigations failed to show a restriction in passive lateral flexion.

Several recommendations have been made toward the prevention of brachial plexus injury and the use of functional cervical collars. Some researchers have suggested that the braces should be mandatory to lessen the frequency of injury for athletes who experience recurrent episodes, or have experienced an isolated severe injury or a single injury in a high-risk playing position.[12] Based on the mechanism of injury and the data from the limited studies, prevention of injury may involve more than just functional bracing techniques. Some researchers recommend a comprehensive rehabilitation program consisting of strength, flexibility, and neuromuscular exercises for the neck and shoulder girdle.[4,7]

Critical Thinking Question 2

A freshman defensive back on the intercollegiate football team suffers a grade one brachial plexus injury during a tackling drill in preseason practice. His medical history reveals chronic episodes of the injury in high school. He used a foam roll functional brace in high school and is currently wearing a similar design. An evaluation with the team physician concludes with a discussion of preventive bracing techniques.

▶ **Question: What bracing techniques are appropriate for the player's return to activity?**

SLINGS

▶ **Purpose:** Slings provide support and immobilization when treating thorax and spine injuries and conditions.
  • Use sling technique one (see Fig. 8–11) when treating pectoralis major strains and brachial plexus injury.

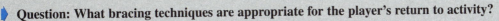

Padding Techniques

A variety of off-the-shelf padding techniques can be used to prevent and treat injuries and conditions of the thorax, abdomen, and spine. Custom-made pads may also be constructed from thermoplastic material and foam. Padding of the thorax, abdomen, and spine is required in several interscholastic and intercollegiate sports. These padding techniques will be discussed further in Chapter 13.

OFF-THE-SHELF Figures 12–12, 12–13

▶ **Purpose:** Off-the-shelf padding techniques are available in a variety of designs to provide shock absorption and protection. Use these techniques when preventing and treating rib, abdominal, kidney, pulmonary, genital, breast, and coccygeal contusions; Cooper's ligament sprains; rib, coccygeal, and stable cervical fractures; and costochondral and brachial plexus injury. Following is a description of two basic designs.

Soft, Low-Density

> ○ **DETAILS**
>
> Soft, low-density pads are commonly used to provide shock absorption to the thorax, abdomen, and spine of athletes in sports such as baseball, basketball, fencing, field hockey, football, ice hockey, lacrosse, soccer, skiing, softball, volleyball, and wrestling. The pads can be used in combination with mandatory protective equipment, among different sports, or worn alone. Use the pads with work and casual activities. These pads may be washed and reused.

▸ **Design:**
- These universal fit designs are available in predetermined sizes based on chest or waist circumference measurements or age of the individual.
- Shirt designs are manufactured of polyester/spandex materials with thermal foam pads incorporated in the inner lining over the ribs, kidney, and spine to provide shock absorption.
- Padded shorts are constructed of nylon/spandex materials with a mesh covering.
- These designs contain EVA foam incorporated in the inner lining over the coccyx and spine area.
- The shorts extend from the mid thigh area to the waist; most have an elastic waistband.
- Bra and top designs are manufactured of nylon/spandex materials with additional foam incorporated to support and protect the breast.
- Individual pad designs are constructed of varying thicknesses of low-density open- and closed-cell foams; viscoelastic polymer or gel materials are available in a variety of sizes to provide shock absorption of the thorax, abdomen, spine, and coccyx.

▸ **Position of the individual:** Standing with the arms at the side of the body.

▸ **Preparation:** Apply shirts, shorts, bras, tops, and individual pads directly to the skin. Individual pads may also be applied under tight-fitting clothing or within athletic clothing.

▸ **Application:**

STEP 1: To apply a padded shirt, place the shirt over the head and insert the arms through the sleeves. Pull the shirt and pads onto the thorax, abdomen, and spine (Fig. 12–12A). Adjust the pads if needed.

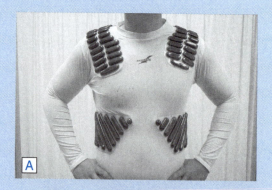

STEP 2: When using short designs, place the feet into the shorts and pull in a proximal direction until positioned on the waist (Fig. 12–12B). Adjust the pads over the coccyx and spine.

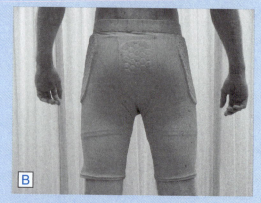

Figure 12-12

STEP 3: Apply the bra and top designs by placing them over the head and arms (Fig. 12–12C). Position the pads over the breasts.

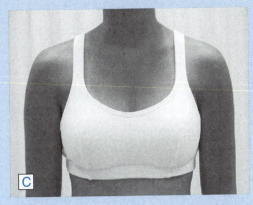

Figure 12-12 *continued*

STEP 4: Attach an individual, closed-cell foam pad to the spine and/or coccyx by placing the pad underneath tight-fitting clothing or within athletic girdles (see Fig. 7–18F).

STEP 5: Apply other closed-cell foam designs over the head and shoulders and anchor under the axillae with elastic straps or around the chest with Velcro straps (see Fig. 8–18G).

STEP 6: Attach viscoelastic polymer or gel material pads to the inner lining of football shoulder pads (see Fig. 8–18F). The pads may also be anchored with elastic material or with the contusion/fracture taping technique or circular wrapping technique.

RESEARCH BRIEF

Soft, low-density padding has been used to prevent brachial plexus injury. Skeleton, viscoelastic polymer, or gel pads attached underneath football shoulder pads may reduce the incidence of injury.[6,15] Use these pads to improve shoulder pad fit, lessen pressure on the cervical spine, and provide additional shock absorption.[38,39]

Hard, High-Density

DETAILS

Hard, high-density pads are commonly used to provide shock absorption to the thorax, abdomen, and spine of athletes in sports such as baseball, basketball, fencing, field hockey, football, ice hockey, lacrosse, skiing, soccer, softball, volleyball, and wrestling. Use the pads in combination with mandatory sports equipment or wear the pads alone. The pads may be used in work and casual activities, and reused.

DETAILS

Football shoulder pads can provide protection of the anterior and posterior upper thoracic and cervical areas. However, these pads do not protect the lower rib cage and abdominal areas from injury.[1,13]

▶ **Design:**

• Universal fit designs are available in predetermined sizes based on chest circumference measurements or age of the individual (Fig. 12–13).

• Rib vests or jackets (flak jacket) are constructed of a high-density plastic material outer shell pre-molded to the contours of the thorax and abdomen. The outer shell is lined with open-cell foam.

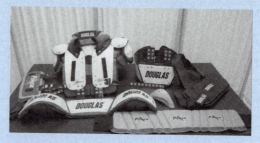

Figure 12-13 Variety of hard, high-density pads.

○ **DETAILS**

The term "flak," an abbreviation for *Flugzeugabwehrkanone*—aircraft attack gun— was used to describe German antiaircraft fire during World War II.[11] The name flak jacket originates from an armored jacket worn by Allied troops and air crews for protection against bullets and shell fragments.

• The pads are available in various lengths and widths depending on the size of the individual and the area to be protected.

• Some designs are attached directly to football shoulder pads with zippers, bolts, and/or nylon straps.

• Other pads are incorporated and attached to the thorax and abdomen with adjustable elastic suspenders.

• Most rib vest/jacket designs are anchored over the anterior thorax/abdomen with laces or Velcro closures.

○ **DETAILS**

Vests/jackets designed as mandatory equipment for one sport may be used for another sport. For example, use lacrosse rib pads for an athlete participating in baseball or basketball.

• Another pad design uses a high-density plastic plate lined with open-cell foam.

• These plates are attached directly to football shoulder pads with zippers, bolts, and/or nylon straps over the anterior and/or posterior thorax, abdomen, and spine.

• Athletic cups are constructed of high-density, flexible plastic materials pre-molded to the contours of the genital area. The edges of these designs are covered with closed-cell foam to prevent irritation.

• Designs are available for males and females and are typically used in combination with an elastic supporter.

• Another cup design is manufactured of low-density polyethylene plastic materials. This cup is designed for female breasts and is used in combination with bras and tops.

▶ **Position of the individual:** Standing with the arms at the side of the body.

▶ **Preparation:** Apply these designs directly to the skin, over or under tight-fitting clothing, or within athletic clothing.

▶ **Application:**

STEP 1: Begin application of some rib vests/jackets and plates by attaching the designs to football shoulder pads (Fig. 12–13B). Apply and anchor the shoulder pads.

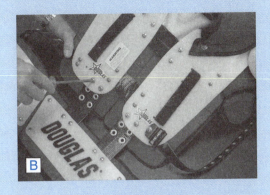

STEP 2: Next, position the vest/jacket or plate over the thorax, abdomen, and/or spine. With most designs, anchor the pads snugly over the anterior thorax/abdomen with laces or Velcro closures (Fig. 12–13C). Adjust the laces or closures if needed to prevent constriction of chest movement and breathing patterns.

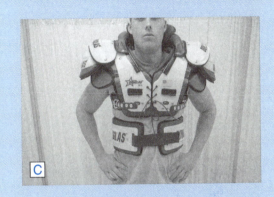

STEP 3: Apply other vests/jackets by placing the suspenders over the shoulders. Position the pads around the thorax, abdomen, and/or spine, and anchor (Fig. 12–13D).

STEP 4: When using athletic cup designs, place the feet into an athletic supporter and pull in a proximal direction until the supporter is positioned around the waist. Place the head and arms into a bra or top and position over the breasts.

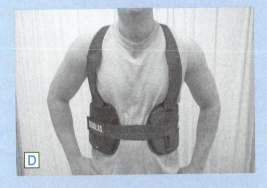

STEP 5: Place most cups in a pocket that is incorporated into the supporter or bra/top (Fig. 12–13E). Cups may also be used under tight-fitting clothing.

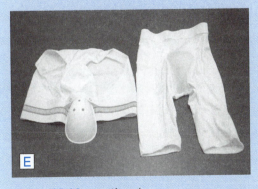

Figure 12-13 *continued*

Critical Thinking Question 3

Near the end of the soccer match, an eight-year-old goalie is struck in the mid to low back area by an opponent's elbow during a shot on goal. His team is participating in a state youth tournament out of town. He is unable to continue play and is taken to a local outpatient medical clinic for evaluation. The physician evaluates the goalie and suspects a first degree kidney contusion. The physician allows a return to play if the area is protected with padding. The team has three matches remaining in the tournament; the goalie's parents will allow him to participate as tolerated. Several parents search the local sporting good stores for padded rib/thorax vests and jackets, but all the designs are too large for the goalie. One of these parents is the coach of the youth football team and commonly carries some of the protective equipment in the back of his van.

▶ **Question: What padding techniques can you apply in this situation?**

CUSTOM-MADE

▶ **Purpose:** Absorb shock and provide protection when preventing and treating rib, abdominal, kidney, pulmonary, genital, breast, and coccygeal contusions; rib and coccygeal fractures; and costochondral injury with thermoplastic material and foam. Use these pads when off-the-shelf designs are not available.

▶ **Materials:**
- Paper, felt tip pen, thermoplastic material, ⅛ inch or ¼ inch foam or felt, a heating source, 2 inch or 3 inch elastic tape, an elastic wrap, soft, low-density foam, rubber cement, taping scissors

▶ **Position of the individual:** Standing with the arms at the side of the body.

▶ **Preparation:** Design the pad with a paper pattern. Cut, mold, and shape the thermoplastic material on the thorax, abdomen, and/or spine over the injured area. Attach soft, low-density foam to the inside surface of the material.

▶ **Application:**

(**STEP 1:**) Place the pad over the injured area and attach with elastic material or with the contusion/fracture taping or circular wrapping technique. Pad all nonpliable materials to meet NCAA[20] and NFHS[21] rules.

(**STEP 2:**) Another option is to attach the custom-made pad to the thorax, abdomen, and/or spine underneath tight-fitting clothing or within athletic clothing .

 Helpful Hint: If off-the-shelf or custom-made padding techniques irritate the nipples, apply a skin lubricant over the area and cover with a wound dressing or adhesive gauze material.

MANDATORY PADDING

Protective equipment is required in several high school and intercollegiate sports. The NCAA[20] and NFHS[21] require that athletes participating in baseball, fencing, field hockey, football, ice hockey, lacrosse, and softball wear protective padding on the thorax, abdomen, and/or spine during all practices and competitions. These pads are typically purchased off-the-shelf; many sport-specific designs are available. A further discussion of these padding techniques can be found in Chapter 13.

Critical Thinking Question 4

A batsman sends a forceful shot to the off side, and a gully is struck in the left anterior ribs with the cricket ball. The gully immediately falls to the ground in pain and is removed from the pitch. An evaluation by a physician, including radiographs, reveals anterior fractures to the sixth and seventh ribs. After several weeks of inactivity, the gully is allowed to return to play.

▶ **Question: What padding techniques can you use to protect the area during play?**

CASE STUDY

During the second quarter of the opening game of the season, John Mariani, a junior wide receiver at Round Top College, jumps to catch a pass. As the ball arrives, the safety collides with John, turning him to a semihorizontal position. John maintains possession of the ball, holding it against his right thorax, and falls toward the ground. Upon landing, John's right shoulder strikes the ground, followed by his thorax on top of the ball, then his lower body. The safety simultaneously falls on John, forcing John's head and neck to the left. John remains on the field; Bernadette Chamberlain, ATC, immediately comes out to the field. John complains of a burning pain and numbness radiating distally in the right arm and pain in the right lateral thorax. Bernadette begins an initial evaluation as the team physician arrives. Following this evaluation, Bernadette and the team physician help John to the sidelines, where they perform further testing. The evaluation reveals pain and paresthesia in the right shoulder and arm, muscle weakness in the right rotator cuff, point tenderness over the lateral aspect of ribs six through nine, and pain with deep inhalation and coughing. John is taken to the locker room for radiographs. The radiographs are negative; the team physician believes John has sustained a grade two right brachial plexus injury, along with a moderate rib contusion. The team physician requests that support, compression, and immobilization be applied for the shoulder and ribs. What wrapping and/or bracing techniques would provide support and immobilization in the immediate management of this case?

John is seen by the team physician in the Athletic Training Room the next day. An evaluation that includes strength, range of motion, nerve root, myotome, and special tests confirms the original diagnosis. John is placed in a therapeutic exercise program with Bernadette and closely followed by the team physician. After many weeks of treatment and rehabilitation, John achieves preinjury strength and range of motion, and is free of neurological symptoms. The team physician allows John to progress back into football activities and discusses with Bernadette protective options for the cervical and thoracic areas. What taping, wrapping, bracing, and padding techniques can you use in this case to limit range of motion of the cervical spine and absorb shock over the thorax?

The return to football activities progresses well, and John enters his first drill since the injury at full speed. John is wearing a functional cervical brace and hard, high-density rib pad. While running deep routes, John notices he is unable to rotate his head completely to the right or left to see the ball, so he drops several passes. He then runs several short, turn-in patterns and easily catches the ball, but cannot secure the ball in his arm against the thorax when running. John becomes frustrated and talks with Bernadette about the possibility of removing the brace and pad. Which bracing and padding techniques are appropriate to allow John improved vision and ball control while providing the necessary protection to allow him to continue football activities?

WRAP UP

- Acute and chronic injuries and conditions to the thorax, abdomen, and spine can be the result of compressive and repetitive forces, excessive range of motion, and overload and violent muscular contractions.
- Elastic material and the contusion/fracture taping and circular wrapping techniques anchor protective padding to the thorax, abdomen, and spine.
- Compression wrap techniques are used to control minimal, moderate, and severe swelling following injury.
- The swathe wrapping and sling bracing techniques provide support and immobilization.
- Rib and sacroiliac belts and lumbar sacral bracing techniques can be used to provide compression

and support, lessen range of motion, and correct structural abnormalities.
- Rehabilitative and functional cervical collar bracing techniques provide support and immobilization, absorb shock, and limit range of motion following injury and surgery.
- Off-the-shelf and custom-made padding techniques constructed of soft, low-density and hard, high-density materials absorb shock and provide protection when preventing and treating injuries and conditions.
- Mandatory protective padding is required by the NCAA and NFHS for the thorax, abdomen, and/or spine in several sports.

WEB REFERENCES

National Athletic Trainers' Association
· Inter-Association Task Force for the Appropriate Care of the Spine-Injured Athlete
http://www.nata.org/spineinjuredathlete/main.htm
· This Web site allows access to the *Prehospital Care of the Spine-Injured Athlete*, which provides guidelines and recommendations for appropriate care of the injured individual.

The Miami Project to Cure Paralysis
http://www.miamiproject.miami.edu/
· This Web site allows access to the research center for information about spinal cord injury and ongoing research to find more effective treatments.

Trauma.Org
http://www.trauma.org/index.html
· This site provides access to an extensive amount of information about the field of trauma, including educational materials, manuscripts, and photographs.

REFERENCES

1. Anderson, MK, Hall, SJ, and Martin, M: Foundations of Athletic Training: Prevention, Assessment, and Management, ed 3. Lippincott Williams & Wilkins, Philadelphia, 2005.
2. Archambault, JL: Brachial plexus stretch injury. J Am Coll Health 31:256–260, 1983.
3. Congeni, J, McCulloch, J, and Swanson, K: Lumbar spondylolysis: A study of natural progression in athletes. Am J Sports Med 25:248–253, 1997.
4. Cramer, CR: A reconditioning program to lower the recurrence rate of brachial plexus neurapraxia in collegiate football players. J Athl Train 34:390–396, 1999.
5. Daniel, JN, Polly, DW, Jr, and Van Dam, BE: A study of the efficacy of nonoperative treatment of presumed traumatic spondylolysis in a young patient population. Mil Med 160:553–555, 1995.
6. Di Benedetto, M, and Markey, K: Electrodiagnostic localization of traumatic upper trunk brachial plexopathy. Arch Phys Med Rehabil 65:15–17, 1984.
7. Gorden, JA, Straub, SJ, Swanik, CB, and Swanik, KA: Effects of football collars on cervical hyperextension and lateral flexion. J Athl Train 38:209–215, 2003.
8. Granhed, H, and Morelli, B: Low back pain among retired wrestlers and heavyweight lifters. Am J Sports Med 16:530–533, 1988.
9. Grod, JP: Diagnosis and evaluation of rib fracture. Topics in Clinical Chiropractic 6:49–61, 1999.
10. Gurtler, R, Pavlov, H, and Torg, JS: Stress fracture of the ipsilateral first rib in a pitcher. Am J Sports Med 13:277–279, 1985.
11. HighBeam Research, http://www.highbeam.com/ref/doc0.asp?DOCID=1P1:100096406&num=1&ctrlInfo=Round18%3AMode18c%3AREFSR%3AResult
12. Hovis, WD, and Limbird, TJ: An evaluation of cervical orthoses in limiting hyperextension and lateral flexion in football. Med Sci Sports Exerc 26:872–876, 1994.
13. Levy, AS, Bassett, F, Lintner, S, and Speer, K: Pulmonary barotraumas: Diagnosis in American football players. Am J Sports Med 24:227–228, 1996.
14. Malanga, GA, and Nadler, SF: Nonoperative treatment of low back pain. Mayo Clinic Proceedings 74:1135–1148, 1999.
15. Markey, KL, Di Benedetto, M, and Curl, WW: Upper trunk brachial plexopathy: The stinger syndrome. Am J Sports Med 21:650–655, 1993.
16. Micheli, LJ: Back injuries in gymnastics. Clin Sports Med 4:85–93, 1985.
17. Moeller, JL, and Rifat, SF: Spondylolysis in active adolescents: Expediting return to play. Physician Sportsmed 29:27–32, 2001.
18. Morita, T, Ikata, T, Katoh, S, and Miyake, R: Lumbar spondylolysis in children and adolescents. J Bone Joint Surg Br 77:620–625, 1995.
19. Motley, G, Nyland, J, Jacobs, J, and Caborn, D: The pars interarticularis stress reaction, spondylolysis, and spondylolisthesis progression. J Athl Train 33:351–358, 1998.
20. National Collegiate Athletic Association, http://www.ncaa.org/library/sports_sciences/sports_med_handbook/2003-04/2003-04_sports_med_handbook.pdf, Sports medicine handbook, 2003–2004.
21. National Federation of State High School Associations. 2004 Football Rules Book. Indianapolis, IN: National Federation of State High School Associations, 2004.
22. O'Kane, J, O'Kane, E, and Marquet, J: Delayed complication of a rib fracture. Physician Sportsmed 26:69–77, 1998.
23. Pezzullo, DJ: Spondylolisthesis and spondylolysis in athletes. Athletic Therapy Today 4:36–40, 1999.
24. Prentice, WE: Arnheim's Principles of Athletic Training, ed 11. McGraw-Hill, Boston, 2003.
25. Quick, G: A randomized clinical trial of rib belts for simple fractures. Am J Emerg Med 8:277–281, 1990.
26. Reyna, JR, Jr, Leggett, SH, Kenny, K, Holmes, B, and Mooney, V: The effect of lumbar belts on isolated lumbar muscle: Strength and dynamic capacity. Spine 20:68–73, 1995.
27. Robertson, WC, Jr, Eichman, PL, and Clancy, WG: Upper trunk brachial plexopathy in football players. JAMA 241:1480–1482, 1979.
28. Sallis, RE, Jones, K, and Knopp, W: Burners: Offensive strategy for an underreported injury. Physician Sportsmed 20:47–55, 1992.
29. Smith, JA, and Hu, SS: Management of spondylolysis and spondylolisthesis in the pediatric and adolescent population. Orthop Clin North Am 30:487–499, ix, 1999.
30. Soler, T, and Calderon, C: The prevalence of spondylolysis in the Spanish elite athlete. Am J Sports Med 28:57–62, 2000.
31. Speer, KP, and Bassett, FH, III: The prolonged burner syndrome. Am J Sports Med 18:591–594, 1990.
32. Standaert, CJ, and Herring, SA: Spondylolysis: A critical review. Br J Sports Med 34:415–422, 2000.
33. Starkey, C, and Ryan, JL: Evaluation of Orthopedic and Athletic Injuries, ed 2. FA Davis, Philadelphia, 2002.
34. van Poppel, MN, Koes, BW, Smid, T, and Bouter, LM: A systematic review of controlled clinical trials on the prevention of back pain in industry. Occup Environ Med 54:841–847, 1997.
35. van Poppel, MN, Koes, BW, van der Ploeg, T, Smid, T, and Bouter, LM: Lumbar supports and education for the prevention of low back pain in industry: A randomized controlled trial. JAMA 279:1789–1794, 1998.
36. Vegso, JJ, Torg, E, and Torg, JS: Rehabilitation of cervical spine, brachial plexus, and peripheral nerve injuries. Clin Sports Med 6:135–158, 1987.
37. Walsh, NE, and Schwartz, RK: The influence of prophylactic orthoses on abdominal strength and low back injury in the workplace. Am J Phys Med Rehabil 69:245–250, 1990.
38. Watkins, RG: Neck injuries in football players. Clin Sports Med 5:215–246, 1986.
39. Watkins, RG, and Dillin, WM: Cervical spine and spinal cord injuries. In Fu, FH, and Stone, DA (eds): Sports Injuries: Mechanisms, Prevention, Treatment. Williams & Wilkins, Baltimore, 1994, pp 854–859.
40. Woodhouse, ML, McCoy, RW, Redondo, DR, and Shall, LM: Effects of back support on intra-abdominal pressure and lumbar kinetics during heavy lifting. Hum Factors 37:582–590, 1995.

Protective Equipment and Padding

1. Describe the legal issues, manufacturing standards, and testing procedures of protective equipment and padding.
2. Discuss the different types of protective equipment and padding used to prevent, treat, and rehabilitate injuries in interscholastic and intercollegiate sports and in recreational activities.
3. Demonstrate how to apply protective equipment and padding in order to prevent, treat, and rehabilitate injuries.
4. Explain and demonstrate the ability to select appropriate protective equipment and padding to prevent, treat, and rehabilitate various injuries.

LIABILITY ISSUES SURROUNDING PROTECTIVE EQUIPMENT

Legal issues plague the design, manufacture, fit, application, and use of protective equipment and padding. The responsibility to ensure appropriate design and use is shared by the individuals who manufacture, purchase, fit, apply, and use the equipment and padding. For example, manufacturers may be found liable if an individual is injured while using their products or if the products are found to be defective or unfit for their designed purpose. Manufacturers may also be found liable if **foreseeable,** or anticipated, risks associated with the use of the products were not lessened or eliminated.[46]

Health-care professionals have a duty to fit and apply the protective equipment according to manufacturers' guidelines and intended uses. Modifications to or use of equipment or padding in ways other than the intended purpose can place the liability on the health-care professional and/or individual using the equipment and padding. Modifications that result in injury to the individual may lead to liability for the health-care provider.

Health-care professionals and others involved with protective equipment and padding can use the following recommendations to mitigate vulnerability to liability:

- Select and purchase only high-quality equipment and padding from reputable manufacturers.

- Become familiar with the warning labels and intended purposes for all equipment and padding purchased.
- Read and follow the manufacturer's instructions when fitting the equipment and padding to the individual. Do not attempt to modify and/or alter any equipment and padding.
- Instruct the individual on the use, application, and care of the equipment and padding.
- Ensure that individuals read the warning labels and understand the use and care of the equipment or padding. Have individuals sign a form stating they understand the warning labels and risks involved with the sport or activity.
- Continually monitor the use of and inspect the condition of the equipment and padding.
- Perform regular maintenance on the equipment and padding as recommended by the manufacturer.

Legal issues surrounding protective equipment leave some questions for the health-care professional. Can health-care professionals be held liable if they don't monitor the equipment regularly or schedule regular reconditioning? Are they liable if they don't fully instruct the individual on the uses of the equipment? Further discussion on these liability issues can be found elsewhere. For more complete information, see the Web References.

Critical Thinking Question 1

During batting practice prior to a weekend intercollegiate baseball series, the center fielder picks up his batter's helmet and notices that the open- and closed-cell foam inner lining is partially missing. He brings you the helmet and asks if you can replace the padding. The team is away from home this weekend, and no one on the team wears the same size helmet.

▶ **Question: What can you do in this situation to provide protection for the center fielder and avoid legal problems?**

STANDARDS AND TESTING

Many national and international agencies and organizations have been established to protect the individual from ineffective and poorly designed and constructed protective equipment and padding.[2] In response to the high incidence of various acute injuries in sport, recreational, and work activities, these agencies and organizations have developed standards and testing procedures for the manufacturing, maintenance, and use of equipment and padding. The National Operating Committee on Standards for Athletic Equipment (NOCSAE), the Hockey Equipment Certification Council (HECC), ASTM International, the Canadian Standards Association (CSA), the Protective Eyewear Certification Council (PECC), the American National Standards Institute (ANSI), and the U.S. Consumer Product Safety Commission (CPSC) currently set standards and conduct testing and research for protective equipment and padding.

NOCSAE was formed in 1969 with the purpose "to commission research on and, where feasible, establish standards for protective athletic equipment."[42] Consisting of representatives from the American College of Sports Medicine, American College Health Association, American Orthopaedic Society for Sports Medicine, Athletic Equipment Managers' Association, National Athletic Trainers' Association, National Athletic Equipment Reconditioners' Association, National Association of Secondary School Principals, Sporting Goods Manufacturers' Association, and the College Football Association, NOCSAE strives to improve the quality of protective equipment and lessen the occurrence of injury associated with participation in athletic activity through the development of voluntary testing standards.

At the request of USA Hockey in 1978, **HECC** was formed. HECC currently evaluates the needs and recommendations of amateur hockey-governing bodies in relation to protective equipment and safety.[51] HECC promotes and sponsors research focusing on the prevention and reduction of injuries associated with participation in ice hockey. Equipment certification testing serves to validate manufacturers' certifications and is based on standards developed by other organizations such as ASTM and CSA.

Originally known as the American Society for Testing and Materials, **ASTM International** is a voluntary standards development organization consisting of members from the government, academia, consumers, and manufacturers.[4] Formed in 1898, ASTM International strives to develop standards to direct the production of safer, more efficient and cost-effective products and services. The organization has developed standards directly related to protective equipment, specifically the certification of ice hockey equipment and athletic mouth and eye guards.

CSA develops standards to address the needs of business, industry, government, and consumers.[10] The organization serves as a neutral third party to provide a structure and forum for standards development, including safety and prevention. CSA has developed standards for the design and manufacture of ice hockey helmets, face guards, and visors.

PECC strives to reduce eye injuries through certification of eye guards that comply with ASTM standards.[52] A third-party laboratory is used to validate the guard manufacturer's conformance with the standards. A PECC seal is placed on all guards that meet the certification requirements.

Currently, there are published NOCSAE, HECC, ASTM, and CSA standards for several types of equipment: football, baseball, softball batter's and catcher's, lacrosse, ice hockey, and polo helmets and appropriate face guards; ice hockey face protectors and visors; and mouth and eye guards. The following provides an overview of testing methods for a sample of required helmet and face guard designs.

Football Helmets

Football helmets, excluding face guards and face guard hardware, are tested with the NOCSAE drop test method,[42] conducted in-house by helmet manufacturers and reconditioners of used, originally certified helmets. In the drop test, the helmet is placed on a headform (model head) and dropped onto a cylindrical rubber pad. The test is scored on a pass/fail basis and produces a Severity Index (SI), which is described as "a measure of the severity of impact with respect to the instantaneous acceleration experienced by the headform as it is impacted."[42]

The helmet is exposed to ambient temperatures and dropped once on the front and side from heights of 36 and 48 inches. The test continues with two successive drops from a 60-inch height onto the front, side, front/side, rear/side, rear, and top areas of the helmet. An additional two drops are conducted from a 60-inch height on random areas of the helmet. Next, the helmet is exposed to hot temperatures and dropped twice from a height of 60 inches onto the side of the helmet. The SI is calculated for each drop; helmets that do not exceed the limit of 1200 SI, and that meet construction and material requirements, pass.

Football helmets that meet the NOCSAE standards must be permanently and legibly marked with the manufacturer's name, model, and size. On the exterior of the shell, there should be an easily readable warning label and a NOCSAE seal.[42] The warning label states:

WARNING

NO HELMET CAN PREVENT ALL HEAD OR ANY NECK INJURIES A PLAYER MIGHT RECEIVE WHILE PARTICIPATING IN FOOTBALL.

DO NOT USE THIS HELMET TO BUTT, RAM OR SPEAR AN OPPOSING PLAYER. THIS IS IN VIOLATION OF THE FOOTBALL RULES AND SUCH USE CAN RESULT IN SEVERE HEAD OR NECK INJURIES, PARALYSIS OR DEATH TO YOU AND POSSIBLE INJURY TO YOUR OPPONENT.

NOCSAE does not perform surveillance to determine adherence to the football helmet standard. The responsibility to ensure the condition of the helmet falls on the purchaser and wearer. NOCSAE does recommend the implementation of a reconditioning and recertification program for all helmets originally certified when manufactured. The frequency of reconditioning and recertification of helmets should be based on the amount and intensity of usage.[42] Reconditioning and recertification involves the repairing, cleaning, and retesting of helmets. At high competition levels, such as intercollegiate and professional football, for example, helmets are reconditioned and recertified at the conclusion of each season. The NOCSAE standard is not a warranty against injury and resulting liability, but most helmet manufacturers provide a separate 3- to 5-year warranty on the helmet shell.

DETAILS

NOCSAE standards were initiated in response to football injuries. In 1970, NOCSAE developed a helmet standard, which was published in 1973 and implemented in 1974 with new helmet models. The standard has resulted in shell size changes, softer construction materials, a reduction of models being manufactured from 85 in 1972 to 25 in 1992, and improved quality control during manufacturing.[42]

Baseball and Softball Batter's Helmets

Newly manufactured baseball and softball batter's helmets undergo a projectile impact test to meet the NOCSAE standard.[42] The impact test produces an SI and is scored with pass/fail criteria. The helmet is fit on a headform attached to a sliding table top; the test involves an air cannon assembly launching a baseball (used by Major League Baseball) at the helmet from a 24-inch distance.

After exposing the helmet to ambient temperatures, a baseball is launched at a speed of 60 miles per hour (mph), striking the helmet on the front, right front/side, right side, right rear/side, and rear areas. One random impact area is also tested. The helmet is then exposed to high temperatures and impacted once on the right side. At impact in each testing condition, the SI is calculated; helmets that do not exceed the limit of 1200 SI, and meet construction and material requirements, pass.

Baseball and softball batter's helmets meeting the NOCSAE standard must be permanently and legibly labeled with the manufacturer's name, model, and size. A NOCSAE seal and the warning label,[42] similar to the football helmet label, must be placed on the exterior shell. A reconditioning and recertification program, as recommended by the manufacturer, should also be used with NOCSAE-certified baseball and softball batter's helmets.

Baseball and Softball Catcher's Helmets with Face Guards

NOCSAE standards for new baseball and softball catcher's helmets with attached face guards consist of the drop test method and projectile impact tests.[42] The face guard must be attached to the helmet during all testing.

The helmets and face guards are exposed to ambient temperatures and dropped onto a steel anvil from a height of 36 inches onto the right side, right rear/side, and rear of the helmet. Two additional random drops are also conducted. After the helmets and face guards are exposed to hot temperatures, two drops are performed from a 36-inch height onto the right side of the helmet. SI measures are calculated; helmets that do not exceed the limit of 1200 SI pass.

The impact test, with a baseball launched at 60 mph, is performed on the right side, right rear/side, and rear of the helmet, followed by a random impact after the helmet is exposed to ambient temperatures. One impact is conducted to the right side of the helmet after the helmet is exposed to hot temperatures. Helmets that do not exceed the limit of 1200 SI pass.

A face guard is placed on a catcher's helmet following the manufacturer's guidelines and subjected to the projectile impact test with a baseball launched at 70 mph.[42] The face guards are exposed to ambient temperatures, and impact tests are conducted at the front, side, ocular, and one random area of the guard. After the face guards are exposed to hot temperatures, impact tests at the front and side areas are performed. A paste, applied to the headform, is used to verify ball or guard contact during testing.

Baseball and softball catcher's helmets that meet the standard must be marked with a NOCSAE seal and a warning label[42] in the same manner as batter's helmets. Catcher's helmets, sold by manufacturers without a face guard, must also have a warning statement permanently placed on the exterior shell.

Face guards with stand-alone padding must be sold with manufacturer's guidelines indicating which helmet should be used with the guard. A warning statement[42] must be affixed to the mask.

Lacrosse Helmets with Face Guards

Test standards for new lacrosse helmets with compatible face guards include a helmet stability and retention, drop method, and projectile impact test.[42] During all tests, face guards certified by NOCSAE must be attached to the helmets.

In the stability and retention test, the helmet is exposed to ambient temperatures and placed on a headform connected to a stability stand with the retention system fastened. The back edge of the helmet is attached to a hook on the stand, and a weight, connected to the hook, is dropped from a height of 2.78 feet. During the test, the headform is canted downward; to pass, the helmet must remain on the headform throughout the test.

Drop tests are performed with impacts occurring on a cylindrical rubber pad. After the helmets are exposed to ambient temperatures, the helmets are dropped once from a height of 24 inches onto seven different areas, from 48 inches onto seven areas, and from 60 inches onto seven areas. Three random drops are then conducted.[42] Next, helmets not previously tested are exposed to high temperatures and dropped from a 60-inch height onto two areas.

Impact tests are conducted with the helmet using a NCAA-approved lacrosse ball launched at 75 mph. Impacts are conducted on four areas after the helmets are exposed to ambient temperatures and one area after the helmets are exposed to hot temperatures.

Lacrosse helmets with face guards meeting the NOCSAE standard must be permanently marked with the manufacturer's information. A NOCSAE seal and a warning statement[42] must be placed on the exterior shell.

Lacrosse Helmet Face Guards

Lacrosse helmet face guards manufactured for use with NOCSAE-certified helmets undergo a projectile impact and penetration test.[42] A different guard is used for each impact test.

Impact tests are performed with the air cannon aimed at the nose, at one eye, and at a random area with the headform in different positions after the helmet and face guard are exposed to ambient temperatures. After the helmet and guard are exposed to cold temperatures, impacts are conducted to the nose and eye areas. The air cannon launches a lacrosse ball at 70 mph for all tests. Paste is used to verify ball or guard contact.

The penetration test is performed with the helmet mounted on a headform. A rigid, semicircle blade is placed into the openings of the guard in the attempt to contact the blade with the face. No contact is allowed.

Lacrosse face guards that meet the NOCSAE standard[42] must be permanently labeled with the manufacturer's information and include instructions on which helmet should be used with the guard and how to attach the guard.

Ice Hockey Helmets

Newly manufactured ice hockey helmets are subjected to retention, stability, drop method, and projectile impact tests to determine certification according to the NOCSAE standard.[42] During all tests, helmet face guards and face guard hardware are removed.

The retention test evaluates the dynamic strength of the chin strap(s) and is conducted by first exposing the helmet to hot temperatures, then placing it on a head-shaped platform attached to a strength and extension apparatus.[42] The retention system is fastened on the helmet and placed under a metal fixture on the apparatus. A weight is dropped 1.5 feet, elongating the retention

system. The system must remain fastened without stretching more than 1.25 inches.[42] Next, the weight is dropped from 3 feet. The retention system must release, allowing removal of the helmet. These same tests are repeated after the helmet is exposed to cold temperatures.

The stability, drop method, and projectile impact tests for ice hockey helmets are similar to the lacrosse helmet tests. The stability test with ice hockey helmets is identical to the procedure performed with lacrosse helmets, except the height of the drop is 2 feet. Similarities also exist in the drop method testing for these two helmets. After the helmets are exposed to ambient temperatures, the drop heights and repetitions are identical. Two additional drops are performed for high and low temperature tests. Impact tests are performed with an International Ice Hockey Federation standard hockey puck launched at 63 mph. Impact locations at ambient temperatures are identical to those used with lacrosse helmets. An additional location is used for a test at hot temperatures. Ice hockey helmets meeting the NOCSAE standard are permanently marked with the manufacturer's information, a NOCSAE seal, and a warning label.[42]

HECC also evaluates new ice hockey player helmets using the ASTM F1045 standard. Helmets are fit on headforms and undergo retention system, drop method, and penetration tests at ambient, hot, and cold conditions.[51] Helmets that meet the standard must be marked on the exterior shell with a HECC label.

CSA Standard CAN/CSA-Z262.1 also applies to helmets intended for use in ice hockey.[10] Impact, penetration, strength and durability, and assembly tests are performed on the helmets. Helmets meeting the standard are labeled with a CSA seal.

Ice Hockey Helmets with Face Guards

Newly manufactured ice hockey goalkeeper's helmets with face guards are evaluated by HECC to the ASTM F1587 standard.[51] The helmet is placed on a headform, and penetration and retention system tests are conducted. After the helmets and face guards are exposed to cold temperatures, projectile impact tests using an ice hockey puck launched at 80 mph are conducted. Drop method tests are performed after the helmets and guards are exposed to ambient, hot, and cold temperatures. Helmets meeting the standard must be marked with a HECC label.

Ice Hockey Helmet Face Guards and Visors

Ice hockey helmet face guards manufactured for use with NOCSAE-approved helmets are subjected to projectile impact and penetration tests.[42] The helmets are exposed to ambient temperatures and impacted using the same testing procedures as the lacrosse helmet face guard standard, except that hockey pucks are launched at 63 mph. After the helmets and guards are exposed to cold temperatures, impacts are performed at the nose and eye. Different guards are used for each impact test. The penetration test procedure is identical to the lacrosse helmet face guard standard, although a different sized blade is used to accommodate the smaller openings in the guard. Ice hockey face guards meeting the NOCSAE standard[42] must be permanently labeled in the same manner as the lacrosse face guard standard.

Using ASTM F513 standard, full face guards (except goalkeepers') are subjected to penetration and projectile impact tests to determine HECC certification.[51] The face guards are mounted on certified helmets, then placed on headforms. For the impact test, the launch speed of the hockey puck varies, 32 mph for youth guards and 63 mph and 74 mph for all other guards (except goalkeepers'). Impact tests are performed in ambient and cold temperatures. Full face guards that meet the standard are marked with a HECC seal.

New ice hockey visors manufactured for use with certified helmets are subjected to penetration and projectile impact tests by HECC with CSA Standard CAN/CSA-Z262.2.[51] Visors are mounted on certified helmets and positioned on headforms. Impact testing is similar to the procedure used with full face guards, with differences in impact locations and speeds. Hockey pucks are launched at 22 mph and 63 mph. The tests are conducted in ambient and cold conditions. Visors meeting the standard are marked with a HECC label.

CSA Standard CAN/CSA-Z262.2 applies to face guards and visors intended for use in ice hockey.[10] Area of coverage, optical requirements, stability, impact, penetration, and assembly tests are performed. Face guards and visors that meet the standard are marked with a CSA seal.

DETAILS

The governing bodies of interscholastic, intercollegiate, and amateur athletics may require different testing standards for approved protective equipment used in practices and competitions. For example, the NCAA and NFHS require the use of HECC and/or ASTM Standards for ice hockey helmets and face masks, although NOCSAE performs testing on ice hockey helmets. To ensure compliance, read and follow the governing bodies' regulations prior to purchasing and using protective equipment.

...IF/THEN...

IF a helmet is worn incorrectly or the individual uses it for purposes other than those designed or intended, **THEN** a manufacturer or health-care professional most likely will not be held liable for injuries sustained while wearing the helmet.

PROTECTIVE EQUIPMENT AND PADDING

Protective equipment and padding are available in many designs, based on the sport, the playing position, the activity, the individual, or the objective of the technique. The designs are constructed from a variety of materials. Some pads are manufactured from soft, low-density materials such as open- and closed-cell foams, while others are made of hard, high-density polycarbonate, Kevlar, or ABS plastic materials. Several designs are constructed from both soft, low-density and hard, high-density materials. For example, football shoulder pads have a high-density outer shell lined with open- and closed-cell foams. Proper fitting and application of the equipment and padding are critical; carefully follow manufacturers' instructions to prevent injury to the individual and to avoid liability. The following general fitting guidelines apply to most designs.

- Baseball, softball, and soccer shin guards and field hockey shin and leg guards and kickers are manufactured in individual and universal fit designs in predetermined sizes corresponding to lower leg length measurements or age of the individual.
- Ice hockey and lacrosse shoulder pads are available in individual fit designs in predetermined sizes based on chest circumference measurements.
- Baseball, field hockey, football, and softball glove designs are constructed in individual fit, right- and left-handed designs in predetermined sizes corresponding to tip of the third finger to the wrist length measurements.
- Baseball, field hockey, and softball chest protectors are manufactured in predetermined sizes based on chest circumference and length measurements.
- Baseball and softball batter's and catcher's, field hockey, football, ice hockey, and lacrosse helmets and wrestling ear guards are constructed in individual fit designs in predetermined sizes corresponding to head circumference measurements. For most designs, circumference measurements are taken 1 inch above the eyebrows.

Critical Thinking Question 2

You are performing outreach services through the hospital to a local senior league ice hockey team. During a practice, the coach asks if you could replace a face guard on a helmet so he can continue to work with the team on the ice. The coach provides you with the helmet, a new face guard, and tools.

▶ **Question: Can the face guard be replaced without jeopardizing NOCSAE and/or HECC certification?**

• Baseball, field hockey, lacrosse, and softball throat guards are available in universal fit designs in predetermined sizes.

The governing bodies of interscholastic, intercollegiate, and amateur athletics have established rules that govern the use of mandatory equipment and padding. The National Collegiate Athletic Association (NCAA), the National Association of Intercollegiate Athletics (NAIA) the National Federation of State High School Associations (NFHS), the United States Olympic Committee (USOC), and individual state high school athletic associations require equipment/padding in several sports. For our purposes, we will focus on protective equipment and padding required by the NCAA[33] and NFHS.[34–41,55]

Regardless of the requirements, many athletes wear equipment and padding that are not required. For example, the NCAA does not require baseball catchers to wear a chest protector or shin guards. Catchers nonetheless voluntarily wear the equipment because participation without the padding increases the risk of injury. This section discusses mandatory protective equipment and other standard equipment commonly worn by athletes during participation in practices and competitions. Eye and mouth guards are discussed at the end of the section.

Baseball

Mandatory Equipment

On deck, batting, and base running (NCAA and NFHS)
Retired runners, players/students in coach's boxes, nonadult bat/ball shaggers (NFHS)

• Helmet with double ear-flap design, NOCSAE Standards

Catcher

• Helmet, NOCSAE Standards (NCAA)
• Helmet and face mask with dual ear-flap design, NOCSAE Standards (NFHS)
• Throat guard (NCAA and NFHS)
• Body protector, shin guards, protective cup (NFHS)

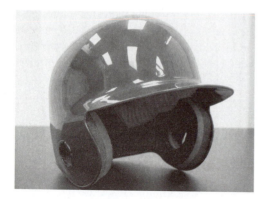

Figure 13-1 Double ear-flap batter's helmet.

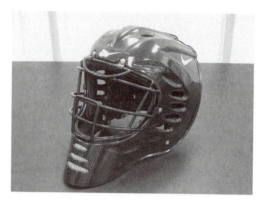

Figure 13-2 One-piece catcher's helmet.

Standard Equipment
Batting

• Gloves

Batter's helmets are manufactured of a pre-molded ABS, polycarbonate, or polyethylene plastic material outer shell with a front bill and double ear flaps and an open- and closed-cell foam inner lining. Several designs are available with a mechanism that allows for adjustments in fit; other designs are manufactured with hardware to attach a chin strap or cup and/or metal face guard (Fig. 13–1).

Catcher's helmets and **face guards** are available in a one- or two-piece style. One-piece designs are constructed of a pre-molded fiberglass resin, polymer nylon, Kevlar, or ABS plastic material outer shell lined with open- and closed-cell foam. The face guard is attached to the outer shell; most face guards are manufactured of metal and/or steel compound materials (Fig. 13–2). Several designs are available with adjustable posterior plates and chin straps for adjustments in fit. Two-piece designs consist of an individual helmet and face guard, which are used in combination with one another. The helmets are manufactured similarly to batting helmets, with or without a bill and ear flaps. Face guards are constructed of a tubular steel or hollow wire frame. Removable soft padding covered with polyurethane, leather, and/or synthetic leather materials is attached to the wire frame with metal snaps or Velcro closures. Most face guards are anchored over a helmet by a three-way, adjustable elastic harness (Fig. 13–3).

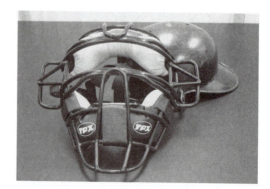

Figure 13-3 Two-piece catcher's helmet.

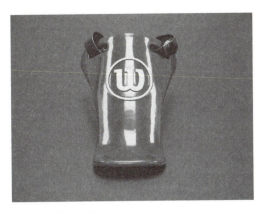

Figure 13-4 Throat guard.

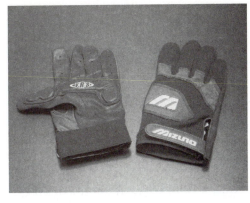

Figure 13-6 Batting gloves.

Throat guards are manufactured of rigid plastic materials; most throat guards attach to the distal face guard with laces or ties (Fig. 13–4). Many one-piece catcher's helmets/face guards and individual face guards are constructed with extensions over the throat and neck.

Chest protectors are constructed in individual fit, right- and left-handed designs and are manufactured of open- and closed-cell foam, covered with a nylon mesh material outer lining. Some designs are available with wings or extensions that protect the upper arm and genitalia. The protectors are contoured to allow for unrestricted shoulder and arm range of motion and are attached with an adjustable harness and straps with Velcro and/or D-ring closures (Fig. 13–5).

Shin guards are constructed of multiple polycarbonate or other rigid material outer shells incorporated in an inner shell of synthetic leather or nylon material lined with open- and closed-cell or EVA foam, air bladder, or rubber padding materials. Shin guards are attached with adjustable nylon straps with metal closures (see Fig. 13–5).

Protective athletic cups used in baseball and softball were discussed in Chapter 12 in the Padding section (see Fig. 12-13).

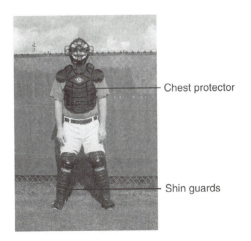

Chest protector

Shin guards

Figure 13-5 Catcher in protective equipment. Chest protector and shin guards.

Batting gloves are constructed of leather materials; most batting gloves have spandex, Lycra, and/or neoprene material finger, thumb, and knuckle gussets. Most designs are manufactured with spandex, Lycra, and/or neoprene materials over the dorsal hand for comfort; some gloves have foam and/or gel material padding incorporated in this area to absorb shock. Batting gloves are anchored with an elastic nylon strap with Velcro closures (Fig. 13–6).

Field Hockey

Mandatory Equipment
Goalkeeper

- Helmet with full-face design (NCAA and NFHS), no protruding visor (NFHS)
- Throat guard (NCAA and NFHS)
- Chest protector (NFHS)
- Elbow pads (NCAA)
- Gloves (NCAA and NFHS)
- Leg guards (NFHS)
- Kickers (NFHS)

Kicking back (NCAA)

- Helmet
- Throat guard
- Chest protector

Field athletes (NFHS)

- Shin guards

All athletes (NCAA and NFHS)

- Mouth guard

Standard Equipment
Goalkeeper

- Pants

Helmets are manufactured of a pre-molded fiberglass resin, polyethylene, or polycarbonate plastic material outer shell with an open- and closed-cell foam inner lining. Many designs extend over the throat. A carbon steel wire face guard is attached to the outer shell. The helmets are anchored with an adjustable strap (Fig. 13–7).

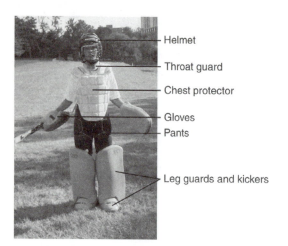

Figure 13-7 Goalkeeper in protective equipment. Helmet, throat guard, chest protector, gloves, leg guards and kickers, and pants.

Helmet
Throat guard
Chest protector
Gloves
Pants
Leg guards and kickers

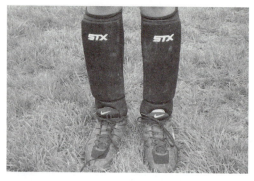

Figure 13-8 Shin guards.

Throat guards are manufactured of a rigid plastic material inner lining with a pre-molded foam outer shell covered with cotton and/or nylon materials. These guards wrap around the neck and are anchored with Velcro closures (see Fig. 13–7).

Chest protectors are manufactured in individual and universal fit designs and are constructed of open- and closed-cell and/or EVA foam with a nylon mesh outer lining. Most wrap-around designs have a nylon mesh back. Some designs have additional padding over the thorax; many have detachable pads around the shoulder. Chest protectors are anchored with an adjustable harness and straps with Velcro and/or D-ring closures (see Fig. 13–7).

Arm and **elbow pads** are constructed in individual fit designs in predetermined sizes corresponding to mid upper arm to mid forearm length measurements. These pads are manufactured of a spandex and/or nylon material outer shell with a neoprene and/or EVA foam inner lining. Pre-molded polycarbonate or rigid plastic materials are incorporated in the outer shell over the elbow and forearm. Arm and elbow pads are attached with adjustable nylon straps with Velcro closures.

Gloves are manufactured of leather materials with spandex or Lycra material finger, thumb, and knuckle gussets with foam and/or gel padding material incorporated throughout the glove. Several designs are available for athletes, excluding the goalkeeper, to protect the nondominant stick hand with foam and/or gel padding material incorporated in the dorsal hand. The gloves are anchored with elastic nylon straps with Velcro closures (see Fig. 13–7).

Leg guards and **kickers** are constructed of pre-molded laminate foams and are attached with nylon straps and plastic closures (see Fig. 13–7).

Mouth guards are discussed at the end of this section (see Figs. 13–29, 13–30, and 13–31).

Goalkeeper's pants are manufactured of nylon/Lycra materials with high- and low-density foam padding incorporated over the thigh, hip, pelvis, genitalia, abdomen,

and back. Most designs are available with an adjustable belt (see Fig. 13–7).

Shin guards consist of a pre-molded rigid plastic material outer shell with a soft foam inner lining. Some designs are manufactured of thermoplastic or fiberglass materials that allow for custom-fitting. Other guards extend over the medial and lateral malleoli to provide additional protection. Most shin guards are attached with Velcro straps (Fig. 13–8). Some guards have nylon foot stirrups to lessen migration during activity.

Football

Mandatory Equipment
All athletes

- Helmet, NOCSAE Standards, risk of injury warning label, attached face mask (NCAA and NFHS), four- or six-point chin strap (NCAA), fastened chin strap (NFHS)
- Shoulder pads (NCAA and NFHS)
- Hip, thigh, and coccyx pads (NCAA and NFHS), thigh pad must have at least ¼ inch thick outside and ⅜ inch thick inside surface (NFHS)
- Knee pads (NCAA and NFHS), at least ½ inch (NCAA, NFHS) or ⅜ inch thick (NFHS)
- Mouth guard, intraoral design covering all upper teeth (NCAA and NFHS), readily visible color (not white or transparent) with FDA-approved base materials (FDCS) (NCAA)

Standard Equipment
All athletes

- Gloves

Helmets are manufactured of a polycarbonate alloy or ABS plastic material outer shell. Some designs use one or two crown air bladder(s) and dual-density foam as an inner liner. Other designs use multiple individual pads constructed of an air bladder and dual-density foam. Inflation ports located on the outer shell allow for adjustments of air pressure within the bladders. The foam is available in varying thickness and firmness for adjustments in fit. The air bladders and/or foam padding of most designs are removable for replacement and maintenance.

Helmets are anchored with chin straps in a variety of designs. Chin straps are available in two-, four-, and six-point or snap designs. The straps are constructed of cotton materials with a vinyl coating and are anchored to the helmet with plastic or metal snaps. Some designs consist of a soft chin cup while others have a polycarbonate cup. Many designs are available with a foam inner lining.

Face guards are available in a variety of designs and sizes based on playing position and desired level of protection. Face guards are constructed of carbon steel or titanium with a vinyl coating or thermoplastic materials. The guards are attached directly on the helmet using plastic grommets and screws .

Shoulder pads are constructed in individual fit designs in predetermined sizes based on chest circumference, AC joint to AC joint, or lateral shoulder to lateral shoulder length measurements. The pads are available for each playing position in two basic designs: cantilever and flat. Both designs consist of a two-piece, high-density plastic material arch or outer shell pre-molded to the contours of the thorax. Pre-formed, high-density plastic epaulets and caps or cups, covering the shoulder and upper arm, are attached to the outer shell. Cantilever designs have a high-density plastic arch or bridge located underneath the outer shell over the AC joint. Cantilevers are used to disperse impact forces away from the shoulder and AC joint to the

> **Helpful Hint:** When the face guard hardware of a football helmet becomes rusted as a result of environmental conditions and/or perspiration, replace the hardware with parts that meet or exceed original manufacturer specifications.[42] Regular maintenance increases protection and allows for removal of the face guard in an emergency situation.

DETAILS

General Football Helmet Fitting Guidelines[16]

- Place the athlete in a standing position with the hair at a length worn during the season. Wet the hair to simulate perspiration.
- Use a helmet manufacturer's caliper or measuring tape and measure the circumference of the head above the ears to determine helmet shell size (Fig. 13–9A).
- Select the appropriate helmet shell size. Remove the jaw pads and deflate all air bladders.
- Have the athlete place the helmet on the head.
- Inspect the jaw area to determine what size pads are needed. Select and fit the proper jaw pads (see Fig. 13–9B). The pads should feel firm against the face. When using some designs, inflate the jaw pads with air.
- Inflate crown air bladder(s) through holes in the exterior shell so that the helmet rises to the proper position just above the eyebrows, approximately one to two finger widths (see Fig. 13–9C).
- Center the chin strap cup over the chin. Adjust the chin straps on the side of the helmet to provide equal tension in each strap and anchor (see Fig. 13–9D).
- If air bladders are present, inflate side and back air bladders.
- Check for proper fit. The helmet should be fit to snugness rather than comfort or too tight over the crown, front, back, and sides.
- The helmet should cover the base of the skull, but not prevent normal range of neck extension.
- The helmet ear holes should align with the ears.
- The face guard should be positioned approximately two to three finger widths from the nose and forehead and allow for unrestricted vision (see Fig. 13–9E).
- Continue to check for proper fit by having the athlete maintain a rigid head and neck position.
- Apply downward pressure on the crown of the helmet with the hands (see Fig. 13–9F). The helmet should not move.
- Grasp the face mask and pull downward (see Fig. 13–9G). The helmet should not move.
- Place the hands on the sides of the helmet, then on the front and back, and attempt to rotate the helmet (see Fig. 13–9H). The helmet should not rotate.
- Remove the helmet, apply shoulder pads, then reapply the helmet. Have the athlete move through several position-specific movements to check for proper fit. The helmet should not move at any time and allow for upper body range of motion.

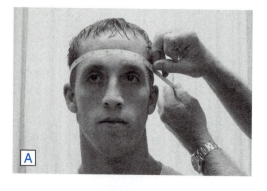

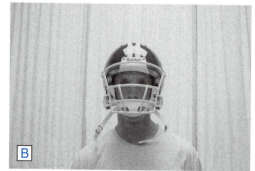

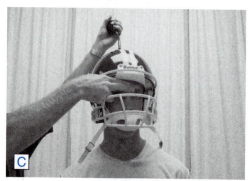

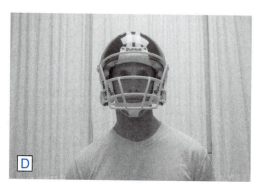

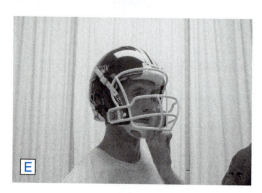

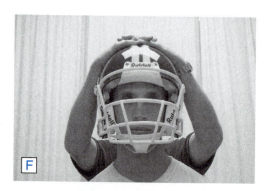

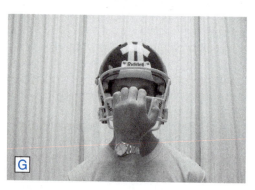

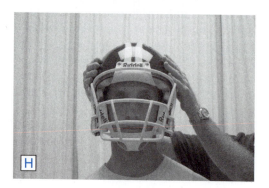

Figure 13-9

RESEARCH BRIEF

Helmets are mandatory in several NCAA and NFHS sports; these designs are certified according to NOCSAE, HECC, ASTM, and/or CSA standards. Although these helmets are effective in reducing injuries,[22,31] refinement and verification of current testing methods continue. Several investigators have suggested that the testing methods performed in the laboratory setting rarely duplicate conditions experienced on the field during actual use.[21,22] Changing weather conditions such as humidity and external temperature levels, density of the playing surface and equipment, and the direction, speed, and amount of force typically found on the field are absent in the existing testing procedures. Regardless, the use of certified helmets should be enforced to protect the athlete against injury.

What type of protection does a certified helmet provide for the athlete? Helmets are designed primarily to prevent catastrophic injuries such as skull fractures and intracranial hematomas. Helmets appear to have minimal effect on the prevention of concussions and catastrophic cervical spine injuries.[21–23] After examining football players, researchers have found a decrease in the incidence of fatalities and nonfatal catastrophic injuries following the introduction of helmet standards, rule changes eliminating spearing, increased player education and awareness, limitation of contact in practice, and improved assessment and treatment techniques following injury.[11,32] After examining athletes participating in ice hockey, researchers have found that the use of helmets with full face shields resulted in significantly less time missed from practices and games following a concussion than helmets with half face shields.[5,6] The researchers suggested that full face shield helmets may disperse and absorb greater amounts of force and remain in place on the head more effectively because of the additional chin strap. Headbands for soccer athletes have been developed in response to the repetitive blows sustained to the head

with ball and opponent contact during play. Currently, research findings do not support the use of headbands to attenuate impact during simulated soccer heading.[21,43] Some researchers have stated that headband use may increase the incidence of injury due to a false sense of protection and more aggressive play.[21] Researchers have examined the ability of contemporary and traditional lacrosse helmets to attenuate impact and found differences among the designs.[12] Overall, traditional designs appeared to attenuate more force at the front drop site, and contemporary designs were more effective at the right rear boss drop site. Both helmet designs decreased in the ability to dissipate force over 10 drops.

Injuries to the head may occur through several mechanisms. Two basic types are linear and rotational acceleration. Linear acceleration, acceleration along a line,[22] is used in standard testing methods; a certified helmet meets the established values. Standards and test values for rotational acceleration, angular or nonlinear acceleration, have not been established; some researchers suggest that helmets would not prevent injuries from these forces because contact is not required.[22] Other researchers have stated that axial loading resulting in catastrophic cervical spine injury can neither be caused nor prevented by standard equipment.[9,23,53,54,59]

NOCSAE, HECC, ASTM, and/or CSA certified helmets are not designed to prevent all head injuries, but should be recommended for athletes when appropriate. Helmets should be maintained in their original form and constantly monitored for wear. Use a certified reconditioner to evaluate and repair helmets at regular intervals and adhere to manufacturer recommendations. Lastly, athletes should be educated about the proper use of the helmet, safe sport techniques such as blocking and tackling, and the signs and symptoms of acute and chronic trauma to the head and neck.

thoracic surfaces of the pads. Cantilever pads provide the greatest amount of protection, but are bulky and restrict glenohumeral joint range of motion. These designs are commonly used by linemen, linebackers, and running backs. Flat pads do not use a cantilever and are less bulky, provide a more contoured fit, and allow greater glenohumeral joint range of motion, but provide less protection. These designs are commonly worn by quarterbacks, receivers, and defensive backs, but can be used with any position.

Construction of the inner lining depends on the specific pad design. Most designs use a combination of open-

and closed-cell foams covered with a moisture-resistant nylon material in various individual patterns and sizes. The individual inner lining pads are attached to the outer shell with Velcro or zippers; most designs allow for adjustments in fit. The inner lining forms a channel over the shoulder and AC joint to disperse forces to the thoracic padding. One design uses plastic tubes incorporated in the inner lining to release cool, compressed air to the thorax to lower core body temperature. Shoulder pads are anchored with adjustable anterior and/or posterior laces, elastic straps with T-hook closures, and/or polyurethane belts with buckle closures.

DETAILS

General Football Shoulder Pad Fitting Guidelines[17]

- Place the athlete in a standing position without a shirt or only wearing a T-shirt. Perform an assessment of the athlete that includes body weight and height, medical history, playing position, and chest circumference and/or shoulder length measurements.
- Match the body type, past injury concerns (AC joint sprain, upper arm contusions, etc), playing position, and chest/shoulder measurements with a corresponding shoulder pad design. Refer to the manufacturer's sizing chart.
- Place the shoulder pads on the athlete and anchor the laces, straps, and/or belts to achieve a snug fit.
- Next, conduct an anterior, lateral, and posterior visual assessment.
- Anterior: The pads should fully cover the clavicles, AC joints, pectoralis and trapezius muscles, and extend ½ inch over the deltoid. The collar should provide a comfortable range of motion to the neck, and arms raised overhead should not cause pinching of the neck. The caps/cups should fit snugly over the deltoid muscle. The outer shell should meet evenly with no overlap, and the laces should be tight and centered over the anterior thorax (Fig. 13–10A).
- Lateral: The inner lining should form a channel over the AC joint and not make contact with the AC joint. The caps/cups should cover the deltoid muscle (see Fig. 13–10B).
- Posterior: The outer shell should extend below the inferior angle of the scapula, covering the scapula and trapezius, rhomboids, and latissimus dorsi muscles. If present, the laces should be tight and centered over the posterior thorax. The collar should not cause pinching of the neck (see Fig. 13–10C).
- The last assessment is conducted following application of a helmet and jersey. Have the athlete assume several different upper and lower body movements required by the playing position.
- A properly fitted shoulder pad should be snug over the entire thorax and shoulder, but still allow for upper body range of motion.
- The pads should return to the thorax and shoulder after movement.
- A properly worn jersey and sleeves should assist in anchoring the pads to the shoulder, thorax, and upper arm.

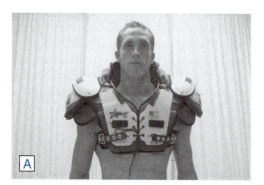
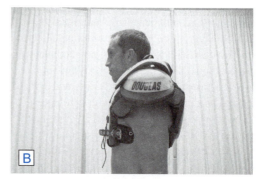
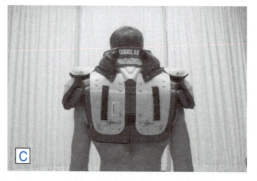

Figure 13-10

Knee, hip, thigh, and **coccyx pads** are manufactured in individual and universal fit designs in predetermined sizes based on circumference measurements of the thigh or waist, or age of the individual. Universal fit pads are constructed of varying thicknesses of high-impact or high-density, open- and closed-cell foams (see Fig. 7–18A). Some designs are coated with vinyl. Most thigh pads are manufactured with a rigid plastic insert. The individual fit hip and thigh pads are larger in size with additional padding than the mandatory designs and are commonly used following injury to provide additional protection (see Figs. 7–18B–C). Mandatory knee, hip, thigh, and coccyx pads are available from most manufacturers in a complete set. These pads are attached in pad pockets of nylon/polyester/Lycra girdles (see Fig. 7–18F). Some pads are placed into pad pockets of football pants.

Mouth guard designs for use in football are illustrated in Figs. 13–29, 13–30, and 13–31.

Gloves are constructed of leather, synthetic leather, and/or vinyl materials for specific playing positions. Receiver, tight end, running back, linebacker, and defensive back gloves are lightweight designs with spandex, Lycra, or neoprene material finger, thumb, and knuckle gussets. The leather or synthetic leather covering the palmar aspect of the fingers, thumb, and hand on most designs is treated to provide an adherent surface for athletic equipment. Some gloves are available with foam padding. These gloves are anchored with elastic nylon straps with Velcro closures (Fig. 13–11A). Some designs are available without straps or closures. Linemen gloves are heavyweight designs with reinforced leather, synthetic leather, and/or vinyl materials and foam, gel, or viscoelastic polymer padding. Several designs have spandex, Lycra, or neoprene finger and thumb gussets. Most line-

men gloves are manufactured with an adherent surface on the palmar aspect. The gloves are anchored with a wide, elastic nylon strap with Velcro closures (Fig. 13–11B).

Ice Hockey

Mandatory Equipment

All athletes

- Helmet attached with chin strap, HECC Standards (NCAA), HECC-ASTM Standards (NFHS)
- Face mask, HECC–ASTM F 513-95 Eye and Face Protective Equipment for Hockey Players Standard (NCAA and NFHS)
- Mouth guard, intraoral design (NCAA and NFHS), covering all upper teeth (NCAA), covering teeth of one jaw, colored, non-clear material, attached to face guard (NFHS)
- Gloves (NFHS)

Goalkeeper

- Leg guards, not to exceed 12 inches in width (NCAA and NFHS)
- Gloves, not to exceed 8 inches in width and 16 inches in length (NFHS)
- Throat guard, separate, commercially manufactured (NFHS)

Standard Equipment

All athletes except goalkeepers

- Elbow pads
- Shin guards
- Pants
- Shoulder pads

Goalkeepers

- Chest pads

Helmets are manufactured of a pre-molded polycarbonate or polyethylene plastic material outer shell and dual-density and/or EVA foam or air bladder inner lining. Many designs are constructed of a two-piece outer shell allowing for adjustments in fit. The helmets are available with or without face guards. Most face guards are manufactured of a carbon steel or titanium wire pattern extending over the jaw, permanently attached to the superior outer shell. These helmets are anchored with an adjustable two- or four-point cotton or nylon chin strap (see Fig. 13–12). Many designs have a soft chin cup.

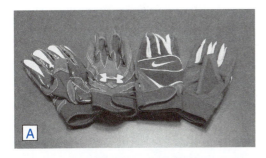

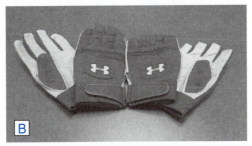

Figure 13-11 **A** Receiver, tight end, running back, linebacker, and defensive back gloves. **B** Linemen gloves.

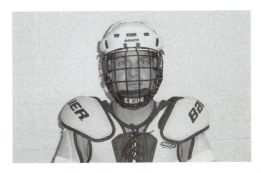

Figure 13-12 Helmet with attached face guard.

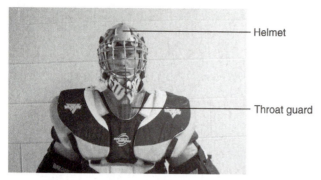

Figure 13-13 Goalkeeper's helmet with attached throat guard.

Goalkeeper's helmets and **face guards** are available in a two-piece style constructed of a pre-molded Kevlar, fiberglass resin, or polymer nylon material outer shell. An adjustable plate incorporated in the posterior outer shell allows for adjustments in fit. Dual-density foam and gel materials are used for the inner lining. Face guards constructed of carbon steel wire are attached to the outer shell. Goalkeeper's helmets are attached with an adjustable elastic or nylon chin strap and/or chin cup (Fig. 13–13).

Leg guards or **pads** for goalkeepers are manufactured in individual fit designs in predetermined sizes based on the sum of instep to knee and patella to distal thigh length, and skate size measurements. The designs are constructed of a thick, laminated foam material outer shell covered with synthetic leather and nylon materials. The outer shell is incorporated in a laminated foam inner lining consisting of vertical rolls and wings that extend around the knee, lower leg, ankle, and foot. Most designs are anchored with leather and/or nylon straps with plastic or metal closures (Fig. 13–14).

Player's gloves are manufactured in individual fit and right- and left-handed designs, in predetermined sizes in various lengths corresponding to fingertip to mid forearm length measurements, or from the fingertips to the distal edge of the elbow pad. The gloves are constructed of a multiple-piece leather or synthetic leather outer shell lined with a nylon mesh material. Most designs have leather incorporated in the palmar hand, finger, and thumb gussets. Multidensity foam or air bladder padding and polyethylene or Kevlar inserts incorporated throughout the dorsal fingers,

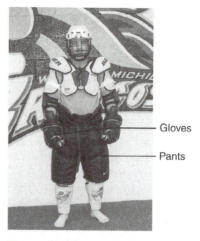

Figure 13-15 Player's gloves and pants.

thumb, and hand and around the wrist absorb shock and provide protection. These gloves are constructed with two- or three-piece flared or winged cuffs to provide additional protection. Most gloves are anchored with leather straps with Velcro closures (Fig. 13–15).

Goalkeeper's gloves consist of a catcher and blocker design. Catchers and blockers are available in individual fit, right- and left-handed designs in predetermined sizes identical to player's gloves. Catchers are worn on the non-stick hand and are manufactured of a multiple-piece leather, synthetic leather, and/or nylon outer shell with a moisture-resistant mesh material inner lining with individual finger and thumb stalls. A leather or synthetic leather mesh pocket is incorporated in the outer shell. Contoured, high-density foam and/or air and polyethylene inserts are incorporated throughout the glove for protection and improved fit. Catchers are anchored with multiple Velcro straps (Fig. 13–16). Blockers are worn on the stick hand and are constructed of dual-density foam with a leather, synthetic leather, or nylon outer shell. A foam padded glove is incorporated in the inner surface of the blocker.

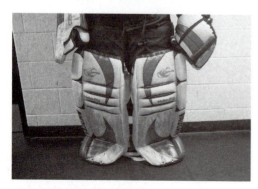

Figure 13-14 Goalkeeper's leg guards.

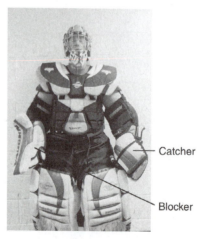

Figure 13-16 Goalkeeper's gloves. Blocker and catcher.

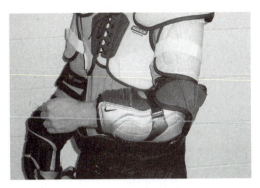

Figure 13-17 Left arm and elbow pad.

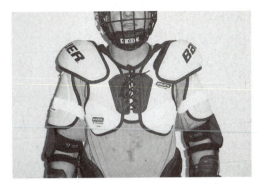

Figure 13-19 Shoulder pads.

Pre-molded, high-density foam and polyethylene inserts provide protection for the first finger, thumb, and wrist. Most designs have finger, thumb, and palmar hand gussets and a strap to anchor the glove. Blockers are attached through various straps with webbing or lace closures.

Throat guards are available in individual fit designs in predetermined sizes corresponding to neck circumference measurements. Most guards are constructed of a pre-molded, high-density foam material collar and bib with a ballistic nylon material covering. These throat guards are anchored with adjustable elastic straps with Velcro closures. Other throat guards are manufactured of rigid plastic materials and attach to the distal helmet and face guard with laces or ties (see Fig. 13–13).

Mouth guards are discussed in Figures 13–29, 13–30, and 13–31.

Arm and **elbow pads** are manufactured in universal and right- and left-handed styles in predetermined sizes based on mid upper arm to mid forearm length measurements, or from the distal edge of the shoulder pads to the proximal glove. Most pads are constructed of a polycarbonate or plastic outer shell incorporated in a vinyl, nylon, or woven fabric material inner shell with open- and closed-cell foam padding. The pads are anchored with adjustable nylon straps with Velcro or buckle closures (Fig. 13–17).

Shin guards are available in individual and universal fit designs in predetermined sizes based on superior patella to top of the skate length measurements. The designs are manufactured of a polycarbonate or other rigid material outer shell incorporated in an inner shell constructed of various foams. The outer and inner shells are covered

with polyester mesh, nylon, or thermoregulatory materials. The inner shell and padding of some designs can be removed and/or adjusted to allow for additional protection and custom-fitting. Most designs are anchored with adjustable nylon straps with Velcro closures (Fig. 13–18).

Pants are constructed of water-resistant nylon/spandex materials with high- and low-density foams or air bladder padding incorporated in the inner and/or outer lining over the thigh, hip, pelvis, abdomen, and back. Some designs allow for adjustments or removal of padding materials for an individual fit. Most pants are available with a contoured waistband and adjustable belt (see Fig. 13–15).

Shoulder pads are manufactured with an outer shell constructed of varying thicknesses of open- and closed-cell and EVA foams covered with a nylon/polyester material. Most designs have a moisture-resistant inner lining. These pads have rigid polyethylene plastic plates and rounded caps incorporated in the outer shell over the spine, thorax, shoulder, and upper arm. Some designs have a polyethylene plate over the clavicle; other designs have a detachable abdominal pad. Shoulder pads are anchored with adjustable nylon straps with Velcro closures (Fig. 13–19).

Chest pads are available in individual fit designs in predetermined sizes corresponding to chest circumference measurements. The designs are manufactured of open- and closed-cell block foam pads arranged in various patterns covered with nylon materials. The chest pads have pre-molded polyethylene plastic plates and caps incorporated over the thorax, shoulder, upper arm, and elbow. Chest pads are anchored with an adjustable harness and straps with Velcro and/or D-ring closures (Fig. 13–20).

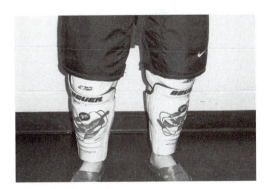

Figure 13-18 Shin guards.

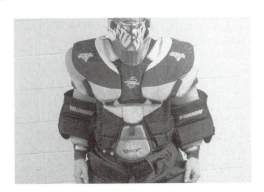

Figure 13-20 Goalkeeper's chest pads.

Lacrosse

Women's and Girls' Lacrosse

Mandatory Equipment

All athletes

• Eye guard, ASTM F803-03 Standard, PECC Certified (NCAA and NFHS)
• Mouth guard (NCAA and NFHS), intraoral design covering all upper teeth (NCAA)

Goalkeeper

• Helmet with attached face mask (NCAA and NFHS)
• Chest protector (NCAA and NFHS)
• Throat protector (NCAA and NFHS)

Men's and Boys' Lacrosse

Mandatory Equipment

All athletes

• Helmet, NOCSAE Standards, risk of injury warning label (NCAA and NFHS), chin strap and chin pad (NFHS), cupped four-point chin strap with high-point hookup, chin pad (NCAA)
• Face mask, NOCSAE Standards (NCAA), fixed, center bar from top to bottom (NCAA and NFHS), horizontal openings not to exceed 1½ inches (NFHS)
• Gloves (NCAA and NFHS)
• Mouth guard, intraoral design covering all upper teeth (NCAA and NFHS), yellow or any other highly visible color, clear color may be used if head coach certifies that it must be clear for a medical reason (NCAA)
• Shoulder pads, except goalkeeper (NCAA), optional for goalkeeper (NFHS)
• Arm pads, except goalkeeper (NCAA), optional for goalkeeper (NFHS)

Goalkeeper

• Chest protector (NCAA)
• Throat protector, lacrosse design (NCAA)

Helmet designs are constructed of a polyethylene or polycarbonate plastic material outer shell with an inner lining of dual-density foam. A visor is incorporated in the outer shell. The face guard is manufactured of carbon steel and is anchored to the outer shell. A rigid plastic chin guard is attached to the distal face guard and extends downward. Most helmets and face guards are anchored with a four-point adjustable chin strap with a chin cup (Fig. 13–21).

Shoulder pads can serve as a chest protector and are manufactured of an open- and closed-cell and EVA foams or viscoelastic gel material outer shell covered with a mesh material lining. Most pads have an inner lining of moisture-resistant material. In most designs, polyethylene plastic plates and caps are incorporated in the outer shell over the thorax, shoulder, and upper arm. Some designs use a wire mesh material incorporated in the outer shell over the shoulder to provide additional protection.

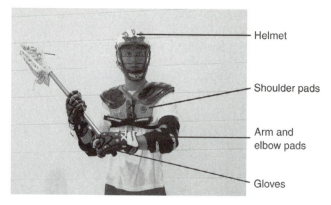

Figure 13-21 Field player in protective equipment. Helmet, shoulder pads, arm and elbow pads, and gloves.

Shoulder pads are attached with adjustable nylon straps with Velcro closures (Figs. 13–21 and 13–22).

Arm and **elbow pads** are manufactured, fit, and attached in the same manner as ice hockey designs (see Fig. 13–21).

Gloves are available in individual fit and right- and left-handed designs in various lengths and predetermined sizes based on length measurements identical to ice hockey designs. The multi-piece designs consist of a contoured leather, synthetic leather, and/or vinyl outer shell; moisture-resistant inner lining; finger and thumb gussets; leather or mesh surface on the palmar hand; and flared or winged wrist cuffs. The gloves have multi-density foam and polyethylene inserts incorporated throughout the dorsal finger and hand surface for protection and stability. Most gloves are attached with laces (see Fig. 13–21).

Throat guards are constructed of rigid plastic material or high-density foam. The guards attach to the distal face guard with laces or nylon straps with metal snaps (see Fig. 13–22).

Eye guards for use in lacrosse are discussed at the end of this section (see Fig. 13–28).

Mouth guard designs for lacrosse are illustrated in Figures 13–29, 13–30, and 13–31.

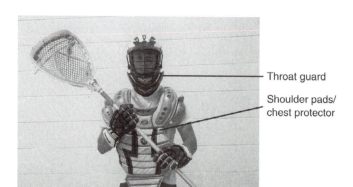

Figure 13-22 Goalkeeper in protective equipment. Shoulder pads/chest protector and throat guard.

Critical Thinking Question 3

During the second half of a soccer match, a forward is tackled and falls to the ground on her left posterior elbow, sustaining a moderate contusion. Following an evaluation by the team physician and several days of treatment, she is allowed to return to play if properly protected.

▶ **Question: What padding technique can you use to provide adequate protection?**

Soccer

Mandatory Equipment

All athletes

- Shin guards, professionally manufactured, age and size appropriate, no alterations (NCAA and NFHS), bottom edge no higher than 2 inches above the ankle (NFHS)

Standard Equipment

Goalkeeper

- Gloves

Shin guards are manufactured of a pre-molded rigid or semirigid plastic material outer shell. Some designs use thermoplastic materials for a custom-fit. The outer shell of the guards is lined with soft, EVA, or closed-cell foam. Many designs are manufactured with padding over the medial and lateral malleoli. Some guards are covered with a nylon mesh material and others with a cotton sock or elastic sleeve. Most shin guards are attached with adjustable nylon straps with Velcro closures (Fig. 13–23). Some designs have nylon foot stirrups.

> **...IF/THEN...**
>
> **IF** soccer shin guards do not provide adequate protection of the anterior lower leg, **THEN** consider purchasing a larger size or a thermoplastic design; the larger size should extend coverage over the area, and thermoplastic designs can be custom fit.

Gloves are manufactured in individual fit, right- and left-handed designs in predetermined sizes corresponding to hand, excluding the thumb, circumference measurements. The designs are manufactured of a latex, contact, or EVA foam outer shell on the palmar surface of the hand. In some designs, an irregularly textured surface is provided with a waffle or dimple pattern to improve grip. Some gloves are constructed with a nylon mesh material covering the dorsal hand. Other designs use metal plates or pre-molded metal wire incorporated in the dorsal fingers to prevent hyperextension. Most gloves have finger and thumb gussets and are anchored with an elastic strap and Velcro closure (Fig. 13–24).

Softball

Mandatory Equipment

On deck, batting, and base running (NCAA and NFHS)
Retired runners, players/students in coach's boxes, nonadult bat/ball shaggers (NFHS)

- Helmet with double ear-flap design, NOCSAE Standards (NCAA and NFHS), risk of injury warning label (NFHS)

Catcher

- Helmet, NOCSAE Standards (NCAA and NFHS)
- Face mask, NOCSAE Standards (NCAA and NFHS)
- Throat guard (NCAA and NFHS)
- Chest protector (NCAA)
- Shin guards, foot to knee (NCAA)
- Body protector, shin guards, protective cup (male catcher), while warming up pitcher (NFHS)

Standard Equipment

Batting

- Gloves

Helmet, face mask, throat guard, chest and body protector, shin guard, protective cup, and **glove designs** are identical to baseball equipment (see Figs. 13–1, 13–2, 13–3, 13–4, 13–5, and 13–6).

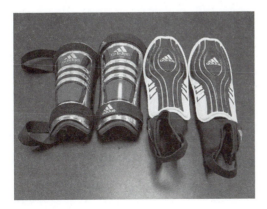

Figure 13-23 Shin guards.

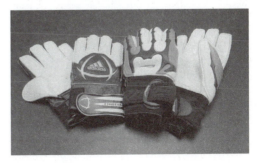

Figure 13-24 Goalkeeper's gloves.

RESEARCH BRIEF

The majority of injuries sustained during participation in soccer occur to the lower extremities,[13,30,47] and include minor trauma, such as contusions and high-impact trauma such as fractures.[19] Several investigations have been conducted to examine the effectiveness of shin guards in reducing trauma to the lower leg.

Some researchers have suggested that shin guards may lessen the occurrence of minor trauma,[28,50] while others have demonstrated that guards may protect against lower leg fractures. Among recreational and intercollegiate soccer athletes, using shin guards was shown to prevent lower leg fractures.[8,13] Using fiberglass[18] and metal rod[7] lower leg models, other researchers found significant reductions in peak forces at the proximal and distal ends of the models during controlled impact-loading testing. At a 50-cm

drop height, a 6% to 21%[18] and 40% to 77%[7] reduction was demonstrated with the guarded model compared to the unguarded. The differences in reductions may be attributed to the different leg models.[18] Although not significant, peak forces were also reduced with the guarded model at drop heights of 20, 30, and 40 cm.[18]

The results of these limited studies appear to support the use of shin guards to prevent lower leg injuries. However, the level of protection may depend on the size and construction of the guard. Although heavier, thicker, and longer guards most likely provide greater protection, soccer participants prefer lower profile and lighter designs for fit and comfort.[18] Future research is needed to design the optimal shin guard that provides maximal protection and comfort.

Wrestling

Mandatory Equipment

All athletes

• Ear guard (NCAA and NFHS), worn at all times (NCAA)

Ear guards are available with an outer shell constructed of various nylon and/or neoprene straps with a polypropylene and/or air bladder guard incorporated in the straps over the ears. Most ear guards are lined with EVA foam and/or neoprene materials. Some designs use a padded nylon guard that attaches to the outer shell to protect the forehead. Ear guards are anchored with adjustable nylon and/or neoprene straps with Velcro closures (Fig. 13–25). Some designs are available with a chin cup.

Eye Guards

Eye guards are available in individual fit designs in predetermined sizes corresponding to head circumference measurements and helmet and face guard style. The guards are manufactured in three designs: glasses, shields, and

goggles. Eye guards are mandatory in only one NCAA and NFHS sport, women's and girls' lacrosse, but can provide protection for athletes participating in baseball, basketball, fencing, field hockey, football, ice hockey, rifle, skiing, softball, swimming, volleyball, and water polo. Baseball, fencing, field hockey, football, ice hockey, lacrosse, and softball helmets, face guards, and masks, by design, also provide some protection of the eyes.

Glasses are used for protection in baseball, basketball, field hockey, football, ice hockey, lacrosse, and softball. Most designs are manufactured of polycarbonate plastic material lenses and are available with ultraviolet (UV) protection, anti-fog, anti-glare, and anti-scratch coatings, as well as prescription vision corrections. The lenses are incorporated in one- or three-piece polycarbonate or other plastic material frames that extend across the eyes and lateral face. The nose piece is padded with foam or viscoelastic materials; some frames are lined with these materials for additional protection. Glasses are attached with temples behind the ears and/or adjustable elastic nylon straps (Fig. 13–26). ♪

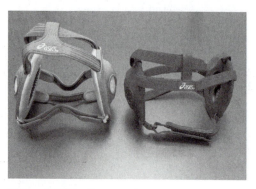

Figure 13-25   Ear guards.

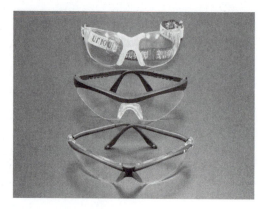

Figure 13-26   Glasses.

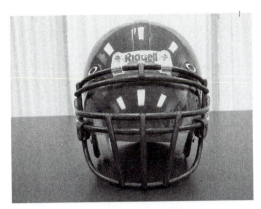

Figure 13-27 Shield attached to a football helmet.

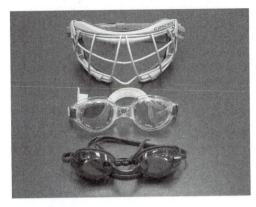

Figure 13-28 Goggles.

Helpful Hint: Protective eye guards should fit snugly. To test for proper fit, lightly run a finger around the outside perimeter of the eye guard. No gaps large enough to allow a finger to lightly touch the eye should be present.[52]

Shields are designed to be used in combination with baseball and softball catcher's, field hockey, football, ice hockey, and lacrosse helmets and face guards to provide protection. These shields are manufactured from polycarbonate or other plastic materials and are coated to provide UV and scratch protection and resist fogging and glare. The shields extend the width of the face guard; most shields are attached on the inside surface of face guards with plastic grommets or wire or plastic ties (Fig. 13–27).

Goggles are used to provide protection in lacrosse, skiing, swimming, and water polo (Fig. 13–28). Most designs are constructed of polycarbonate lenses with UV, anti-scratch, anti-fog, and anti-glare protection. Prescription goggles are also available. Some lacrosse designs are constructed of a foam-lined, light wire frame with adjustable elastic straps. Skiing goggles are used in combination with helmets and are attached over the helmet with adjustable nylon straps. Swimming and water polo designs are manufactured in a cup style that fits snugly over the eye socket with watertight silicone, neoprene, or closed-cell foam gaskets and a flexible nose bridge. Most designs are anchored with adjustable silicon straps.

RESEARCH BRIEF

A risk of injury to the eye is present in any sport that involves a stick or racquet, a ball or other projectile, or body contact. The risk of eye injury does not correlate with the common classifications of collision, contact, and noncontact sports, in which collision and contact sports typically possess the highest risk of injury. With eye injuries, the risk is proportional to the chance of receiving a blow significant enough to result in injury.[56] Sports with a high risk of eye injury include baseball, basketball, boxing, fencing, field hockey, ice hockey, lacrosse, martial arts, paintball, racquetball, softball, squash, and street hockey. However, at least 90% of eye injuries can be prevented by using off-the-shelf eye guards.[26,29,49]

Several studies have demonstrated a high incidence of eye injury in athletic activities. Among intercollegiate basketball athletes, it has been estimated that 5.5% suffer an injury each season.[44] Likewise, an incidence rate of 0.03 injuries per 1,000 practice and game sessions was found among 6,229 intercollegiate football athletes.[64] From these data, the researchers suggested that the average intercollegiate football athlete sustained a significant injury once during every 62 weeks of participation. Other researchers demonstrated a 6.2% to 9.9% incidence of face, eye, and tooth injuries among women's lacrosse athletes.[57]

Choosing the correct eye guard to lessen the risk of injury involves three steps.[56] First, conduct an eye medical history and vision screening to identify potential concerns. Second, only select and use eye guards that meet ASTM, ANSI, NOCSAE, and PECC standards. Athletes wearing eye guards that met ASTM F803 standards have reported no eye injuries during several million player-years of use.[56] Also, more than one million athletes since 1978 wearing a full hockey face shield certified by HECC or CSA have been injury-free. Lastly, have an experienced ophthalmologist, optometrist, optician, or other health-care professional select and fit the guards. Glasses should consist of polycarbonate lenses and high-impact plastic frames.[58] Contact lenses alone do not provide protection; wearers should use glasses, shields, or goggles for protection.[56]

The high risk of eye injury in sports, and the high success in injury prevention when using eye guards, indicates that athletic associations and organizations should consider mandating the use of certified eye guards in high risk sports.

Critical Thinking Question 4

The fullback on the football team requires the use of contact lenses during all practices and competitions. Several times during preseason practices, dirt and grass were thrown through the face guard into his eyes, damaging the lenses, but fortunately not his eyes. A polycarbonate shield was attached to his helmet and face guard to provide protection. Although the shield protected against large objects entering through the face guard, the debris continued to reach his contact lenses and eyes.

▶ **Question: What techniques can you use to prevent debris from entering the face guard and eyes?**

Mouth Guards

The ASTM[1] has categorized mouth guards based on the fitting process and the level of comfort and protection provided. The categories include Type I stock, Type II mouth-formed, and Type III custom-fabricated. Stock, mouth-formed, or custom-fabricated mouth guards are mandatory in NCAA and NFHS field hockey, football, ice hockey, and lacrosse, but can be used in any sport.

Stock mouth guards are available in predetermined sizes based on mouth circumference measurements (Fig. 13–29). These guards are constructed of pre-molded rubber or polyvinyl materials, are ready to be used upon purchase, and do not allow for customization. Stock mouth guards are anchored by clenching the teeth together and commonly interfere with speech and breathing. Some designs are available with loop straps to attach the guard to a face guard.

Mouth-formed designs are manufactured in predetermined sizes corresponding to mouth circumference measurements (Fig. 13–30A). This design is the most commonly used guard. Some designs, referred to as boil and bite guards, are constructed of a thermoplastic material shell, while other designs consist of a rigid material outer shell and an ethyl methacrylate material inner lining. These guards are heated in boiling water and intraorally shaped to the contours of the mouth and teeth, preferably by a dentist. Mouth-formed guards are anchored to the teeth if properly fit; most are available with a face guard strap.

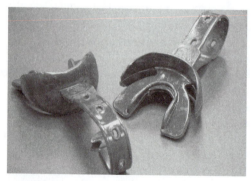

Figure 13-29 Stock mouth guards with loop straps.

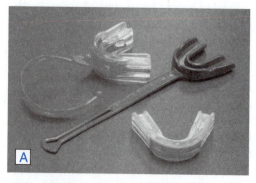

Figure 13-30A Mouth-formed mouth guards. (Left and middle) With loop straps. (Right) Without loop strap.

DETAILS

Mouth-Formed Fitting Process

- Hold the mouth guard by the face guard strap and insert the guard into boiling water until the guard becomes pliable (Fig. 13–30B). For most designs, 20 to 30 seconds is recommended.
- Remove the guard from the water and allow the excess water to drain for approximately 5 seconds.
- Place the guard directly into the mouth. For most designs, position the guard over the upper arch (see Fig. 13–30C). Center the guard over the teeth using the strap as a guide.[2]
- Press the lips together to create a tight seal and aggressively suck the guard against the upper arch to obtain a contoured fit (see Fig. 13–30D). For most designs, 15 to 30 seconds is recommended.
- During the forming process, do not bring the upper and lower jaw together or bite into the guard.
- Remove the guard from the mouth and rinse in cold water.
- Cutting the posterior ends or trimming the edges next to the gums lessens the protective properties and increases the risk of injury (see Fig. 13–30E).[48]
- If the guard requires re-forming, begin the fitting process with a new guard.

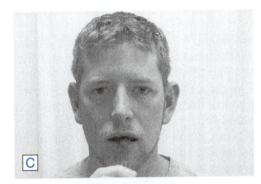
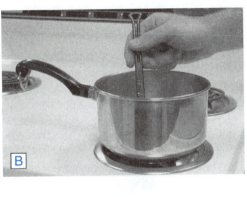
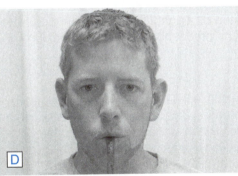
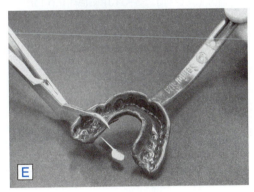

Figure 13-30 *continued*

Custom-fabricated guards are manufactured in individual fit designs corresponding to an upper or lower arch model (Fig. 13–31A). Some guards are constructed of thermoplastic materials using a vacuum process. Other designs are manufactured of thermoplastic or laminated resin materials using a pressure-formed lamination process. These guards are typically manufactured in a dental office or laboratory, but can be constructed in-house. Although rarely needed because of the custom-fit, a face guard strap can be incorporated in these designs.

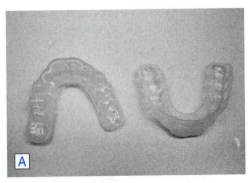

Figure 13-31A   Custom-fabricated mouth guards.

DETAILS

Custom-Fabrication Positive Pressure Process

• To form the impression, place alginate material into tray (Fig. 13–31B). The material is available in regular or fast set mix.

• Insert the tray into the mouth and press into the arch (see Fig. 13–31C). An upper or lower arch impression can be made. The tray is held in the mouth for approximately 90 seconds or until there is a firm set.

• Remove the tray and wrap in a wet paper towel until ready to pour the die stone mix into the impression.

• To form the model, mix die stone powder with water (see Fig. 13–31D). Remove the paper towel from the impression and spray the impression with surfactant.

• Place the impression on a heavy duty vibrator and carefully pour the die stone mix into the impression (see Fig. 13–31E). This takes approximately 20 to 30 seconds. The vibration will allow the mix to slowly flow throughout the impression and lessen the formation of air pockets in the mix.

• Remove the impression from the vibrator. Form a patty with the remainder of the mix and invert the model on the patty to form the base for the model (see Fig. 13–31F). Set aside for approximately 1 hour to cure.

• Gently remove the impression from the die stone model (see Fig. 13–31G).

• Using a model trimmer, trim the model of any imperfections and/or air bubbles to produce a finished model (see Fig. 13–31H).

• Paint the model with separating medium to prevent adherence of mouth guard material to the model. Allow the model to dry 15 to 20 minutes. The model may be heated at 200 F° for approximately 5 to 10 minutes to dry.

• To fabricate the mouth guard, center the model on the metal plate of the positive pressure forming machine (see Fig. 13–31I).

• Place a piece of pre-cut 3-mm-thick silicon thermoplastic guard material in the bottom section of the flip-top and anchor (see Fig. 13–31J). Start the forming machine. The heating element, located on the upper section of the flip-top, will begin to heat.

• When the heating element is ready, commonly indicated by a light, flip the element down over the thermoplastic material (see Fig. 13–31K). Generally, the preset heating time is approximately 105 seconds .

 Helpful Hint: Heating times of thermoplastic and laminated resin mouth guard materials vary. Specific instructions for heating are included by the manufacturer when the materials are purchased. Carefully follow the guidelines to prevent overheating of the materials and to avoid lessening the thickness of the guard during the pressure process.

• When the material is heated, flip the heating element to its starting position (see Fig. 13–31L). Turn the bottom section of the flip-top holding the thermoplastic material onto the model (see Fig. 13–31M).

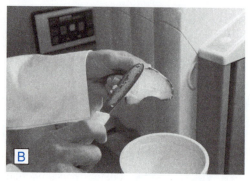

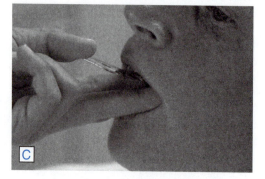

Figure 13-31   *continued*

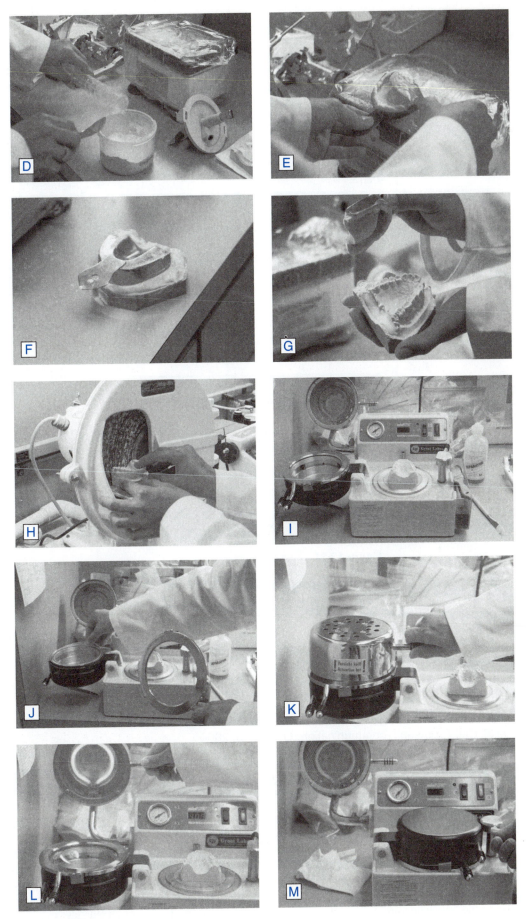

Figure 13-31 *continued*

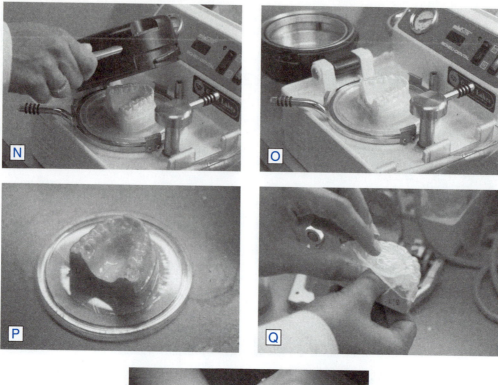

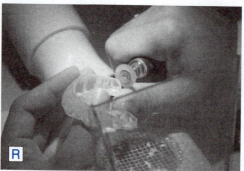

Figure 13-31   *continued*

- The heated thermoplastic guard material is shaped to the mold through the positive pressure process (see Fig. 13–31N). The process takes approximately 2 minutes.
- When the process ends, return the bottom flip-top to its starting position (see Fig. 13–31O).
- Remove the model and thermoplastic guard material from the bottom flip-top and place in an upright position on a counter for approximately 2 minutes to cool (see Fig. 13–31P).
- With scissors, cut the excess material off the model and carefully separate the guard from the model (see Fig. 13–31Q).
- Continue to trim the guard with a small grinder to remove sharp edges (see Fig. 13–31R).
- Thoroughly clean the guard and store in a plastic container.

T. Russ and R. Salko, personal communication, October 8, 2004

RESEARCH BRIEF

Participation with mouth guards in athletic activities is mandatory for several sports, but the type of design used is often the choice of the institution and/or athlete. The term mouth guard encompasses many different types of designs, from one-size-fits-all to custom-fabrication. These guards are typically categorized by the fabrication process and include stock, mouth-formed, and custom, or by design, such as single-arch or dual-arch.[1,63] Single-arch designs cover only one arch of the teeth, commonly the maxillary, while dual-arch designs cover the maxillary and mandibular arches.[20] The choice and use of the appropriate design may determine the amount of protection provided.

A review of the literature demonstrates that mouth guard use may lessen the risk of injury.[3] The guards have been shown to reduce lacerations of the tongue, lips, and cheek caused by tooth edges,[14] lessen jaw fractures from blows to the chin,[27] reduce chipping and fractures to the teeth,[14] and lessen concussions occurring from an anterior or inferior blow to the mandible.[14,24,27] A properly fitted mouth guard should be resilient, tear resistant, tasteless, and protective.[48] The guard should also be comfortable, have minimal effects on speech and breathing patterns, and maintain retention and fit.

The choice and use of mouth guard designs appear to be based on general beliefs and perceptions rather than clinical effectiveness.[61] It has been reported that more than 90% of guards currently used are off-the-shelf designs, with the remaining 10% custom-fabricated.[48] Most off-the-shelf guards in use today are bulky, uncomfortable, and affect speech and breathing, perhaps supporting the belief and perception that all designs are the same. Most researchers agree that stock and mouth-formed guards are unsatisfactory and should be used with caution.[45,48,60]

The effectiveness of a mouth guard is dependent on its thickness and on the materials used in the construction process. Some researchers have suggested that labial[15] and/or posterior occlusal[62] thicknesses are important factors in the protective capabilities of a guard, with an optimal thickness of 3 mm.[25] Guards constructed of materials with high-stiffness characteristics appear to redistribute loads and offer more protective effects under soft-object collisions. Low-stiffness materials deform under stress, providing shock absorption under hard-object collisions.[15]

Although more expensive than off-the-shelf designs, custom-fabricated vacuum and pressure-laminated guards appear to offer more protection and comfort. Several dual-arch jaw joint protectors have been introduced recently and should assist in the continued development of the optimal mouth guard.

...IF/THEN...

IF an athlete continually bites through a boil and bite mouth guard during use, **THEN** consider replacing the guard with a rigid outer shell mouth-formed or custom-fabricated design.

CASE STUDY

Three weeks prior to the start of practice for the upcoming season, the Lions, a local youth baseball team, lost their sponsorship by the bank. Then, 2 weeks later, their coach of five years received a work promotion and moved to another town. Bill Munch has a son on the team and agreed to take over as coach of the Lions. Bill immediately began sorting through the equipment to take an inventory. He discovered that several batter's helmets had cracks in the ear flaps and the steel/wire frames of the catcher's face guards were bent. As a result of losing their sponsorship, the Lions cannot purchase new equipment at this time. Bill is employed at the local home improvement store and believes fiberglass tape strips and epoxy can be applied to the ear flaps to repair the cracks. He also plans to use a vise to straighten the wire/steel frames of the face guards. Are there implications in making modifications and/or repairs to protective equipment? What other possible solutions exist to provide protective equipment for the Lions in the management of this case?

During the second offensive series of the game, Mike Short, the fullback on the McCallum High School football team, was handed the ball on a third down play. Mike ran across the line of scrimmage and was immediately hit in the left thorax by the middle linebacker, causing Mike to fall backward. As he was falling to the ground, Mike was struck again in the anterior thorax and throat by a defensive back, causing extension of his neck. The motion of his head and the force of the blow resulted in a laceration to Mike's chin. Mike got to his feet and began to walk off the field. Lynne Mary, ATC, came onto the field, applied direct pressure, and assisted him to the bench. The team physician evaluated Mike on the sidelines, then took him into the locker room for treatment. In the locker room, the team physician cleansed the wound and closed it with sutures. As Lynne returned to the locker room at halftime, Mike asked if he could return to the game. The team physician will allow Mike to return if his chin is properly padded and the helmet is securely anchored. What padding techniques could be used to provide protection to allow Mike to return to the game?

Protective Equipment and Padding

WRAP UP

- Individuals who design, manufacture, purchase, fit, and use protective equipment and padding share a legal responsibility to ensure safety.
- Purchase only high-quality equipment and padding, follow manufacturer's instructions, do not make modifications, and monitor and perform regular maintenance.
- NOCSAE, HECC, ASTM, CSA, and PECC have established safety standards and testing procedures for the manufacturing, maintenance, and use of protective equipment and padding.
- Baseball, football, lacrosse, ice hockey, and softball helmets and face guards that meet NOCSAE, HECC, ASTM, and/or CSA testing standards are permanently branded or stamped with a seal or label.

- The NCAA and NFHS require mandatory protective equipment and padding for athletes participating in many sports.
- Athletes voluntarily wear many protective equipment and padding designs that are not required during practices and competitions.
- Off-the-shelf equipment and padding techniques are available in a variety of universal and custom-fit designs to absorb shock and provide protection.
- Although protective equipment and padding are not designed to prevent all injuries, using such equipment and padding is recommended when appropriate.

■ WEB REFERENCES

American Association of Oral and Maxillofacial Surgeons
http://www.aaoms.org/
- This Web site allows you access to information about the prevention and treatment of oral sport injuries.

Canadian Standards Association
http://www.csa.ca/Default.asp?language=english
- This Web site allows you to search and purchase standards developed for protective athletic equipment.

Cornell Law School Legal Information Institute
http://www.law.cornell.edu/
- This Web site allows access to information about sports law and product liability.

Douglas
http://www.douglaspads.com/pc/about.asp
- This Web site is an online catalog for the manufacturer and provides sizing and ordering information for football, baseball, and ice hockey equipment.

Great Lakes Orthodontics, Ltd.
http://www.greatlakesortho.com/index.php
- This Web site provides information about equipment for the custom-fabrication of mouth guards.

MegaLaw.com
http://www.megalaw.com/index.php
- This site provides access to sport law topics, including sports law federal decisions and sports law statutes and regulations.

National Collegiate Athletic Association
http://www2.ncaa.org/
- This Web site allows access to online rules and guidelines for each sponsored sport in regard to mandatory and recommended protective equipment.

National Federation of State High School Associations
www.nfhs.org/ScriptContent/Index.cfm
- This site provides you information about ordering sponsored sport rules and guidelines, which include mandatory and recommended protective equipment.

National Operating Committee on Standards for Athletic Equipment
http://www.nocsae.org
- This site provides access to standards, certifications, and testing procedures for protective equipment.

Riddell
http://www.riddell.com/
- This site is an online catalog for the protective equipment manufacturer and provides technical, fitting, and ordering information.

Schutt Sports
http://www.schutt-sports.com
- This site provides access to sport-specific catalogs containing protective equipment.

The Hockey Equipment Certification Council Inc.
http://www.hecc.net/home.html
- This Web site provides information about the testing and certification of ice hockey equipment.

The Protective Eyewear Certification Council
http://www.protecteyes.org/
- This site provides you recommendations about appropriate eye guards to prevent sport-related eye injuries.

Williams Sports Group
http://www.footballshoulderpads.com/football-shoulder-pads.asp
- This site allows access to information about the Temperature Management System (TMS) used in the construction of football shoulder pads.

■ REFERENCES

1. American Society for Testing and Materials: Standard Practice for Care and Use of Mouthguards. Designation: F 697-80 (Reapproved 1992). American Society of Testing and Materials. Vol. 15.07: 418, 1999.
2. Anderson, MK, Hall, SJ, and Martin, M: Foundations of Athletic Training: Prevention, Assessment, and Management, ed 3. Williams & Wilkins, Philadelphia, 2005.
3. Andreasen, JO: Traumatic Injuries of the Teeth, ed 2. Munksgaard, Copenhagen, 1981.
4. ASTM Internal, Inc, http://www.astm.org/cgi-bin/SoftCart.exe/index.shtml?E+mystore, 2005.
5. Benson, BW, Mohtadi, NGH, Rose, MS, and Meeuwisse, WH: Head and neck injuries among ice hockey players wearing full face shields vs half face shields. JAMA 282:2328–2332, 1999.
6. Benson, BW, Rose, MS, Meeuwisse, WH, Kissick, J, and Roberts, WO: The impact of face shield use on concussions in ice hockey: A multivariate analysis/commentary. Brit J Sports Med 36:27–32, 2002.
7. Bir, CA, Cassatta, SJ, and Janda, DH: An analysis and comparison of soccer shin guards. Clin J Sport Med 5:95–99, 1995.
8. Boden, BP, and Garrett, WE: Tibia and fibula fractures in soccer players. Knee Surg Sports Traumatol Arthrosc 7:262–266, 1999.
9. Burstein, AH, Otis, JC, and Torg, JS: Mechanisms and pathomechanics of athletic injuries to the cervical spine. In Torg, JS (ed): Athletic Injuries to the Head, Neck, and Face. Lea & Febiger, Philadelphia, 1982, pp 139–154.

10. Canadian Standards Association, http://www.csa.ca/Default.asp?language=english, 2004.

11. Cantu, RC, and Cantu, RI: Neurologic Athletic Head and Spine Injuries. WB Saunders, Philadelphia, 2000, p 243.

12. Caswell, SV, and Deivert, RG: Lacrosse helmet designs and the effects of impact forces. J Athl Train 37:164–171, 2002.

13. Cattermole, HR, Hardy, JRW, and Gregg, PJ: The footballer's fracture. Br J Sports Med 30:171–175, 1996.

14. Chapman, PJ: Mouthguards and the role of sporting team dentists. Aust Dent 34:36–43, 1989.

15. Cummins, NK, and Spears, IR: The effect of mouthguard design on stresses in the tooth-bone complex. Med Sci Sports Exerc 34:942–947, 2002.

16. Davidson, M: Helmets. Annual Athletic Equipment Managers Association Convention, Kansas City, MO, June 9, 2004.

17. Davidson, M: Shoulder pads. Annual Athletic Equipment Managers Association Convention, Kansas City, MO, June 9, 2004.

18. Francisco, AC, Nightingale, RW, Guilak, F, Glisson, RR, and Garrett, WE, Jr: Comparison of soccer shin guards in preventing tibia fracture. Am J Sports Med 28:227–233, 2000.

19. Gainor, BJ, Piotrowski, G, Puhl, JJ, and Allen, WC: The kick: Biomechanics and collision injury. Am J Sports Med 6:185–193, 1978.

20. Gusenbauer, A, http://www.wipss.com/Med_dentistryToday.htm, Brain injury in sports related to trauma to the lower jaw, 2002.

21. Guskiewicz, KM, Bruce, SL, Cantu, RC, Ferrara, MS, Kelly, JP, McCrea, M, Putukian, M, and McLeod, TC: National Athletic Trainers' Association position statement: Management of sport-related concussion. J Athl Train 39:280–297, 2004.

22. Halstead, PD: Performance testing updates in head, face, and eye protection. J Athl Train 36:322–327, 2001.

23. Heck, JF, Clarke, KS, Peterson TR, Torg, JS, and Weis, MP: National Athletic Trainers' Association position statement: Head-down contact and spearing in tackle football. J Athl Train 39:101–111, 2004.

24. Hickey, JC, Morris, AL, Carlson, LD, and Seward, TE: The relation of mouth protectors to cranial pressure and deformation. JADA 74:735–740, 1967.

25. Hoffmann, J, Alfter, G, Rudolph, NK, and Göz, G: Experimental comparative study of various mouthguards. Endod Dent Traumatol 15:157–163, 1999.

26. Jeffers, JB: An ongoing tragedy: Pediatric sports-related eye injuries. Semin Ophthalmol 5:216–223, 1990.

27. Johnsen, DC, and Jackson, EW: Prevention of intraoral trauma in sports. Dent Clin North Am 35:657–666, 1991.

28. Kujala, UM, Taimela, S, Antti-Poika, I, Orava, S, Tuominen, R, and Myllynen, P: Acute injuries in soccer, ice hockey, volleyball, basketball, judo, and karate: Analysis of national registry data. BMJ 311:1465–1468, 1995.

29. Larrison, WI, Hersh, PS, Kunzweiler, T, and Shingleton, BJ: Sport-related ocular trauma. Ophthalmology 97:1265–1269, 1990.

30. Lindenfield, TN, Schmitt, DJ, Hendy, MP, Mangine, RE, and Noyes, FR: Incidence of injury in indoor soccer. Am J Sports Med 22:364–371, 1994.

31. Mueller, FO, and Blyth, CS: An update on football deaths and catastrophic injuries. Phys Sportsmed 14:134–142, 1986.

32. Mueller, FO, and Cantu, RC: Nineteenth Annual Report of the National Center for Catastrophic Sports Injury Research: Fall 1982-Spring 2001. National Center for Catastrophic Sports Injury Research, Chapel Hill, 2002.

33. National Collegiate Athletic Association, http://www.ncaa.org/library/sports_sciences/sports_med_handbook/2003-04/2003-04_sports_med_handbook.pdf, Sports medicine handbook, 2003–2004.

34. National Federation of State High School Associations: 2004 Baseball Rules Book. National Federation of State High School Associations, Indianapolis, 2004.

35. National Federation of State High School Associations: 2004–05 Field Hockey Rules Book. National Federation of State High School Associations, Indianapolis, 2004.

36. National Federation of State High School Associations: 2004 Football Rules Book. National Federation of State High School Associations, Indianapolis, 2004.

37. National Federation of State High School Associations: 2004–05 Ice Hockey Rules Book. National Federation of State High School Associations, Indianapolis, 2004.

38. National Federation of State High School Associations: 2004 Boys Lacrosse Rules Book. National Federation of State High School Associations, Indianapolis, 2004.

39. National Federation of State High School Associations: 2004–05 Soccer Rules Book. National Federation of State High School Associations, Indianapolis, 2004.

40. National Federation of State High School Associations: 2004 Softball Rules Book. National Federation of State High School Associations, Indianapolis, 2004.

41. National Federation of State High School Associations: 2004–05 Wrestling Rules Book. National Federation of State High School Associations, Indianapolis, 2004.

42. National Operating Committee on Standards for Athletic Equipment, http://www.nocsae.org, 2005.

43. Naunheim, RS, Ryden, A, Standeven, J, Genin, G, Lewis, L, Thompson, P, and Bayly, P: Does soccer headgear attenuate the impact when heading a soccer ball? Acad Emerg Med 10:85–90, 2003.

44. Powell, JW: National Athletic Injury/Illness Reporting System: Eye injuries in college wrestling. Int Ophthalmol Clin 21:47–58, 1981.

45. Ranalli, DN: Prevention of craniofacial injuries in football. Dent Clin North Am 35:627–645, 1991.

46. Ray, R: Management Strategies in Athletic Training, ed 2. Human Kinetics, Champaign, 2000.

47. Sadat-Ali, M, and Sankaran-Kutty, M: Soccer injuries in Saudi Arabia. Am J Sports Med 15:500–502, 1987.

48. Sports Dentistry, http://www.sportsdentistry.com/mouthguards.html, Types of athletic mouthguards, 2002.

49. Strahlman, E, and Sommer, A: The epidemiology of sports-related ocular trauma. Int Ophthalmol Clin 28:199–202, 1988.

50. Tenvergert, EM, Ton Duis, HJ, and Klasen, HJ : Trends in sports injuries, 1982–1988: An in-depth study on four types of sport. J Sports Med Phys Fitness 32:214–220, 1992.

51. The Hockey Equipment Certification Council, Inc, http://www.hecc.net/home.html, 2005.

52. The Protective Eyewear Certification Council, http://www.protecteyes.org/PECC%20Injuries%20prevention.pdf, The mechanisms and prevention of sports eye injuries, 2004.

53. Torg, JS, Truex, Jr, R, Quedenfeld, TC, Burstein, A, Spealman, A, and Nichols, III, CE: The National Football Head and Neck Injury Registry: Report and conclusions, 1978. JAMA 241:1477–1479, 1979.

54. Torg, JS, Vegso, JJ, O'Neill, MJ, and Sennett, B: The epidemiologic, pathologic, biomechanical, and cinematographic analysis of football-induced cervical spine trauma. Am J Sports Med 18:50–57, 1990.

55. United States Lacrosse, http://www.uslacrosse.org/the_sport/womens_rules.phtml, Women's condensed lacrosse rules, 2005.

56. Vinger, PF: A practical guide for sports eye protection. Phys Sportsmed 28:49–50,55–56,59,63–66,69, 2000.

57. Vinger, PF: The eye and sports medicine. In Tasman, W, Jaeger, EA (eds): Duane's Clinical Ophthalmology. JB Lippincott, Philadelphia, 1994, pp 1–103.

58. Vinger, PF, Parver, L, Alfaro, III, DV, Woods, T, and Abrams, BS: Shatter resistance of spectacle lenses. JAMA 277:142–144, 1997.

59. Watkins, RG: Neck injuries in football players. Clin Sports Med 5:215–246, 1986.

60. Welburry, RR, and Murray, JJ: Prevention of trauma to teeth. Dent Update 17:117–121, 1990.

61. Westerman, B, Stringfellow, PM, and Eccleston, JA: Forces transmitted through EVA mouthguard materials of different types and thickness. Aust Dent J 40:389–391, 1995.

62. Winters, JE: Commentary: Role of properly fitted mouthguards in prevention of sport-related concussion. J Athl Train 36:339–341, 2001.

63. Woodmansey, KF: Athletic mouthguards prevent orofacial injuries: A review. Gen Dent Jan–Feb:64–69, 1999.

64. Zemper, ED: Injury rates in a national sample of college football teams: A 2-year prospective study. Phys Sportsmed 17:100–105, 1989.

CHAPTER 1 SOLUTIONS

Case Study Solution

A delivery service driver has sustained an inversion ankle sprain. Applying non-elastic or elastic tapes, elastic or cloth wraps, or functional ankle braces will provide support and protection from further injury.

A football running back has suffered an anterior thigh contusion. Applying a hard, high-density pad constructed of plastic or thermoplastic material will provide protection from further injury upon a return to activity. An elastic or self-adherent wrap or elastic or neoprene sleeve will provide compression and support following activity.

Critical Thinking Question Solutions

1. To lessen irritation of the skin, correctly position the individual and clean and dry the skin prior to application. You can use adherent tape spray, pre-tape material, and thin foam pads to reduce irritation. When applying tape, be sure to follow the normal contours of the body, overlapping each strip, avoiding gaps, wrinkles, or inconsistent roll tension, and following the sequence of steps in the technique.

2. Use a 3 or 4 inch width elastic or 1½, 2, 2¾, or 3 inch width self-adherent wrap for compression. You can also use an elastic sleeve.

3. First, remove the brace and clean and dry the skin. Then, reapply the brace, following the step-by-step procedure. You can also use a neoprene sleeve under the brace if the fit of the brace allows. Applying adherent tape spray may lessen migration. Contact the brace manufacturer, if needed.

4. Cover the semirigid cast with high-density, closed-cell foam or similar material of at least ½ inch thickness to meet NCAA and NFHS rules. The on-site referee or official must approve the padding prior to competitive play. You may need written verification of the injury and cast from the physician to obtain approval.

CHAPTER 2 SOLUTIONS

Case Study Solution

A PT/ATC is performing outreach services with a local high school. She has been asked to design the application area in the athletic training room as part of a renovation project. She must first consider the current number of athletes who require daily technique application and the time available for application. Future needs may include additional facility renovations and the addition of staff or sport teams.

The design of the application area must address the overhead ventilation duct, cracked tile floor, vertical support beam, and overall dimensions. Move the taping table to an area away from the ventilation duct to allow for proper height clearance. Replace the individual cracked tile pieces or the entire floor. The cracked tile may be filled in with grout or cement and covered with non-slip plastic, rubber, or carpet runners or mats. Build or

purchase a custom-made taping table or bench to fit around the vertical support beam or into a corner to utilize the restricted space. Design the application area within the dimensions given.

Critical Thinking Question Solutions

1. Purchase or construct tables with varying heights, between 30 and 40 inches, to accommodate you and your staff. Design the tables with adequate storage and countertop space to provide easy access to materials during application.

2. Store all non-elastic, elastic, and cast tapes; self-adherent wraps; braces; and hard, high-density pads in the well-ventilated area. Elastic wraps and soft, low-density pads can be stored in taping tables and benches.

3. First, examine the location of the application area in your facility. The area should be located near an entrance and exit to allow easy access. Second, if possible, have adequate health-care professionals, tables, and benches available during this time for application of techniques. Third, using a seating area may lower the congestion.

CHAPTER 3 SOLUTIONS

Case Study Solution

A basketball athlete has bilateral plantar fasciitis. The application of the "X," loop, or weave arch, Low-Dye, or plantar fascia strap taping technique will support the longitudinal arch and should lessen pain levels during practices and competitions. Night splints will provide a static stretch to the plantar fascia while the athlete is sleeping and should lessen pain upon initial weight-bearing in the morning. Soft orthotic designs such as heel cups or full-length neoprene, silicone, or viscoelastic polymer insoles may be used to absorb shock and support the rearfoot during athletic and casual activities. These orthotic designs can be used alone or in combination with the "X," loop, or weave arch, Low-Dye, or plantar fascia strap taping techniques during athletic activities. Off-the-shelf or custom-made semirigid orthotics constructed of thermoplastic, cork, leather, and foam materials can be used to absorb shock and support the forefoot and/or rearfoot during athletic and casual activities, eliminating the need for daily application of tape. Using the longitudinal arch padding technique during athletic and casual activities provides support of the longitudinal arch. If heel cups are not available, use the heel pad technique to absorb shock and lessen pain by compressing the fat pad under the calcaneus during athletic and casual activities.

Critical Thinking Question Solutions

1. Using only non-elastic tape, the circular, "X," loop, or weave arch techniques support the longitudinal arch and should lessen the pain.

2. Place a piece of adhesive gauze material over the abraded area or completely cover the toe to treat the

abrasion. Apply a skin lubricant over the tape and adjacent toes to prevent irritation of the skin.

3. Place a soft orthotic design such as a full-length neoprene, silicone, or viscoelastic polymer insole inside each boot to provide shock absorption.

4. A walking or cast boot will provide support and allow for a normal gait.

5. Place a soft heel cup in each shoe or apply a donut, heel, or viscoelastic polymer pad to each heel to reduce stress over the injured area.

CHAPTER 4 SOLUTIONS

Case Study Solution

A volleyball/softball athlete suffers a moderate inversion ankle sprain. The application of the posterior splint or walking boot will provide immobilization and support to the ankle. Using rigid cast tape will not allow for daily removal and treatment. The open basketweave, compression wrap, elastic sleeve, or soft cast techniques can be applied under the splint or boot to assist in controlling swelling and effusion. During volleyball activities, the closed basketweave, Spartan Slipper, and subtalar sling taping techniques and lace-up, semirigid, air/gel, and wrap bracing designs will provide support. Combinations of the taping and bracing techniques can also be applied. The restriction of plantar flexion and dorsiflexion with the use of the taping and lace-up and wrap bracing techniques may affect her vertical jump height and should be closely evaluated. For softball activities, the closed basketweave, Spartan Slipper, and subtalar sling will provide support and limit dorsiflexion. Lace-up, semirigid, air/gel, and wrap brace techniques can be used, but only lace-up and wrap designs will limit dorsiflexion. The combination of taping and bracing techniques can also be applied to provide maximal support and limit dorsiflexion.

Critical Thinking Question Solutions

1. Provide extra support to the ankle with the basketweave variations. Using moleskin or thermoplastic stirrups will reduce inversion and eversion at the subtalar joint and allow available plantar flexion and dorsiflexion at the talocrural joint. Restricting plantar flexion may decrease vertical jump height. Elastic or semirigid cast tape heel locks will provide additional support, but may further reduce plantar flexion.

2. You can apply the closed basketweave with elastic or semirigid cast tape heel locks, moleskin or thermoplastic stirrups, or subtalar sling or the Spartan Slipper technique to support the subtalar and talocrural joints.

3. An elastic wrap, elastic sleeve self-adherent wrap, elastic tape compression wrap, or soft cast technique will provide additional compression to assist in controlling swelling and effusion.

4. Bracing techniques would perhaps offer the best solution. The availability of a health-care professional to apply taping techniques and the associated cost of the taping materials are two issues that must be addressed. If permitted, the athlete can be fitted for a brace and be given application instructions for use over the summer. Lace-up, semirigid, and air/gel bladder braces could be used. However, to lessen the restrictions in range of motion caused by the taping techniques, a semirigid brace may be more effective. The brace limits inversion, eversion, and rotation and allows normal plantar flexion and dorsiflexion.

5. Determine proper fit by ensuring that the heel is positioned firmly in the brace, the eyelets are less than 2 inches apart, and the straps are correctly applied. If stirrups are included with the brace design, you can provide additional support by using plastic or thermoplastic stirrups. You can also use the brace in combination with several taping techniques.

6. You can place a viscoelastic polymer or foam or felt donut pad over the lateral malleolus under the brace to lessen shearing forces.

CHAPTER 5 SOLUTIONS

Case Study Solution

A female investment banker training for a marathon has developed medial tibial stress syndrome. Applying the circular, "X," loop, weave, and Low-Dye taping techniques will support the longitudinal arch and forefoot and correct excessive pronation. The spiral lower leg technique can provide compression. If necessary, rigid cast tape or a walking boot will provide support and complete immobilization. Use soft orthotic designs, such as heel cups and full-length neoprene, silicone, and viscoelastic polymer insoles, to provide shock absorption. Semirigid and rigid orthotic designs will support and correct excessive pronation. A neoprene sleeve may be used for compression and support. Using the heel pad technique will provide shock absorption to lessen repetitive stress to the lower leg. Use the medial wedge pad to correct excessive pronation or the longitudinal arch pad to support the arch.

Critical Thinking Question Solutions

1. Prior to technique application, carefully determine the range of dorsiflexion that produces pain. Position the foot in a pain-free range and monitor this position, preventing any movement into dorsiflexion during application. Apply adherent tape spray, apply the technique directly to the skin, and/or use the inferior knee anchor to lessen migration.

2. Apply compression wrap technique one to provide compression over the foot, ankle, and lower leg. Use a foam or felt pad over the proximal contusion under the wrap to assist in venous return. If swelling is present over the lateral and/or medial malleoli, the horseshoe pad can provide additional compression.

3. Use the spiral lower leg taping technique or the elastic sleeve compression wrap technique to provide

compression and support. Monitor for an increase in pain following application.

4. To temporarily immobilize the foot and ankle, apply a posterior splint. Use this technique if the individual is to be seen by the surgeon in a few days. The team physician might apply a short-leg cast with rigid cast tape. A walking boot will also immobilize the foot and ankle. Regardless of the technique, crutches are required for non–weight-bearing ambulation.

5. Use an off-the-shelf shin guard and supplement this design with additional open-cell foam attached to the inside surface. Cut a hole in the foam to disperse any impact force. Use thermoplastic materials to mold and shape a custom-made design to the lower leg. Attach both designs with 2 inch or 3 inch elastic tape or self-adherent wrap or place under a knee-high sock.

CHAPTER 6 SOLUTIONS

Case Study Solution

A member of a cycling club has been experiencing anterior knee pain as a result of the development of patellofemoral stress syndrome. After determining static and dynamic patellar orientation, using the McConnell taping technique can lessen pain and correct patellofemoral malalignment. The patellar tendon strap taping and bracing techniques can reduce the tension of the patellar tendon on the inferior pole of the patella and/or the tibial tubercle, thereby reducing pain. The Low-Dye taping technique can provide support and correct excessive foot pronation. Using a neoprene sleeve with an open patella can provide compression and mild support. Use a neoprene sleeve with buttress bracing technique to reduce friction and stress, provide compression, and support and correct patellofemoral malalignment. Semirigid and rigid orthotic designs can support and correct excessive foot pronation.

Critical Thinking Question Solutions

1. The patellar tendon strap taping technique one should prove effective in this situation. Heavyweight elastic tape, which is thicker and possesses more tensile strength than other tapes, is used to provide maximal tension over the patellar tendon. The application of ½ inch non-elastic tape will also allow for adjustments of tension. If tension lessens during workouts, reapply the ½ inch non-elastic tape.

2. Use a compression wrap with the compression wrap pad technique to lessen the swelling. Being in the 103 lb weight class, it is likely the athlete has an ectomorph body type with bony prominences. The open-cell foam pad will conform to the prepatellar region and maintain uniform pressure when placed under a 5 yard or 10 yard length elastic wrap. An elastic sleeve may also be used with the compression pad.

3. Use bracing techniques to provide stability and protection for the knee. Prophylactic braces can be used to protect the knee, but only from valgus and hyperextension forces. The MCL has connections with the medial joint capsule and medial meniscus and MCL laxity may lead to damage of these structures from valgus and rotary forces. Functional braces will provide greater stability and protection from valgus, varus, hyperextension, and rotary stresses. In this situation, the functional brace serves both a functional and prophylactic role.

4. The collateral "X" taping technique or the neoprene sleeve with hinge bars bracing technique will provide support and protection to the LCL during activity. To apply the collateral "X" technique, you will need adherent tape spray, 3 inch heavyweight elastic tape, and perhaps pre-tape material. On average, you can purchase adherent tape spray (4 oz can) for $3.80, pre-tape material (roll) for $0.60, and heavyweight 3 inch elastic tape (roll) for $3.73. Over the 2-week period (10 practices and two competitions), using three rolls of elastic tape per application, your costs will include adherent tape spray ($3.80), five rolls of pre-tape material ($3.00), and 36 rolls of elastic tape ($134.28) for a total of $141.08. You can purchase an off-the-shelf neoprene sleeve with hinge bars brace for $52–$132. The taping technique is single use, but the bracing technique, following washing, can be reused. Adjustments in fit can be made with the brace, but may be troublesome with the taping technique.

5. Compression wrapping techniques will reduce swelling and effusion. The compression wrap technique two, which incorporates the foot, ankle, lower leg, and knee, may provide the most effective mechanical pressure for the ACL injury. Use a rehabilitative brace with adjustable hinges to provide support and control of range of motion. The hinges allow you to modify the range of motion to the individual's tolerance.

6. Place a donut pad over the inflamed area, most likely the inferior fibular head, to lessen the compression on the peroneal nerve. Attach the pad to the knee under the off-the-shelf knee pad with adhesive gauze material or elastic tape.

CHAPTER 7 SOLUTIONS

Case Study Solution

A hockey athlete has suffered a third degree quadriceps contusion. In the acute management of the case, apply compression wrap technique two to control swelling. A third degree contusion can produce severe swelling; the compression wrap, extending from the proximal toes to the proximal thigh, will assist in preventing distal migration of the swelling. Consider using a foam or felt pad over the inflamed area underneath the compression wrap.

For a return to activity, use off-the-shelf or custom-made padding techniques to provide protection and prevent reinjury. Off-the-shelf ice hockey pants are available with thigh pads incorporated, but these pads are not sufficient in this particular situation. A pad with a high-density shell is required. Purchase individual, universal, or postinjury designs off-the-shelf, or construct custom-made designs. Attach the pad to the thigh with elastic tape, an elastic wrap, neoprene straps, or underneath tight-fitting clothing.

To achieve the team physician's recommendations, apply compression wrap technique one, two, or three, or a neoprene sleeve or pair of shorts to provide compression to control swelling. Cut and place a foam or felt pad over the inflamed area under the wrap or elastic or neoprene sleeve to provide additional compression. These compression techniques, excluding technique two, may be used during athletic and casual activities. Several techniques are available to provide additional padding. Consider using a larger pad or purchasing a design specifically constructed for use following injury. Mold and attach thermoplastic material to an existing pad to provide additional protection. Also consider attaching open-cell foam to the inside of an existing pad with a hole cut in the foam over the injured area to disperse any impact force.

Critical Thinking Question Solutions

1. Use a neoprene sleeve or neoprene shorts during aquatic therapy to provide support. Neoprene will absorb minimal amounts of water and will not become saturated. Elastic wraps and tape will become saturated. This can result in the addition of weight to the leg and loss of compression and support, and can cause irritation to the skin. The adhesive properties of most tapes are also lost in water.

2. Consider several techniques in this situation. First, additional elastic tape circular patterns may be applied over the elastic wrap with moderate roll tension. Second, apply the quadriceps strain technique two. Encircling the waist with the elastic wrap and tape should assist in maintaining compression and support. Third, using a neoprene sleeve, neoprene shorts, or a thigh, hip, and pelvis combination brace will allow the individual the opportunity to adjust the brace during work activities to maintain effectiveness.

3. Because of the limited amount of time left in the game, an off-the-shelf padding technique would be indicated. When on the bench, if the athlete is wearing tight-fitting shorts, place the pad underneath or use a strap design and anchor the neoprene straps with Velcro. When on the bench or in the locker room, use the circular thigh taping technique or quadriceps strain wrapping technique one or two to attach the pad.

CHAPTER 8 SOLUTIONS

Case Study Solution

A tire carrier for a racing team has suffered a GH joint dislocation. Using sling technique one with an accompanying swathe, or the swathe wrapping technique, or the

4S wrapping technique will provide support and immobilization in the immediate treatment of the GH dislocation. For the extended period of immobilization, the application of sling technique one with a swathe or sling technique two with a small pad or low inflated pillow can be used. For a return to activity, choose a shoulder stabilizer brace that will limit abduction and external rotation in the desired ranges of motion. Several torso vest designs are available and can be worn underneath the team uniform. The uniforms worn on race day are constructed of flame retardant materials; consideration of brace construction may be needed. In a hot and humid environment, a torso vest constructed of canvas and leather may cause dehydration concerns. However, the effectiveness of the design to limit range of motion should be the main concern in brace selection. For the remainder of the season, monitor the existing brace for effectiveness and comfort. Another design can be purchased if loosening permits excessive range of motion or if irritation of the skin occurs.

Critical Thinking Question Solutions

1. To lessen skin irritation, apply the existing pad directly to the skin or over a neoprene sleeve and anchor with the shoulder spica wrapping technique. Also consider purchasing another off-the-shelf design, such as the viscoelastic polymer, gel, skeleton, or closed-cell foam pad, designed to be used in combination with mandatory protective equipment.

2. Use sling technique one and an accompanying swathe, or the swathe wrapping technique to support and immobilize the shoulder and arm during workouts. The sling, swathe, and elastic wrap can be washed and reused daily. This will lessen soiling and excessive wear of the post-operative sling and swathe.

3. After anchoring the strap around the upper arm, apply an elastic wrap or self-adherent wrap or elastic tape with moderate roll tension over the pad in a circular pattern to lessen migration. Also, examine the jersey worn by the athlete. Do not allow the sleeve to be cut on the involved shoulder and upper arm. The sleeve covers the pad and can be tied around the upper arm to assist in lessening migration of the pad.

4. Most off-the-shelf AC joint pads are anchored to the shoulder with neoprene straps. These straps may restrict normal range of motion and the throwing motion. Construct a custom-made thermoplastic material pad to provide protection and allow unrestricted range of motion. Anchor the pad directly to the skin with the shoulder pointer/AC joint sprain taping technique; and if the pad is used daily, monitor the area for irritation.

CHAPTER 9 SOLUTIONS

Case Study Solution

A bull rider sustains a posterolateral elbow dislocation. Support and immobilize the bull rider's left elbow in 90°

of flexion with the posterior splint technique one or two or a rehabilitative bracing technique. Consider using sling technique one with the splint or brace. Use compression wrapping technique one, four, or five to control swelling and effusion.

A rehabilitative or off-the-shelf functional bracing technique will provide support and stability and prevent further injury from valgus and hyperextension stress during rehabilitation. Since upper arm and forearm atrophy may have occurred, a custom-made functional design is not indicated at this time. Control persistent swelling and effusion by applying compression wrapping technique one, four, or five.

Provide stability to the elbow during the return to bull riding activities with an off-the-shelf or custom-made functional bracing technique. The left arm is the free hand during bull riding and is subjected to violent flexion and extension at the elbow. Proper brace application and fit is important.

Use compression wrapping technique one, four, or five with the compression wrap padding technique to reduce swelling and effusion associated with olecranon bursitis. Protect the olecranon bursa with an off-the-shelf or custom-made padding technique. A hard, high-density pad is required in this situation and can be worn in combination with the functional brace. Anchor the pad over the brace with the figure-of-eight elbow taping technique, circular elbow wrapping technique, or nylon straps.

Critical Thinking Question Solutions

1. Several options are available. With the use of hyperextension taping technique one or two, crease or pinch the edges of the "X" or longitudinal strips to prevent tearing. Consider using hyperextension taping technique three with a heavy resistance exercise band. Off-the-shelf hyperextension brace designs are also available with adjustable hinges to limit range of motion.

2. During practice, apply compression wrap technique four with an open-cell foam pad over the posterior elbow to provide additional compression and prevent distal migration of the swelling. Use an off-the-shelf hard, high-density or custom-made pad over the wrap to absorb shock. Away from practice, use compression wrap technique one or five with an open-cell foam pad over the posterior elbow to provide compression.

3. Use an off-the-shelf or custom-made functional design or neoprene sleeve with a hinged bar brace to provide support to the elbow. Because of the demands of his work and risk of re-injury, a custom-made design may be the most appropriate.

4. Perspiration and normal wear can cause the neoprene or foam composite materials to stretch over time. Hand washing and air drying may return the brace to its original size. Consider purchasing the off-the-shelf braces in smaller sizes. As the braces become worn and loose, the smaller braces will allow for further tightening to achieve the appropriate tension.

5. The use of hard, high-density pads is recommended for rollerblading. Check the fit of the pads with the upper arm, forearm, or elbow joint circumference measurements or age of the individual and the application of the straps with the manufacturer's instructions. Consider applying elastic tape around the upper arm and/or forearm to provide additional anchors. It is possible to use the figure-of-eight taping technique or circular elbow wrapping technique to anchor the pad. Last, cut and apply soft, low-density padding to the inside surface of the pads to achieve proper fit.

CHAPTER 10 SOLUTIONS

Case Study Solution

An in-line skater suffers a second degree wrist sprain. Provide support and immobilization of the wrist with the posterior splint taping or rehabilitative or custom-made bracing techniques. Use the brace anchor or figure-of-eight taping or figure-of-eight wrapping technique to anchor the custom-made brace. Use the compression wrap technique to provide compression and lessen swelling. If needed, use sling technique one to provide support and immobilization.

A rehabilitative or custom-made bracing technique will provide support and immobilization and limit range of motion during the two-week period. If needed, the compression wrap technique can be used to provide compression. The posterior splint taping technique may be used, but a bracing technique may prove more comfortable. If necessary, continue to use sling technique one during this period.

A rehabilitative or custom-made bracing technique can be used for night splinting. When using a custom-made design, use the brace anchor taping or figure-of-eight taping or wrapping technique to anchor the brace. For in-line skating and soccer activities, provide support to the wrist with the fan, strip, or "X" taping or functional bracing techniques. One of the taping techniques may be used in combination with the functional brace to provide additional support. As strength and flexibility return to preinjury levels, the circular wrist or figure-of-eight taping techniques can be applied for support. Consider using prophylactic bracing techniques to prevent further injury during in-line skating and soccer activities.

Critical Thinking Question Solutions

1. Because of the previous sprain, use a taping technique in combination with the off-the-shelf brace to provide stability. The fan, strip, or "X" technique will provide moderate support and should be used in this situation. The circular and figure-of-eight taping techniques, when used alone, may not provide the necessary support and protection from further injury in this situation.

2. The individual may be suffering from an allergic reaction. Use the following techniques to manage the

situation; if the symptoms persist, refer the individual to a physician. Cut and apply a piece of nonallergic stockinet or apply one layer of self-adherent wrap to the thumb, hand, and wrist underneath the brace. The brace may be washed or another brand or style of brace may be purchased. If the physician allows, discontinue use of the existing brace for several days and apply a taping technique to immobilize the thumb, hand, and wrist.

3. First determine whether any changes have been made to work and casual activities that may have caused the return of symptoms. Next, examine the brace for excessive wear and proper fit. Damage to the dorsal and/or palmar stabilizing bar(s) of the brace may have occurred during the trip, placing the wrist into excessive flexion or extension. For most brace designs, simply remold the bar(s) to the desired range of motion. Last, if remolding is unsuccessful, consider purchasing another brace.

4. Use a viscoelastic polymer sleeve or foam, felt, or viscoelastic polymer donut pad to absorb shock and lessen compression over the cyst. Although the exact causative factors of ganglion cysts are unknown, repetitive wrist extension during blocking and weightlifting activities may be associated and should be addressed. Using a functional wrist bracing technique and/or the fan, strip, or "X" taping technique will provide stability and lessen excessive wrist extension.

CHAPTER 11 SOLUTIONS

Case Study Solution

A football defensive lineman has sustained contusions to the dorsal aspect of his hands and PIP joints of fingers two, three, and four. Applying the hand or boxer's wrap compression technique will assist in reducing inflammation in the dorsal hand. Because of the irregular surface of the dorsal hand, consider using the compression wrap pad to provide additional compression. Use elastic tape, self-adherent wrap, or a finger sleeve to assist in controlling swelling over the PIP joints. These techniques can be worn throughout the day and be removed for treatment.

Upon a return to activity, the boxer's wrap technique, in combination with a viscoelastic polymer or foam padding technique for the hand, may reduce his risk of further injury to the area. Using viscoelastic or foam sleeves over the PIP joints of fingers two, three, and four will absorb shock and limit excessive pressure. The boxer's wrap and viscoelastic or foam sleeves can be worn with minimal effect on hand and finger range of motion. Consider using off-the-shelf padded gloves if these techniques prove ineffective.

Critical Thinking Question Solutions

1. Check the width and length of the foam or felt between the fingers to ensure anatomical alignment. Make sure

the circular strips do not cover the joints. If non-elastic tape was used, consider applying the circular strips with elastic tape. The buddy technique may be replaced by the "X" taping or finger sleeve wrapping technique.

2. During postop weeks 3 to 6, use a semirigid thumb spica cast for all practices and competitions to provide support. Construct and apply a thermoplastic hood to protect the fingers and distal thumb. Cover the cast and hood with high-density, closed-cell foam or similar material of at least ½ inch thickness. Following activity, cut and remove the cast for treatment and rehabilitation. The cast may be reused. Apply an off-the-shelf or custom-made thermoplastic thumb brace to provide support with nonathletic activities. During postop weeks 6 to 8, use the basic thumb spica and variation three, four, and/or the anchor taping techniques to protect the MCP joint. These techniques may be applied under or over a glove that is commonly worn by linemen. An off-the-shelf brace can also be used. The semirigid cast can be cut or scaled-down and also used during this period.

3. To provide adequate support for a first degree ulnar collateral ligament sprain, several options are available. Use the basic thumb spica or one of its variations applied directly to the skin or over pre-tape material or self-adherent wrap. A batting glove may be applied over these techniques. For batting and base running, apply an off-the-shelf thumb brace over the taping technique and/or batting glove to provide additional support. The Velcro attachments of the brace allow for quick application and removal between innings.

4. Apply adhesive gauze material or lightweight elastic tape over sterile materials, donut pad, or friction-reducing lubricant, viscoelastic polymer sleeves, caps, pads, or a foam sleeve to lessen pain and reduce pressure over the fingertips.

CHAPTER 12 SOLUTIONS

Case Study Solution

In the immediate management of the case, apply sling technique one to support and immobilize the right shoulder. Use the compression or circular wrapping or rib belt bracing technique to provide compression and support to the thorax and ribs. Monitor the mechanical restriction for tightness and remove the wrap or brace if symptoms worsen.

Provide support, absorb shock, and limit range of motion of the cervical spine during the return to football activities with an off-the-shelf functional bracing technique. A vest, strap, rigid, or foam design can be used in combination with football shoulder pads. Protect the thorax/ribs with an off-the-shelf or custom-made padding technique. A hard, high-density pad is indicated in this situation. Off-the-shelf pads can be attached directly to the shoulder pads or worn underneath. Anchor custom-made pads with elastic material or with the contusion/fracture taping or circular wrapping technique. The pad may also be anchored underneath a tight-fitting shirt.

Prior to making any modifications or eliminating the use of the bracing and/or padding techniques to improve the wide receiver's vision and ball control, consult with the team physician. The objective of the technique and the injury should guide any decisions regarding the techniques' use. With the assistance of a certified athletic equipment manager, first evaluate the design and fit of the helmet and shoulder pads. Second, apply and secure the helmet and shoulder pads. Next, evaluate the effectiveness of several functional cervical braces in limiting the desired ranges of active and passive motion in a controlled setting. Lastly, repeat this procedure to evaluate several padding designs for the thorax. Use caution if modifications are made to off-the-shelf bracing and/or padding techniques and always follow the manufacturer guidelines. Cutting away excess material or reshaping the designs could place the wide receiver at a greater risk of injury.

Critical Thinking Question Solutions

1. Check to determine the proper fit of the rib belt and reapply. If the problems continue, discontinue use of the belt. Consider purchasing another off-the-shelf brace after determining circumference measurements of the thorax. Many designs are contoured for females. Use the circular wrap technique in place of the brace, and, if needed, apply additional circular patterns of elastic tape for support. When applying the brace or wrap, have the individual inhale. As previously mentioned in the chapter, mechanical restriction of the thorax may result in worsening of symptoms for some individuals. A follow-up with the physician may be needed.

2. Functional cervical braces are used in combination with football shoulder pads; proper fit of the pads is critical. First, have a certified athletic equipment manager measure and fit the athlete with the appropriate shell and pad design and provide application and wear instructions. Next, use a vest, strap, rigid, or another foam roll design to limit range of motion. Consider the use of adjustable, rigid plastic materials or various thickness designs. Last, instruction on proper tackling techniques and a comprehensive therapeutic exercise program should lessen the risk of injury.

3. Because the off-the-shelf rib/thorax vests and jackets are too large, attempts to use them may cause additional injury rather than protection. Consider searching through the parent's van for a football thigh pad. These pads consist of a rigid plastic insert covered by varying thicknesses of foam. Fit and apply the pad over the injured area with elastic material or the contusion/fracture taping or circular wrapping technique. Football knee pads are constructed of open- and closed-cell foam and are not appropriate in this situation. If the materials are available, a custom-made pad may be constructed.

4. Several padding options are available for the individual. Off-the-shelf rib vests/jackets or suspender designs will protect the area from further injury. Choosing the appropriate length and width of the pad is important to prevent restriction of batting and fielding movements. A custom-made thermoplastic pad will also protect the area. Anchor the pad with elastic material or the contusion/fracture taping or circular wrapping technique. A soft, low-density padded shirt or individual pad can be used underneath the high-density outer shell of the vest/jacket for additional comfort and protection.

CHAPTER 13 SOLUTIONS

Case Study Solution

A coach for a local youth baseball team is planning to repair several pieces of protective equipment. Do not proceed with the repairs to the helmets and face guards. Contact the manufacturer(s) to determine whether the equipment is still under warranty. A NOCSAE licensed reconditioning firm may also be contacted to inquire about repairs. If the equipment was originally purchased from a reputable manufacturer, the helmets and face guards were most likely certified by NOCSAE standards. Any modifications and/or repairs to the equipment not recommended by the manufacturer will void the certification and may lessen the protection provided, increasing the risk of injury. The coach can be held liable for the repairs and any injuries caused by the modifications if the equipment is used in practices and/or competitions. If the equipment cannot be replaced or repaired as previously mentioned, new helmets and face guards should be purchased. Several strategies such as finding new sponsorship, financial involvement from the players' parents, donations, and/or fundraisers could provide the necessary funding for new protective equipment.

A fullback on the football team has sustained a chin laceration and was treated with sutures. To protect the chin upon a return to play, cover the laceration with a sterile wound dressing and consider applying adhesive gauze material to anchor the dressing. Use a four- or six-point chin strap with a soft or polycarbonate chin cup. When using some designs, apply foam or viscoelastic polymer materials as an inner lining to provide additional protection. A donut pad may be constructed from these materials to disperse the stress away from the laceration. Last, apply the helmet and center the chin cup over the chin. Adjust and anchor the straps to the helmet to produce equal tension in the straps. Check for proper fit of the helmet by repeating the movement tests used in the General Football Helmet Fitting Guidelines.

Critical Thinking Question Solutions

1. Replacement of the inner lining could lessen the protection provided by the helmet, increase the risk of injury to the athlete, and expose you to liability. The batter's helmet was certified in its original condition

from the manufacturer; replacement of the lining could impact the performance on certification tests. Consider asking the home team for a helmet, and, if one is available, notify the umpires prior to use to obtain approval. When you return home, send the helmet to the manufacturer or licensed reconditioning organization for repair of the inner lining.

2. Face guards certified through NOCSAE and/or HECC are mounted on certified helmets and subjected to testing. To comply with the original certification, a replacement guard must be certified and listed by the manufacturer to be used with the specific helmet design. The guard must be mounted on a certified helmet. Follow the manufacturer's instructions when attaching the guard.

3. Use a field hockey, ice hockey, or lacrosse elbow pad design to provide protection and allow for functional range of motion. These pads are designed to protect the posterior, medial, lateral, and/or anterior elbow with a pre-molded polycarbonate outer shell and open- and closed-cell or EVA foam inner lining. A soft, low-density pad will not provide adequate protection. Obtain approval for use from the referee prior to the start of a match. Written verification from the physician regarding the injury may be required.

4. When used alone, contact lenses do not provide protection for the eyes. Using the shield does provide protection, but only against large objects such as fingers entering through the face guard. Small objects such as dirt and grass can enter under the distal edge of the shield and cause injury. Consider using polycarbonate glasses that fit snugly around the eyes to lessen the risk of injury from both large and small objects. Glasses may be used alone or in combination with a shield.

Glossary

A

Achilles tendinitis: Inflammation of the Achilles tendon with possible involvement of the tendon sheath. Pain can be elicited on the posterior heel with passive dorsiflexion.

Acromioclavicular joint (AC): Gliding joint between the distal clavicle and the acromion process.

Adduct: Movement of a body part toward the midline of the body.

Amenorrhea: Absence of menstruation.

Annular ligament: Encircles the radial head and neck and stabilizes the radial head with the radioulnar joint.

Anterior: Front surface of a body part.

Anterior cruciate ligament (ACL): One of two cruciate ligaments in the knee. Attaches from the anterior aspect of the tibia to the medial surface of the lateral femoral condyle and prevents the tibia from moving anteriorly on the femur, internal and external rotation of the tibia on the femur, and hyperextension of the tibia.

Anterior dislocation/subluxation: Complete or partial separation of humerus from glenoid fossa toward the front of the body.

Anterior instability: Ligamentous laxity and muscular weakness of the glenohumeral joint allowing humeral head to translate anteriorly.

Anterior talofibular ligament: Attaches from the lateral talus to the fibular malleolus and resists anterior movement of the talus. The most commonly injured ligament of the ankle.

Anterior tibialis tendinitis: Inflammation of the anterior tibialis tendon. Pain can be elicited in the lace area with passive plantar flexion.

Anterior tibiofibular ligament: Attaches from the distal anterior fibula to the tibia to join the bones.

Application area: Space in a health-care facility dedicated for the application of taping, wrapping, bracing, and padding techniques.

Avulsion fracture: Tearing away of a piece of bone from a larger bone by force.

Axilla: Armpit.

B

Bankart lesion: Avulsion injury causing permanent damage to the anterior rim of the glenoid labrum, often associated with an anterior dislocation and/or instability of the glenohumeral joint.

Bimalleolar fracture: Fracture of the medial and lateral malleoli.

Bloodborne pathogens: Disease-producing microorganisms transmitted through blood and bodily fluids.

Bunion (hallux valgus): Enlargement of the metatarsophalangeal joint of the great toe as a result of inflammation and thickening of the bursa, with the toe often becoming angled toward the second toe.

Bunionette: Enlargement of the metatarsophalangeal joint of the fifth toe as a result of inflammation and thickening of the bursa, with the toe often becoming angled toward the fourth toe.

Burner: Brachial plexus trauma resulting in a burning and/or tingling sensation often associated with numbness.

Bursitis: Inflammation of a bursa.

C

Calcaneofibular ligament: Attaches from the lateral malleolus to the calcaneus and resists talar inversion.

Carpal tunnel syndrome: Compression of the median nerve in the carpal tunnel resulting in pain and tingling in the nerve distribution of the hand.

Charleyhorse (thigh contusion): Contusion to the anterior aspect of the thigh affecting the quadriceps.

Chondral fracture: Fracture of articular cartilage.

Chondromalacia patella: Softening of the articular cartilage possibly caused by compression and shear forces.

Closed-cell foam: Material that does not allow transfer of air from cell to cell, regains its original shape quickly, and provides minimal protection at low impact levels.

Cock-up position: Relating to a position of slight wrist extension.

Contusion: Trauma to soft tissue from a compressive force, a bruise.

Cooper's ligament: Supportive tissues of the breast at the thoracic wall.

D

Deep infrapatellar bursa: Bursa of the knee located between the tibial tubercle and patellar tendon.

Deltoid ligament: Attaches from the medial malleolus to the medial talus, calcaneus, and navicular bone and resists eversion and rotation. A collective term for four medial ligaments.

de Quervain's tenosynovitis: Tenosynovitis of the abductor pollicis longus and extensor pollicis brevis.

Disinfectant: Agents applied on equipment and surfaces to destroy bacteria.

Dislocation: Separation or displacement of joint or articulating surfaces.

Distal: Away from the center of the body.

Distal interphalangeal joint (DIP): Synovial joint between the head of the middle phalanx and the base of the distal phalanx.

Distal-to-proximal: Taping and wrapping technique sequence that begins away from the center of the body and proceeds toward the center.

Dorsal: The back or posterior surface of a body part.

Dorsiflexion: Movement of a body part to the dorsal or posterior surface.

E

Erb's point: An area 2 to 3 cm superior to the clavicle, level and in front of the transverse process of C–6 vertebra.

Eversion: Movement of the foot outward.

Eversion sprain: Trauma to the ankle resulting in an opening between the medial malleolus and talus.

Exertional compartment syndrome: Pain and swelling within the lower leg compartments caused by vigorous exercise and relieved by rest.

Exostosis: Bony growth arising from the surface of a bone.

Extension: Positioning of the distal portion of a joint in line with the proximal portion along an axis.

External rotation: Turning outward of a body part on an axis.

F

Flexion: Bending of a joint in which the distal and proximal parts come together.

Forearm splints: Increased pressure and pain within the compartments of the forearm caused by inflammation as the result of trauma and/or overuse.

Foreseeable: To see or anticipate.

Functional position: Relating to a position that allows an athlete/patient to perform in athletic or work activities.

G

Gamekeeper's thumb: Sprain of the ulnar collateral ligament at the first metacarpophalangeal joint from forceful abduction and hyperextension of the proximal phalanx.

Ganglion cyst: Cystic tumor mass.

Genu valgum: Abnormal abduction of the lower leg in line with the thigh, knock-knee.

Genu varus: Abnormal adduction of the lower leg in line with the thigh, bow-leg.

Glenohumeral joint (GH): Synovial joint between the head of the humerus and the glenoid cavity of the scapula.

Greater trochanteric bursitis: Inflammation of the greater trochanteric bursa causing pain over the greater trochanter with ambulation.

Ground fault interrupter (GFI): A device that interrupts the flow of electricity in an electrical circuit during a power surge of 5 milliamps or more.

H

Hill-Sachs lesion: Small defect in the cartilage of the humeral head on the posterolateral aspect, often associated with an anterior glenohumeral joint dislocation.

Hip pointer (iliac crest contusion): Contusion of the iliac crest and surrounding tissue.

Hyperextension: Extension of a body part beyond its normal limit of extension.

Hyperflexion: Flexion of a body part beyond its normal limit of flexion.

Hypostatic pneumonia: Pneumonia often seen in bedridden individuals who remain in one position for extended periods of time causing alveolar collapse and supporting bacterial growth.

I

Iliotibial band syndrome: Inflammation of the iliotibial band producing pain over the lateral femoral condyle and possibly the tibial insertion.

Inferior: Below or lower.

Inferior dislocation/subluxation: Complete or partial separation of humerus from the glenoid fossa in a downward direction.

Inferior instability: Ligamentous laxity and muscular weakness of the glenohumeral joint allowing the humeral head to translate inferiorly.

Infrapatellar fat pad: Fat pad of the knee located on the anterior aspect between the synovial membrane and patellar tendon.

Interdigital neuroma: Impingement of the interdigital nerves commonly between the third and fourth metatarsals causing pain in the web space between the toes.

Internal rotation: Turning inward of a body part on an axis.

Interphalangeal joint (IP): Synovial joint between two phalanges.

Inversion: Movement of the foot inward.

Inversion sprain: Trauma to the ankle resulting in an opening between the lateral malleolus and talus. The most common type of ankle sprain.

Ipsilateral: Pertaining to the same side of the body.

L

Lateral: Relating to the side, away from the midline of the body.

Lateral collateral ligament (LCL): One of two collateral ligaments in the knee. Attaches from the lateral epicondyle of the femur to the head of the fibula and prevents the tibia from moving inward (varus stress) on the femur and external rotation of the tibia on the femur.

Lateral epicondylitis (tennis elbow): Inflammation of the lateral humeral epicondyle causing pain in the area of the lateral epicondyle with resistive wrist extension.

Lateral (fibular) malleolus: Distal end of the fibula.

Lateral meniscus: O-shaped fibrocartilage attached to the lateral aspect of the tibial plateau.

Longitudinal: Lengthwise to the body or body part.

Longitudinal arch: Arch of the foot in the anteroposterior direction, from the calcaneus to the metatarsal heads.

Lumbar lordosis: Abnormal convex curve of the lumbar spine.

M

Maceration: Softening of the skin by moisture.

Malleable: Having the capacity to be molded, formed, or shaped by pressure.

Mallet finger: Rupture of the extensor digitorum tendon at the distal phalanx caused by forceful flexion of the distal phalanx.

Medial: Relating to the center or midline of the body.

Medial collateral ligament (MCL): Attaches from the medial epicondyle of the femur to the medial tibia and prevents the tibia from moving outward (valgus stress) on the femur and rotational movement of the tibia on the femur.

Medial epicondylitis (golfer's elbow): Inflammation of the medial humeral epicondyle causing pain distal and lateral to the medial epicondyle with resistive wrist flexion and pronation.

Medial (tibial) malleolus: Distal end of the tibia.

Medial meniscus: C-shaped fibrocartilage attached to the medial aspect of the tibial plateau. The medial meniscus is less mobile than the lateral.

Medial tibial stress syndrome (MTSS): Inflammation and pain in the distal third of the posteromedial tibia caused by overload and structural and muscular abnormalities.

Metacarpophalangeal joint (MCP): Synovial joint between the head of the metacarpal and the base of the proximal phalange.

Metatarsal arch: Arch of the forefoot in the medial to lateral direction, from the first to the fifth metatarsal heads.

Metatarsalgia: Pain around the metatarsal heads.

Metatarsophalangeal joint (MTP): Synovial joint between the head of the metatarsal and the base of the proximal phalange.

Myositis ossificans: Inflammation of muscle tissue with the formation of bone.

Multidirectional forces: Injurious forces that occur in more than one plane.

Multidirectional instability: Ligamentous laxity and muscular weakness in more than one plane.

N

Neutral: Relating to an indifferent position, a relaxed anatomical position.

Nonpliable: Not easily bent or shaped, inflexible.

O

Olecranon bursa: Bursa of the elbow located between the olecranon and the skin.

Olecranon: The proximal end of the ulna that extends posteriorly at the elbow.

Oligomenorrhea: Limited blood flow or infrequent menstruation.

Open-cell foam: Material that allows transfer of air from cell to cell, quickly deformed with stress, and provides low levels of shock absorption.

Osgood-Schlatter disease (OSD): Inflammation and degenerative changes of the tibial tubercle at the insertion of the patellar tendon.

Osteitis pubis: Chronic inflammation of the symphysis pubis.

Osteochondral fracture: Fracture of bone and articular cartilage.

Overuse: Cause of injuries and conditions from excessive, repetitive movement; stress; impact; or incorrect anatomical position.

P

Palmar: Relating to the palm of the hand.

Patella alta: High-riding patella.

Patellar tendinitis (jumper's knee): Inflammation of the patellar tendon typically at the inferior pole of the patella or its distal insertion on the tibial tubercle.

Patellofemoral stress syndrome (PFSS): Lateral tracking of the patella in the femoral groove resulting in anterior knee pain.

Periosteum: Outer membrane of blood vessels and connective tissue cells covering bones.

Peroneal retinaculum: Fibrous band located on the posterior aspect of the lateral malleolus holding the peroneal tendon in its groove.

Peroneal tendinitis: Inflammation of the peroneal tendon. Pain can be elicited over the posterior lateral malleolus with weight-bearing movements onto the ball of the foot.

Pes anserinus bursa: Bursa of the knee located beneath the pes anserinus tendons (sartorius, gracilis, and semitendinosus).

Pes anserinus tendinitis: Inflammation of the sartorius, gracilis, and semitendinosus tendons at the distal insertion at the proximal medial tibia.

Pes cavus: Abnormally high longitudinal arch.

Pes planus: Flatfoot, absence of arch.

Plantar: Relating to the bottom or sole of the foot.

Plantar fasciitis: Pain and inflammation of the plantar fascia, commonly present on the medial heel.

Plantar flexion: Movement of the foot in a downward or depressed motion.

Plica: A fold or thickening of the synovial membrane extending into the joint cavity.

Posterior: Back surface of a body part.

Posterior cruciate ligament (PCL): Attaches from the posterior aspect of the tibia to the lateral anterior medial condyle of the femur and prevents the tibia from moving posteriorly on the femur, internal rotation of the tibia on the femur, and hyperextension of the tibia.

Posterior dislocation/subluxation: Complete or partial separation of humerus from glenoid fossa toward the back of the body.

Posterior instability: Ligamentous laxity and muscular weakness allowing the humeral head to translate posteriorly.

Posterior talofibular ligament: Attaches from the posterior talus and posterolateral calcaneus to the lateral malleolus and resists dorsiflexion and inversion.

Posterior tibialis tendinitis: Inflammation of the posterior tibial tendon. Pain can be elicited over the posterior or medial malleolus with active resistive plantar flexion and inversion.

Posterior tibiofibular ligament: Attaches from the distal posterior fibula to the tibia to join the bones.

Prepatellar bursa: Bursa of the knee located between the anterior surface of the patella and the skin.

Pronate: Turning the palm of the hand downward with inward rotation of the forearm.

Prophylactic: Act of guarding or protecting from injury.

Proximal: Nearest the center of the body.

Proximal interphalangeal joint (PIP): Synovial joint between the head of the proximal phalanx and the base of the middle phalanx.

Proximal-to-distal: Taping and wrapping technique sequence that begins from the center of the body and proceeds away from the center.

Pulmonary contusion: Contusion of the heart producing chest pain, shortness of breath, and rapid breathing.

Q

Q angle: Angle formed between the line of force or pull of the quadriceps and the patellar tendon used to determine patellar tracking.

R

Radial collateral ligament: Attaches from the lateral epicondyle of the humerus to the annular ligament and prevents the ulna and radius from moving inward (varus stress) on the humerus.

Radiocarpal joint: Joint formed between the distal radius and scaphoid, lunate, and triquetrum.

Radioulnar joint: Joint formed between the distal ends of the radius and ulna.

Retrocalcaneal bursitis: Inflammation of the retrocalcaneal bursa between the Achilles tendon and calcaneus.

Reverse Hill-Sachs lesion: Small defect in the cartilage of the anterior humeral head often associated with a posterior glenohumeral joint dislocation.

Rotary forces: Injurious twisting forces.

Rotation: Turning of a body part on an axis.

Rotator cuff: Term used to describe the supraspinatus, infraspinatus, teres minor, and subscapularis muscle group of the shoulder.

S

Scoliosis: A lateral curve of the spine.

Semimembranosus bursa (Baker's cyst): Bursa of the knee located in the popliteal fossa beneath the semimembranous tendon.

Sesamoiditis: Inflammation of the sesamoid bones under the first metatarsal head.

Shoulder pointer: Contusion of the distal clavicle and surrounding soft tissue.

Sinding-Larsen Johansson disease (SLJ): Inflammation and pain at the inferior pole of the patella at the origin of the patellar tendon.

Superior labrum anteroposterior (SLAP) lesion: Defect to the superior glenoid labrum of the shoulder that begins posteriorly and extends anteriorly and damages the attachment of the long head of the biceps tendon.

Sternoclavicular joint (SC): Joint formed between the manubrium of the sternum and the proximal clavicle.

Stinger: (See Burner)

Stress fracture: A fracture of insidious nature.

Subluxation: Partial dislocation.

Subtalar joint: Joint formed between the talus and calcaneus at which inversion, eversion, pronation, and supination occur.

Superior: Above or higher.

Supinate: Turning the palm of the hand upward with outward rotation of the forearm.

Syndesmosis sprain: Trauma to the ankle resulting in an opening of the distal tibiofibular joint.

T

Tackler's exostosis: Bony growth arising from the anterolateral aspect of the humerus commonly seen in football linemen.

Tactile: Referring to the sense of touch.

Taping area: (See Application Area)

Talocrural joint: Joint formed between the distal tibia and talus, medial malleolus and talus, and lateral malleolus and trochlea at which plantar flexion and dorsiflexion occur.

Thenar web space: The area of the hand between the thumb and first finger.

Transverse arch: Arch of the midfoot in the medial to lateral direction, from the medial cuneiform to the cuboid bones.

Triangular fibrocartilage complex (TFCC): Complex located between the distal ulnar head and the lunate and triquetrum, including the triangular fibrocartilage.

Turf burn: Abrasion to the posterior elbow and/or ulnar side of the forearm from contact with artificial grass, wood, or rubber playing surfaces.

U

Ulnar collateral ligament (UCL) Elbow: Composed of three bands, the UCL prevents valgus stress or medial opening of the elbow. Attaches from the medial epicondyle of the humerus to the coronoid process of the ulna and prevents the ulna and radius from moving outward (valgus stress) on the humerus.

Ulnar collateral ligament (UCL) Thumb: Attaches from the dorsal side of the first metacarpal to the palmer aspect of the proximal first phalanx and prevents the phalanx from moving inward (varus stress) and outward (valgus stress) on the first metacarpal.

Ulnar styloid process: Small bony projection on the medial and posterior aspect of the ulnar head.

Unidirectional forces: An injurious force that occurs in one plane.

V

Valgus: Distal segment of a joint bent outward, resulting in an opening on the medial aspect.

Varus: Distal segment of a joint bent inward, resulting in an opening on the lateral aspect.

W

Wryneck: Pain and stiffness associated with spasm of the cervical neck musculature.

Index

Page numbers followed by "f" denote figures